Designing and Implementing an Effective Tobacco Counter-Marketing Campaign

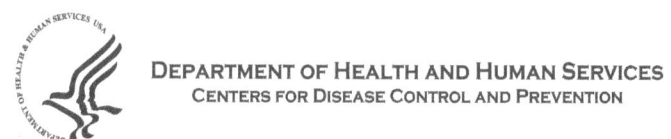

DEPARTMENT OF HEALTH AND HUMAN SERVICES
CENTERS FOR DISEASE CONTROL AND PREVENTION

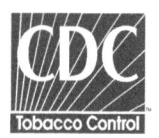

Suggested Citation

Centers for Disease Control and Prevention. *Designing and Implementing an Effective Tobacco Counter-Marketing Campaign.* Atlanta, Georgia: U.S. Department of Health and Human Services, Centers for Disease Control and Prevention, National Center for Chronic Disease Prevention and Health Promotion, Office on Smoking and Health, First Edition October 2003.

Ordering Information

To order a copy of this publication, contact:

Office on Smoking and Health
Media Campaign Resource Center
Mail Stop K-50
4770 Buford Highway, NE
Atlanta, GA 30341-3717
770-488-5705; press 2
e-mail: mcrc@cdc.gov
www.cdc.gov/tobacco/mcrc

Table of Contents

Acknowledgments 5

Introduction: How to Use this Manual 9

Chapter 1: Overview of Counter-Marketing Programs 13

Chapter 2: Planning Your Counter-Marketing Program 21

Chapter 3: Gaining and Using Target Audience Insights 51

Chapter 4: Reaching Specific Populations 87

Chapter 5: Evaluating the Success of Your Counter-Marketing Program 109

Chapter 6: Managing and Implementing Your Counter-Marketing Program 143

Chapter 7: Advertising 163

Chapter 8: Public Relations...201

Chapter 9: Media Advocacy 245

Chapter 10: Grassroots Marketing..267

Chapter 11: Media Literacy...281

Resources and Tools...297

Glossary 331

Appendices 343

    Appendix 2.1: Counter-Marketing Planning Worksheet..343

    Appendix 3.1: Sample Recruitment Screener for Intercept Interviews on Smoking Cessation 349

    Appendix 3.2: Sample Recruitment Screener for Individual Interviews To Test
Advertisements and Ad Concepts 351

    Appendix 3.3: Moderator's Guide for Focus Groups With Smokers 354

    Appendix 3.4: Sample Moderator's Guide for Focus Groups To Test
Advertisements With Youth...360

    Appendix 3.5: Sample Self-Administered Form To Test Fact Sheets 363

    Appendix 3.6 : Sample Intercept Interview Questionnaire 366

    Appendix 5.1: Examples of Inputs, Activities, Outputs, and Outcomes
for Counter-Marketing Programs 374

Appendix 5.2: Key Data Collection Tools and Methods 378

Appendix 5.3: Key Variables and Sample Items to Consider Including in Survey
    of Target Population 381

Appendix 6.1: Key Elements of a Request for Proposals (RFP) for a Media Campaign 386

Appendix 6.2: Questions and Answers on RFPs 394

Appendix 6.3: Elements of a Creative Brief 409

Appendix 6.4: Creative Brief, Florida..413

Appendix 6.5: Creative Brief, Centers for Disease Control and Prevention
    and World Health Organization 415

Appendix 6.6: Creative Brief, Centers for Disease Control and Prevention 418

Appendix 7.1: Sample Advertising Comment Organizer 419

Appendix 7.2: Sample Storyboard—"Carnival" 421

Appendix 7.3: Sample Storyboard—"Drive" 422

Appendix 8.1: Sample Printed Campaign Newsletter 423

Appendix 8.2: Sample Online Newsletter 427

Appendix 8.3: Sample Editorial 431

Appendix 8.4: Sample Letter to the Editor 432

Appendix 8.5: Sample Op-Ed 433

Appendix 8.6: Sample Spokesperson Profile Sheet 435

Appendix 8.7: Sample Pitch Letter 437

Appendix 8.8: Sample News Release 438

Appendix 8.9: Sample Fact Sheet...440

Appendix 8.10: Media Contact Record 445

Appendix 10.1: Georgia Burden of Tobacco Brochure 446

Feedback Form 456

Acknowledgments

The following individuals served as the managing editors for this publication:

Linda Block, MPH, Office on Smoking and Health, National Center for Chronic Disease Prevention and Health Promotion, Centers for Disease Control and Prevention

Karen Gutierrez, Office on Smoking and Health, National Center for Chronic Disease Prevention and Health Promotion, Centers for Disease Control and Prevention

The following individuals are the primary authors of this publication:

Elaine Arkin, Health Communications Consultant

Joan Clayton-Davis, MA, Academy for Educational Development

Susan Middlestadt, Ph.D., Academy for Educational Development

Peter Mitchell, Academy for Educational Development

Anne Marie O'Keefe, Ph.D., JD, Academy for Educational Development

Todd Phillips, MS, Academy for Educational Development

Rose Mary Romano, MA, Academy for Educational Development

Phil Wilbur, MA, Northrop Grumman IT Health and Science Solutions

We thank the following individuals from the Centers for Disease Control and Prevention, for assistance in reviewing and contributing to this document:

Cheri Ahern, Office on Smoking and Health

Stephen Babb, MPH, Office on Smoking and Health

Diane Beistle, Office on Smoking and Health

Galen Cole, Ph.D., Office of Communication

Alyssa Easton, Ph.D., MPH, Office on Smoking and Health

Monica Eischen, Office on Smoking and Health

Reba Griffith, MPH, Office on Smoking and Health

May Kennedy, MPH, Office of Communication

Sharon Kohout, MA, Office on Smoking and Health

Dianne May, MA, MPH, Office on Smoking and Health

Jeff McKenna, MS, Office on Smoking and Health

Patty McLean, M.Ed., Office on Smoking and Health

Rebecca Murphy, Ph.D., Office on Smoking and Health

Claudia Parvanta, Ph.D., Office of Communication

Alpa Patel-Larson, Office on Smoking and Health

Linda Pederson, Ph.D., Office on Smoking and Health

Lisa Petersen, MS, Office on Smoking and Health

Oona Powell, MA, Office on Smoking and Health

Chris Prue, MSPH, Ph.D., Office of Communication

Robert Robinson, Dr.P.H., Office on Smoking and Health

Michael Schooley, MPH, Office on Smoking and Health

Karen Siener, MPH, Office on Smoking and Health

The Office on Smoking and Health thanks the following individuals for their careful review of drafts of this manual:

Debra Bodenstine, Florida Department of Health

Deborah E. Boldt, MPA, Missouri Partnership on Smoking or Health

Nicole Boyd, JD, The Partnership for a Healthy Mississippi

Greg Connolly, DMD, MPH, Massachusetts Department of Public Health

Larry Davis, Global Lead Management Consulting

Peter DeBenedittis, Ph.D., New Mexico Media Literacy Project

Robert Denniston, MA, Office of National Drug Control Policy

Mark Dinneen, Alaska Department of Health

Susan Giarratano Russell, EdD, MSPH, CHES, Health Education and Media Consultant

Sandi Hammond, Massachusetts Department of Public Health

Ann Houston, CHES, North Carolina Department of Health

Lucy Huang, IW Group, Inc.

Mary Jane Mahan, MA, DeKalb County Board of Health

Danny McGoldrick, MA, Campaign for Tobacco-Free Kids

Barbara A. Moeykens, MS, Vermont Department of Health

Mike Pertschuk, JD, Advocacy Institute

Monica Pribil, MA, Nebraska Department of Health and Human Services

Amelie Ramirez, Dr.P.H., Baylor College of Medicine

Janet Reid, Ph.D., Global Lead Management Consulting

Schaelene Rollins, California Department of Health Services

Russell Sciandra, MA, Center for a Tobacco Free New York

David Sly, MS, Ph.D., Florida State University

William D. Snook, MS Ed., Missouri Health Department

Colleen Stevens, MSW, California Department of Health Services

Makani Themba-Nixon, The Praxis Project

Chuck Wolfe, Wolfe Strategies

David Zucker, Porter Novelli

The Office on Smoking and Health thanks the following individuals for support in producing this manual:

Daria Bessom, Northrop Grumman IT Health and Science Solutions

Adjoa Burrowes, Northrop Grumman IT Health and Science Solutions

Sheila E. Coble, Northrop Grumman IT Health and Science Solutions

Vivian Doidge, MA, Northrop Grumman IT Health and Science Solutions

Dee Ellison, MS, Academy for Educational Development

Maxine Forrest, Northrop Grumman IT Health and Science Solutions

Catherine Macapugay, Northrop Grumman IT Health and Science Solutions

Anne Mattison, MA, Northrop Grumman IT Health and Science Solutions

Jennifer Mike, Northrop Grumman IT Health and Science Solutions

Eloisa Montes, MA, Northrop Grumman IT Health and Science Solutions

Don Mullins, MPH, Northrop Grumman IT Health and Science Solutions

Melissa Ratherdale, MA, Academy for Educational Development

Susan Rogers, Ph.D., Academy for Educational Development

Rebecca Rosenthal, Academy for Educational Development

Jeff Roussel, Northrop Grumman IT Health and Science Solutions

Laura Simon, Northrop Grumman IT Health and Science Solutions

Pam Sutton, Academy for Educational Development

Carol Winner, MPH, Northrop Grumman IT Health and Science Solutions

Introduction

How To Use This Manual

This manual is designed to be a comprehensive resource for state health departments and other agencies and organizations in developing and implementing tobacco counter-marketing campaigns. It is designed to help readers who have different levels of experience and are managing programs at different stages of development.

This manual contains a wealth of information on a range of counter-marketing topics. Some of the topics and information may be new to you, while you may already have a good command of other topic areas. This resource is meant to help with activities you're working on currently, as well as projects you undertake in the future. Different chapters will be more helpful at different times.

Don't feel that you have to read the manual from cover to cover. This introduction should give you a sense of the manual's content and organization. We suggest that you begin by reading Chapter 1: Overview of Counter-Marketing Programs. Then feel free to skip some chapters, read other chapters more thoroughly, or move directly to the subjects that are most pertinent to your needs.

What You Will Find in This Manual

The first half of the manual focuses on planning and preparation, and the second half addresses specific counter-marketing techniques. The manual also includes a list of resource organizations, appendices relevant to topics found in individual chapters, and a glossary.

Here's a quick look at each chapter:

- *Chapter 1* provides an overview of tobacco counter-marketing and the key characteristics of a successful tobacco counter-marketing program.

- *Chapter 2* focuses on planning the tobacco counter-marketing program. It describes seven planning steps, from defining the problem through developing the program.

- *Chapter 3* discusses the use of market research to gain insights into your target audience. To create effective messages, it's important to understand the cultures, behaviors, motivations, interests, and needs of the target audiences. This chapter compares and discusses three types of market research methods: qualitative, quasi-quantitative, and quantitative.

- *Chapter 4* focuses on specific populations, which are defined by demographic characteristics such as age, race/ethnicity, income, educational level, and sexual orientation and by epidemiologic data related to health disparities. The chapter discusses cultural context, diversity within and among specific populations, appropriate language, potential audience barriers and how to overcome them, the role of formative research in working with specific populations, and cultural competency.

- *Chapter 5* addresses program evaluation, a critical component in tobacco counter-marketing campaigns. Program evaluation is the systematic collection of data about a program's activities and outcomes, so the program's delivery, efficiency, and effectiveness can be analyzed, better understood, and improved.

- *Chapter 6* explores the key steps in implementing a successful program. It addresses how to manage personnel issues, choose contractors, develop marketing and communication plans, and involve stakeholder organizations.

- *Chapter 7* examines advertising and takes the reader through the four key elements of an advertising campaign: logistics, strategy, creative, and exposure.

- *Chapter 8* focuses on public relations (PR). The first half of the chapter outlines the process for using PR to reach your target audience(s) and key influencers. The second half explains how to implement PR activities, such as managing a PR agency, handling press relations, developing press materials, pitching stories, and responding to media inquiries.

- *Chapter 9* discusses media advocacy. Defined as the strategic use of media and community advocacy to create social or policy change, media advocacy helps communities create long-lasting environmental change.

- *Chapter 10* focuses on grassroots marketing, which includes involving new people in tobacco counter-marketing campaigns, increasing the involvement of those already reached, and using those already engaged to increase an audience's exposure to key messages. Events, community organizing, and partnerships are forms of grassroots marketing, and they are united by their goal to create and use target audience participation.

- *Chapter 11* explains how media literacy relates to and reinforces tobacco counter-marketing campaigns. This chapter highlights the key concepts of media literacy and provides resources for identifying and implementing media literacy programs.

An effective tobacco counter-marketing campaign can make a vital contribution to a comprehensive tobacco control and prevention program. Although the components of counter-marketing are presented separately in this manual, they work synergistically to strengthen the impact of the overall campaign; one or two successful components will not be enough to achieve your program goals. The art of tobacco counter-marketing is in blending and balancing the various components into a coherent, effective whole. We hope the chapters in this manual will help you develop a comprehensive tobacco counter-marketing program that progresses toward achieving your goals.

Chapter 1
Overview of Counter-Marketing Programs

Counter-Marketing: An Art and a Science

With the success of programs in Arizona, California, Florida, Massachusetts, Minnesota, Mississippi, Oregon, and other states in the past decade, it's clear that comprehensive tobacco control programs are a powerful tool for reducing tobacco use. As many studies have shown, an important piece of a comprehensive tobacco control program is a strong counter-marketing program (Centers for Disease Control and Prevention [CDC] 1999; Hopkins et al. 2001). Tobacco counter-marketing is defined as the use of commercial marketing tactics to reduce the prevalence of tobacco use. "Counter-marketing attempts to counter protobacco influences and increase prohealth messages and influences throughout a state, region, or community" (U.S. Department of Health and Human Services [USDHHS] 2000).

Counter-marketing activities can play a role in increasing smoking cessation, reducing smokeless tobacco use, decreasing the likelihood that people will begin smoking cigarettes, and reducing nonsmokers' exposure to secondhand tobacco smoke. Counter-marketing messages can also substantially influence public support for tobacco control interventions and increase support for school and community efforts (USDHHS 2000). Counter-marketing messages work best when they are tied to the activities of local programs throughout a state.

In This Chapter
- Counter-Marketing: An Art and a Science
- What We Are Countering
- Qualities of a Good Counter-Marketing Program
- The Power of Counter-Marketing

What We Are Countering

Tobacco counter-marketing programs play a vital role in countering the influential promotional activities of the tobacco industry, which spends billions of dollars a year on advertising and promotions. The following statistics underscore the importance and necessity of tobacco counter-marketing:

- Total annual spending on cigarette marketing by the six major U.S. cigarette makers rose 16.2 percent from 1999 to 2000, an increase from $8.24 billion to $9.57 billion, the highest figure ever reported to the Federal Trade Commission (FTC 2002).

- In 1999, the five major smokeless tobacco companies in the United States spent $170.2 million on advertising and promotions, an all-time high (FTC 2001).

- The six major U.S. cigarette companies spent more than $949,000 on Internet advertising in 2000, according to the Federal Trade Commission (FTC 2002).

- In 2000, more than 80 percent of young people in the United States were reached an average of 17 times per person by magazine ads for "youth" brands of cigarettes (King and Siegel 2001). (The study defined cigarette brands as "youth" brands if they were smoked by more than 5 percent of the smokers in the 8th, 10th, and 12th grades in 1998.)

- In 2000, about one-third of middle school students and one-fourth of high school students in the United States saw tobacco ads on the Internet (CDC 2001b).

Qualities of a Good Counter-Marketing Program

Best Practices for Comprehensive Tobacco Control Programs (CDC 1999) identifies a number of elements crucial to a comprehensive tobacco control program; one of these elements is counter-marketing. Seven key characteristics apply to all successful counter-marketing campaigns:

1. **A counter-marketing program must be long term.** The tobacco industry took decades to establish brand identity for its products and to normalize tobacco use as a part of our culture. Likewise, tobacco control efforts should be considered long-term commitments to addressing the problems associated with tobacco use, rather than short-term or episodic activities. If a state is developing a branded campaign, it should choose a brand that can stand the test of time and be refreshed as needed with brand extensions. Effective counter-marketing initiatives are intended to make important contributions today toward short-term goals, while also laying the groundwork for meeting long-term goals.

2. **A comprehensive tobacco counter-marketing program should consist of integrated, not isolated, components.** Although they are explained separately in this manual, these components are most effective when they complement and

support one another. A comprehensive counter-marketing program must use a variety of available techniques and components at different times and in different combinations.

3. **The counter-marketing program must be integrated into the larger tobacco control program.** Just as counter-marketing components should be integrated, the counter-marketing program should complement the other elements of the tobacco control program, such as educational efforts, cessation initiatives, enforcement campaigns, and policy campaigns (including those related to secondhand tobacco smoke and price increases for tobacco products). Coordinating your counter-marketing efforts with local programs is a powerful way to extend their effect. In short, you need to tie the counter-marketing goals to the overall strategic goal for your tobacco control program.

4. **A counter-marketing program must be culturally competent.** No single counter-marketing program will be effective for every segment of the population because tobacco use affects socioeconomic groups, age groups, racial/ethnic groups, and other specific populations in varying ways. Messages and strategies should be tailored as needed to be most effective among the campaign's different target audiences.

5. **A counter-marketing program should be strategic.** Successfully managing a counter-marketing program involves making decisions about the overall direction of the program, its target audiences, creative products, implementation, and evaluation. Strategic planning is about setting priorities and making sometimes difficult choices about how program funding will be allocated and how staffing will be organized. These decisions should be based on how these factors will contribute to the program's overall goals.

6. **A counter-marketing program should be evaluated.** This process should begin with two questions: "What information do you or other key stakeholders want to know?" and "How do you obtain and use that information?" Evaluation isn't merely a report that's completed after all the work is finished. Evaluation provides a tobacco control program with continuous updates and insights on what is working, what is not, and what changes might need to be made to ensure that the program is progressing toward achieving its goals and objectives.

7. **A counter-marketing program should be adequately funded.** Tobacco advertising and promotion activities appear to both stimulate adult tobacco consumption and increase risk of youth initiation of tobacco use. Today's average 14-year-old has been exposed to more than $20 billion in imagery, advertising, and promotions since age 6, creating a familiarity with tobacco products and an environment in which smoking is seen as glamorous, social, and normal (CDC 1999). In light of these ubiquitous

and sustained messages promoting tobacco use, counter-marketing efforts of comparable intensity are needed. The Centers for Disease Control and Prevention recommends that, at a mini-mum, states should allocate $1 to $3 per capita annually for a counter-marketing campaign that addresses all program goals in all major media markets in the state (CDC 1999).

The Power of Counter-Marketing

The California Tobacco Education Media Campaign, which began in the late 1980s, is one example of a successful counter-marketing campaign (Independent Evaluation Consortium of The Gallup Organization et al. 2001; Pierce et al. 1998). It uses hard-hitting earned media, grassroots marketing, and paid advertising (television, radio, billboards, transit, and print) to communicate the dangers of tobacco use and secondhand smoke and to counter protobacco messages throughout the state's ethnically diverse communities. California's campaign has demonstrated a strong correlation between its Tobacco Education Media Campaign program and decreased smoking prevalence rates even accounting for all other factors (e.g., increased excise tax):

- A study found that the California antitobacco media campaign reduced sales of cigarettes by 232 million packs between the third quarter of 1990 and the fourth quarter of 1992. This reduction was independent of the decreases in consumption brought about by a tax increase (Hu et al. 1995).

- A report from the University of California, San Diego, covering 1989 to 1993 showed that the proportion of Californians who tried to quit smoking for more than one day rose significantly whenever the media campaign was in effect (Pierce et al. 1994).

Another example of an effective counter-marketing campaign is the Florida Pilot Program on Tobacco Control, which began in 1998 (Bauer and Johnson 2001). Florida's program is a comprehensive, youth-focused campaign that includes a youth-directed media campaign marketing the "truth" brand and slogan, youth and community activities organized as Students Working Against Tobacco (SWAT), school-based education and training, and retailer education and enforcement. From 1998 to 2000, youth tobacco use declined 40 percent among middle school students and 18 percent among high school students, and attitudes among students changed regarding deglamorizing tobacco use and tobacco industry manipulation, which were key campaign themes. Overall program results demonstrated that a comprehensive statewide program can be effective in preventing and reducing youth tobacco use (Bauer and Johnson 2001):

- Current cigarette use dropped among Florida students, from 18.5 percent to 11.1 percent of middle school students and from 27.4 percent to 22.6 percent of high school students. The primary campaign objective, to change attitudes about tobacco, was achieved. The percentage of students committed to never smoking increased from 56.4 percent to 69.3 percent of middle school students and from 31.9 percent to 43.1 percent of high school students. The percentage of students currently experimenting with cigarettes declined from 21.4 percent to 16.2 percent of middle school students and from 32.8 percent to 28.2 percent of high school students. The percentage of students experimenting with tobacco use who indicated they would not smoke again increased from 30.4 percent to 42.0 percent of middle school students and 44.4 percent to 51.0 percent of high school students (Bauer and Johnson 2000).

- Participants surveyed in October 1998 and October 2000 were contacted again in February 2001 to determine their ability to recall specific antitobacco ads and to determine actual changes in smoking behavior. The results showed a strong correlation between confirmed awareness of the "truth" advertising campaign and reduced likelihood of beginning to use cigarettes and increased likelihood of quitting (Sly et al. 2001).

Along with the California and Florida campaigns, successful counter-marketing programs have been implemented in several other states, including Arizona, Massachusetts, Minnesota, Mississippi, and Oregon. In all these states, reductions in smoking consumption or prevalence or both have been attributed to a combination of tobacco control elements, including strong tobacco counter-marketing campaign (CDC 1999; CDC 2003).

The statistics from various state efforts indicate that it is possible to make a significant impact with counter-marketing efforts, but it requires hard work and ongoing commitment to the program. In addition, although many parts of a campaign can be measured and tested, successful counter-marketing remains an art as much as a science. Making the right choices in developing an effective counter-marketing program is often complicated and requires constant strategic focus, coupled with flexibility when needed. This manual presents many of the lessons, subtleties, insights, and experiences of those who have learned firsthand how to create a successful campaign.

Bibliography

American Heart Association. Comments on Cigarette and Smokeless Tobacco Reports: Request for Public Comments. *Federal Register* 2001;66. Available at: http://www.ftc.gov/os/comments/tobaccocomments2/williamsbrian.htm. Accessed July 2, 2002.

Bauer UE, Johnson TM. *Assessing the Impact of Florida's Pilot Program on Tobacco Control, 1998–2000: A Comprehensive Analysis of Data from the Florida Youth Tobacco Survey. Vol. 3, Report* 2. Tallahassee, FL: Florida Department of Health, 2001.

Bauer UE, Johnson TM. Changes in youth cigarette use and intentions: following implementation of a tobacco control program. Findings from the Florida Youth Tobacco Survey, 1998–2000. *Journal of the American Medical Association* 2000;284:723–8.

Biener L. Adult and youth response to the Massachusetts anti-tobacco television campaign. *Journal of Public Health Management and Practice* 2000;6:40–4.

Biener L, et al. Adults' response to Massachusetts anti-tobacco television advertisements: impact of viewer and ad characteristics. *Tobacco Control* 2000;9:401–7.

Centers for Disease Control and Prevention. *Best Practices for Comprehensive Tobacco Control Programs— August 1999.* Atlanta, GA: U.S. Department of Health and Human Services, Centers for Disease Control and Prevention, National Center for Chronic Disease Prevention and Health Promotion, Office on Smoking and Health, August 1999. Reprinted with corrections.

CDC. Cigarette smoking among adults—United States, 1999. *Morbidity and Mortality Weekly Report* 2001a;50(40);869–73.

CDC. *State Programs in Action. Exemplary Work to Prevent Chronic Disease and Promote Health.* Atlanta, GA: USDHHS, CDC, 2003.

CDC. Youth tobacco surveillance—United States, 2000. *Morbidity and Mortality Weekly Report* 2001b;50(SS-4):1–84.

Federal Trade Commission. *Cigarette Report for 2000*; http://www.ftc.gov/os/2002/05/2002cigrpt.pdf, 2002. Accessed April 24, 2003.

FTC. *Report to Congress for the Years 1998 and 1999 Pursuant to the Comprehensive Smokeless Tobacco Health Education Act of 1986*; 2001. http://www.ftc.gov/reports/tobacco/smokeless98_99.htm. Accessed July 19, 2002.

Hopkins DP, Fielding JE, Task Force on Community Preventive Services, editors. The guide to community preventive services, tobacco use prevention and control: reviews, recommendations, and expert commentary. *American Journal of Preventive Medicine Supplement*, February 2001;20(2S).

Hu T, et al. Reducing cigarette consumption in California: tobacco taxes vs. an anti-smoking media campaign. *American Journal of Public Health* 1995;85:1218–22.

Independent Evaluation Consortium of The Gallup Organization, et al. *Interim Report: Independent Evaluation of the California Tobacco Control Prevention and Education Program: Wave 2 Data, 1998; Wave 1 & Wave 2 Data Comparisons, 1996–1998*. Sacramento, CA: California Department of Health Services, Tobacco Control Section, 2001.

King C, Siegel M. The master settlement agreement with the tobacco industry and cigarette advertising in magazines. *New England Journal of Medicine* 2001;345:504–11. http://content.nejm.org/cgi/content/abstract/345/7/504. Accessed July 3, 2002.

Norton GD, Hamilton W. *Sixth Annual Report: Independent Evaluation of the Massachusetts Tobacco Control Program, January 1994 to June 1999*. Prepared for the Massachusetts Department of Public Health. Cambridge, MA: Abt Associates, Inc., 2001.

Pierce JP, et al. *Tobacco Control in California: Who's Winning the War? An Evaluation of the Tobacco Control Program, 1989–1996*. La Jolla, CA: University of California, San Diego, 1998.

Pierce JP, et al. *Tobacco Use in California: An Evaluation of the Tobacco Control Program, 1989–1993*. La Jolla, CA: University of California, San Diego, 1994.

Sly DF, et al. *Florida Anti-Tobacco Media Evaluation (FAME) Follow-up Report*. Tallahassee, FL: Florida Department of Health, Florida Tobacco Pilot Program, University of Miami Tobacco Research and Evaluation Coordinating Center, 2001.

Sly DF, et al. *Florida Anti-Tobacco Media Evaluation 30th Month Report: "truth's" Influence on the Rise and Other Considerations*. Tallahassee, FL: Florida State University, Center for the Study of Population, 2000.

U.S. Department of Health and Human Services. *Reducing Tobacco Use: A Report of the Surgeon General*. Atlanta, GA: USDHHS, Centers for Disease Control and Prevention, National Center for Chronic Disease Prevention and Health Promotion, Office on Smoking and Health, 2000.

Chapter 2

Planning Your Counter-Marketing Program

Planning is the foundation of your counter-marketing program. Although sound planning alone can't guarantee success, it is a very important first step.

Effective planning helps you clarify exactly which aspects of the problem of tobacco use your counter-marketing program can affect and how you can use resources most efficiently to make the greatest impact. Planning helps you set clear objectives that will enable you to select and prioritize activities. Not only does it guide program development, but it also helps you assess progress and make choices that will enhance your program's chances for future success.

Seven Steps for Planning

This chapter describes the steps for planning your program (National Cancer Institute [NCI] 2002; Centers for Disease Control and Prevention [CDC] 2003). Although these steps are described here in sequence, planning is an integrated, not a sequential, process. Become familiar with each of these steps before you start. Planning is also an iterative process; much of the planning you do will incorporate multiple steps at once or require making changes to steps on which you have already worked.

In This Chapter

Seven Steps for Planning Your Counter-Marketing Program

1. Describe the Problem
2. Identify Target Audiences
3. Draft Objectives
4. Determine Approaches, Channels, and Program Strategies
5. Consider Collaboration
6. Plan for Process and Outcome Evaluation
7. Begin Program Development

> **Here are the seven essential steps for planning a counter-marketing program:**
>
> 1. Describe the problem and identify how counter-marketing approaches can address it.
> 2. Identify and learn about target audiences.
> 3. Draft counter-marketing objectives.
> 4. Determine counter-marketing approaches, channels (pathways), and program strategies.
> 5. Consider collaboration.
> 6. Plan for process and outcome evaluation.
> 7. Begin counter-marketing program development.

With so many demands on your time, you may be tempted to skip some steps, but thorough planning will be worth the time invested. A written plan will help you enlist the support of your organization's management, partners, stakeholders, and funding sources, and to respond to critics by defending the choices you have made.

The sample Counter-Marketing Strategic Planning Worksheet (Appendix 2.1) can help you begin. You also may want to review *CDCynergy for Tobacco Prevention and Control*, CDC's CD-ROM-based planning tool that includes several tobacco-related case studies (CDC 2003).

Step 1: Describe the problem and identify how counter-marketing approaches can address it.

Before you start, review the tobacco control goal(s) your program will support. For example, if the overall tobacco control program will focus on adult smoking cessation, then your counter-marketing program shouldn't address smoking cessation in youth. If the overall program goals are to increase adult smoking cessation and to decrease exposure to secondhand smoke, then you'll need to develop counter-marketing plans to address each of these goals.

1a. Describe the problem.

Once you have verified the program's overall goal(s), you can identify the specific problem or issue to address. Make sure that everyone agrees on what the problem is and that you have sufficient information to understand it and describe it. The amount of information needed to develop a description of the problem depends on factors such as the following:

- How much experience your organization has with the issue

- How much information is available on the issue in your area or in a similar locale

- How much research is needed to justify your decision to your organization and to potential critics of your program

Be specific in describing the problem. The problem description should include:

What Works?

Counter-marketing programs with the following characteristics are more likely to succeed (Backer et al. 1992; NCI 2002):

- **Specific outcomes.** Program objectives should be clear and specific. General descriptions don't provide enough direction for program design or evaluation. (See Step 3 for tips on developing objectives that are specific, measurable, achievable, relevant, and time-bound [SMART].)

- **Multiple target audiences.** Many outcomes involve multiple target audiences. For example, if prevention of smoking by adolescents is the goal, you may want to reach teens in different social or age groups, parents, and teen "influencers" (e.g., sports coaches or older siblings) with your program's messages and interventions, assuming the budget is adequate to address all of them.

- **Multiple tactics.** Integrating multiple tactics (e.g., combining advertising with advocacy and media literacy) into a unified counter-marketing campaign can help a program address a problem in different ways and thus enhance its effectiveness.

- **Multiple types of change.** Many outcomes call for changes in individual behavior as well as other types of change (e.g., a shift in policy or environmental norms) that will support or contribute to behavior change.

- **Messages that directly support intended changes.** General awareness or prevention messages (e.g., "don't smoke" or "smoking is harmful") rarely are enough. Messages should be specific and should directly contribute to achieving the intended changes (e.g., encouraging people to call a quitline).

- **Tailored messages and activities.** Appropriate messages and activities are likely to differ for different target audiences and at different times in the program, depending on the perceptions, needs, interests, and behaviors of the audience.

- **Formative research.** Research to glean key insights about target audiences is essential to guide you in program design and to help you determine the most effective strategies, messages, and activities. Research is equally important for programs that target teens, adult smokers, policy makers, or any other targeted group.

- **Consistency.** Although the program's messages and activities are tailored for each audience, they all must support strategies designed to reach the tobacco control program's overall goals.

- **Commitment over time.** Successful programs commit to the long term, recognizing that changes in behavior take time. Initial indicators of progress don't always mean that changes will be maintained.

- **A focus on changing social norms.** Over the long term, changes in social norms that demonstrate acceptance of the desired outcomes are true indicators of the program's success.

- Who is affected and how

- The severity of the problem, along with data used to measure the severity

- Who can positively influence the situation or the affected group

1b. Describe who is affected.

If possible, describe subgroups that may be affected disproportionately by the problem. These subgroups should be sufficiently large and sufficiently different from one another and the general population to justify distinction. Subgroup descriptions can include:

- Demographic information (e.g., age, gender, race/ethnicity, education, and family income)

- Geographic information (e.g., location of residence, school, and work)

- Psychographic information (e.g., attitudes, opinions, intentions, beliefs, and values)

You should become familiar with sources of available data that can help describe the population, the severity of the problem, and the ways to measure change. (See Chapter 5: Evaluating the Success of Your Counter-Marketing Program and the Resources section of this manual for more information.) Individuals in your state programs for chronic disease or health statistics or others with epidemiologic training or experience can help you find relevant data sources. Here are some examples:

- Surgeon General's reports

- Behavioral surveys such as the national Youth Risk Behavior Survey, the Youth Tobacco Survey, and the Behavioral Risk Factor Surveillance System survey

- Consensus statements and recommendations by national organizations, such as the tobacco cessation guidelines published by the Agency for Healthcare Research and Quality

- Web sites that list sources of U.S. government information on tobacco control issues (e.g., http://www.healthfinder.gov and http://www.cdc.gov/tobacco)

- Relevant qualitative and quantitative research that other states or organizations conducted in developing their programs

- Database searches for journal articles and scientific reports (e.g., CDC/OSH's Smoking and Health Database (http://www.cdc.gov/tobacco/search/) and MEDLINE (http://medline.cos.com/)

1c. Refine the problem statement.

As additional information becomes available, refine your problem statement by adding more detailed descriptions of the subgroups affected. For example, if the original problem statement identified a higher rate of adolescent smokers in a certain city, further investigation may reveal that the smokers were 11th and 12th graders in inner-city schools. A review of the scientific literature and of successful tobacco control programs elsewhere may also reveal that their intentions to smoke were influenced by parents, athletic coaches, and peers.

1d. Assess factors that can affect the campaign: strengths, weaknesses, opportunities, and threats (SWOTs).

Before you progress too far in your planning, do a reality check. Assess strengths, weaknesses, opportunities, and threats (SWOTs). First, ask yourself the following questions to determine whether your organization is ready to address the problem:

- Does your organization have the necessary authority or mandate?
- Do you have or can you acquire the necessary expertise and resources?
- Will you be duplicating the efforts of others?
- How much time do you have to address this issue?
- What can you accomplish in that time?

Then identify your assets and your barriers. Consider the following factors:

- Available resources, including funds, time, and personnel and their skills
- The level of your organization's commitment to addressing the issue
- The roles of other concerned or involved groups and whether there is a gap, an opportunity for partnering, or potential overlap in areas being addressed
- Whether sound guidance is available to address the problem
- Political support for, resistance to, or potential criticism of efforts to address the problem
- Policies or lack of policies that can help or hinder your efforts
- Barriers to behavioral or environmental change or both, including activities of adversaries

Also, ask what other states or organizations are doing to address the problem:

- What have they learned?
- Do they have information or advice to help you plan (e.g., advice about targeting, budgeting, and evaluating)?
- From their perspective, what gaps exist in media coverage/advertising, community activities, materials, and target audiences?
- Are there opportunities for collaborative ventures, especially if key goals and target audiences are the same?

Experienced colleagues and contacts at other state health departments can offer suggestions or advice as you conduct this assessment. In addition, CDC's Web-based State Information Forum (http://ntcp.forum.cdc.gov) contains a large collection of state tobacco control documents that you might find useful. Keep all the information gained through this assessment in mind as you develop the counter-marketing program.

1e. Review relevant theories and models.

Your program planning may be helped significantly by a review of theories and models that offer perspective on the target audiences and the steps that might influence them (NCI 1995). Theories can help to explain why problems exist, what you need to know about the target audience, and what you need to do to influence change. Theories and models also can help guide you in choosing realistic objectives, determining effective strategies and messages, and designing an appropriate evaluation. No single theory dominates the design of a counter-marketing program, because issues, populations, cultures, contexts, and intended outcomes vary. Many programs are based on several theories. Best practices in counter-marketing are discussed in this manual. Table 2.1, from the National Cancer Institute's *Theory at a Glance: A Guide for Health Promotion Practice* (NCI 1995), summarizes some key theories.

Step 2: Identify and learn about target audiences.

Understanding the target audience(s) before you plan and develop your program is essential. To be successful in influencing them, you will need to understand the problem and potential changes from the point of view of the target audience(s). Before you start to plan the program, define the audience you want to reach and the results you want to achieve and determine how to measure those results. (See Step 3 for information on defining objectives.) Also, find out about the target audience (e.g., lifestyle, attitudes, environment, culture, knowledge, beliefs, and behaviors), so you can plan appropriate activities while keeping an eye on your program objectives.

In Step 1, you identified who was affected by the problem, but the people affected may constitute a broad population. One or several target audience(s) should be selected on the basis of shared characteristics. For example, if the problem you're addressing is that more middle school students are starting to smoke cigarettes, you may want to target middle school students who are at risk of starting to smoke.

If reliable data on a certain group are not available, you may need to conduct qualitative or quantitative research or both to learn enough to make sound planning decisions. For example, in Massachusetts, the prevalence of cigarette smoking was significantly higher among physically disabled individuals than among other groups, but other descriptive data were lacking, so the state conducted research to further understand this audience. (See Chapter 3: Gaining and Using Target Audience Insights for more information on conducting research.)

In some cases, the target audience(s) may not be the affected population. Let's say you want to decrease illegal tobacco sales to students. Your target audiences might be decision makers, such as school officials, who can set policies about tobacco use on or near school property; community opinion leaders, who can increase community interest in taking action to decrease illegal sales; and merchants, who control access to and availability of tobacco products. If you want to affect

Table 2.1: Summary of Theories: Focus and Key Concepts

Theory	Focus	Key Concepts
Individual Level		
Stages of Change Model	Individuals' readiness to change or attempt to change toward healthy behaviors	• Precontemplation • Contemplation • Decision/determination • Action • Maintenance
Health Belief Model	Individuals' perception of the threat of a health problem and the appraisal of recommended behavior(s) for preventing or managing the problem	• Perceived susceptibility • Perceived severity • Perceived benefits of action • Perceived barriers to action • Cues to action • Self-efficacy
Consumer Information Processing Model	Process by which consumers acquire and use information in making decisions	• Information processing • Information search • Decision rules/heuristics • Consumption and learning • Information environment
Interpersonal Level		
Social Learning Theory	Behavior explained via a three-way, dynamic reciprocal theory in which personal factors, environmental influences, and behavior continually interact	• Behavioral capability • Reciprocal determinism • Expectations • Self-efficacy • Observational learning • Reinforcement

Continues

Table 2.1: Summary of Theories: Focus and Key Concepts (cont.)

Theory	Focus	Key Concepts
Community Level		
Community Organization Theories	Emphasis of active community participation and development of communities that can better evaluate and solve health and social problems	• Empowerment • Community competence • Participation and relevance • Issue selection • Critical consciousness
Organizational Change Theory	Processes and strategies for increasing the chances that healthy policies and programs will be adopted and maintained in formal organizations	• Problem definition (awareness stage) • Initiation of action (adoption stage) • Implementation of change • Institutionalization of change
Diffusion of Innovations Theory	How new ideas, products, and social practices spread within a society or from one society to another	• Relative advantage • Compatibility • Complexity • Trialability • Observability

Source: NCI 1995

pregnant women who smoke, you might target spouses or partners. Changing the behavior of their partners supports the pregnant women's attempts to quit smoking and reduces their exposure to secondhand smoke.

The more specifically you can target an audience, the more likely you are to develop approaches that will be appropriate to the audience's interests and needs. For example, you wouldn't target all middle school students in three counties if you could more specifically and appropriately target those most likely to smoke cigarettes, such as seventh and eighth graders whose parents smoke, who are less likely to be honor roll students, and who are more likely to be on their own in the afternoons.

One exception to this rule may be the targeting of smokers for cessation. A recent global review of smoking cessation campaigns indicated that smokers who are targeted narrowly (e.g., those most ready to stop smoking) may mentally exclude themselves from the category and deny that the message is meant for them, because they know how difficult it can be to stop smoking. Programs found greater success in prompting smokers to call quitlines when all smokers were included in the message's target. Also helpful were messages targeting smokers by undeniable characteristics, such as pregnancy or ethnic background (Schar and Gutierrez 2001).

2a. Clearly define the audience you want to reach and the result to be achieved.

Two steps that will help to set the parameters of your program are defining subgroups of an affected population sharing common characteristics (audience segmentation) and selecting one or more subgroups—your target audience(s). Because no one program can do everything for everyone, choosing a target audience provides a focus for the rest of your planning decisions.

To select your target audience, review the following questions:

- What is the problem?
- What is the solution or desired outcome?
- Who is most likely to be able to make the desired changes happen?
- How specifically can you describe this group or groups—the target audience(s)?
- How large is each group? (Each group should be large enough to make a difference in the problem but should not include so many types of people that you can't tailor your efforts with enough specificity.)

This review may leave you with many options. Answering the following questions will help you to prioritize the audience(s) for the campaign (CDC 2003):

- Which audiences represent the highest priorities for reaching the key tobacco control goals?
- Which audiences can be most easily reached and influenced?
- Which audiences are affected disproportionately by the health problems associated with tobacco use?
- Which audiences are large enough to justify intervention?
- Which audiences are most unique and identifiable?
- Which audiences are most vulnerable to the health problems?
- In which audiences would counter-marketing efforts duplicate the efforts of an existing program or campaign?
- Which audiences, if any, have higher or lower priority because of political considerations?

2b. Find out more about the target audiences.

What "drives" the actions and behaviors of audience members, what interests and appeals to them, and where you can reach them are essential pieces of information for program design. Also, take the time to understand, not simply make assumptions

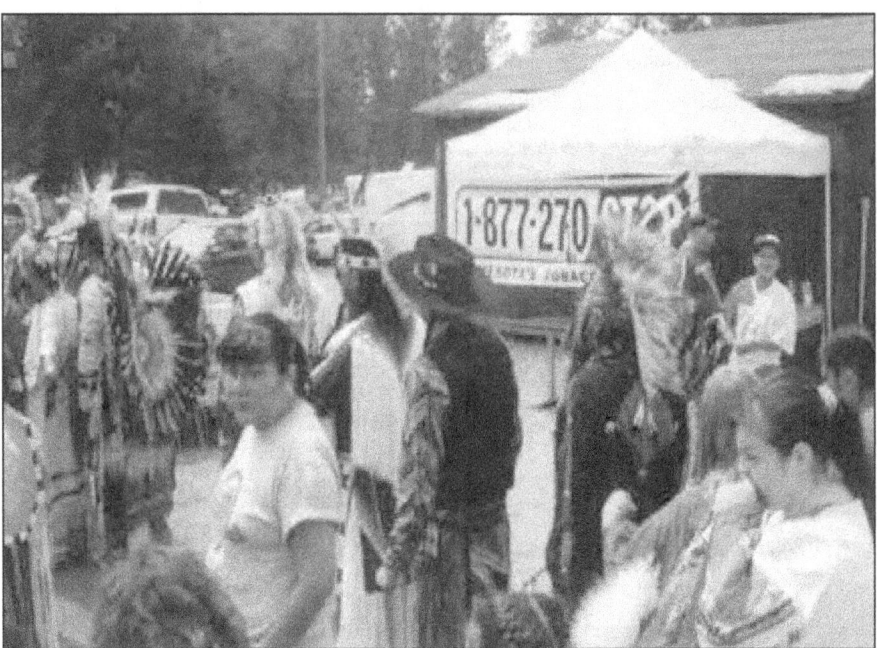

about, cultural contexts that influence how target audiences live, perceive their environment, and make decisions. (See Chapter 4: Reaching Specific Populations for more information on these groups.)

Chapter 3: Gaining and Using Target Audience Insights discusses a variety of methods for conducting market research to learn more about your audience(s). You'll need to answer the following questions about the target audiences to plan an effective program:

- What are the attitudes and beliefs of the target audience about problems and behavior associated with the tobacco control problem? Are there misconceptions that need to be corrected?

- What other attitudes and beliefs could influence behavior related to tobacco use (e.g., perceptions of "cool" that include tobacco use, openness to seeking professional help for medical problems, and feelings about the importance of individual rights over group rights)? If tobacco use is perceived as beneficial, what barriers to change must be addressed?

- Are there social, cultural, and economic factors to consider? For example, does a high percentage of the target audience report that it is difficult to turn down a cigarette offered at a party? Do some individuals use cigarettes as a positive symbol because of cultural beliefs and practices? Does the price of cigarettes influence the number of cigarettes smoked? Do some smokers find ways around pricing changes, such as stealing, getting cigarettes from friends and family, or buying "loosies" (single cigarettes typically sold at small convenience stores or on the street)?

- Where can audience members be reached? In the community? In school? At home? Through television? Radio? Print? Interactive media? (It helps to know about a typical day in the life of an audience member.)

- What are the audience's preferences in terms of learning styles, appeals, language, and tone of messages? Some people learn through reading and contemplation; others prefer discussion. Some may be motivated by positive appeals; while others may be more influenced by fear and other negative emotions. For example, the promise of a healthy baby might motivate a pregnant woman to quit smoking, while the threat of serious heart disease might move a middle-aged man with borderline hypertension to quit.

- What are the audience's preferences in terms of activities, vehicles, and involvement in the issue of tobacco? Some smokers may prefer to quit on their own; others may welcome access to a quitline counselor.

Your counter-marketing plan should include the following information about each of your target audiences:

- Demographics (e.g., gender, age, educational attainment, occupation, income, family situation, and location of residence, work, and school)

- Community norms and cultural and lifestyle characteristics (e.g., language preferences and proficiencies, religion, ethnicity, generational status, family structure, degree of acculturation, and lifestyle factors such as food and activity preferences)

- Preferences, including places where they might be receptive to activities; media use; and types of messages, sources, or sponsors perceived as credible

- Behaviors, knowledge, attitudes, values, and feelings that indicate the audience's willingness to accept and act on the information provided (i.e., their readiness to change)

Step 3: Draft counter-marketing objectives.

Defining your counter-marketing objectives will help you to determine the messages you'll use and to set priorities among possible strategies and activities. Your objectives serve as a kind of contract or agreement about your program's purpose, and they establish the outcomes that should be measured.

Objectives should reflect the results expected from the counter-marketing program within the given time frame and within the context of a comprehensive tobacco control program. In general, counter-marketing programs can:

- Raise awareness about the problem of tobacco use and about the tobacco counter-marketing campaign

- Build knowledge about the specifics of the issues associated with tobacco use and prevention

- Shape or shift individual attitudes or values, contributing to behavior change

- Change community norms

- Result in simple actions (e.g., asking for help or information)

- Win broad public support for tobacco control issues

More specifically, counter-marketing activities designed to support health policy or enforcement of health-related laws, such as a ban on tobacco sales to minors, might be expected to:

- Frame a health policy issue to make it relevant to more people

- Reward retailers who refrain from selling tobacco products to minors

- Increase support for a tobacco control policy

Counter-marketing activities designed to support tobacco cessation or other tobacco-related health services might be expected to:

- Communicate the benefits of cessation or the risks of continuing to use tobacco

- Increase support for coverage of smoking cessation programs under private and public insurance

- Prompt use of population-based counseling services, such as quitlines

Your objectives also should specify the impact you want the program to have on the tobacco-related problem and should support your organization's broader goals for tobacco control. You should write objective(s) that answer these questions:

- What specific effect do you hope to have related to the tobacco problem, and among which affected or influential populations?

- How much change do you expect? By when? (Include intermediate milestones that will help you identify progress.)

Setting achievable objectives is important. Many efforts fail because of unreasonable objectives. For example, achieving anywhere near 100 percent change is generally impossible. If you plan to specify a numerical goal for a particular objective, an epidemiologist, statistician, or advertising or marketing expert can offer guidance on reasonable rates of change. (For example, commercial marketers often consider a 2- to 3-percent increase in sales to be a great success.) Also, you should bring your evaluator into the process when you are ready to draft objectives for the counter-marketing program.

Don't let fear of failure keep you from setting measurable or achievable objectives. Without them, you have no way of showing that you have succeeded or are making progress, which could reduce support for your program.

Chapter 5 offers more information on developing objectives, but here are some SMART tips:

- **Specific.** Be as specific as possible. For example, state that the program will "increase by 10 percent the number of health care providers who counsel pregnant women to quit smoking," rather than stating that it will "increase smoking cessation among pregnant women." Use specific verbs such as "improve," "increase,"

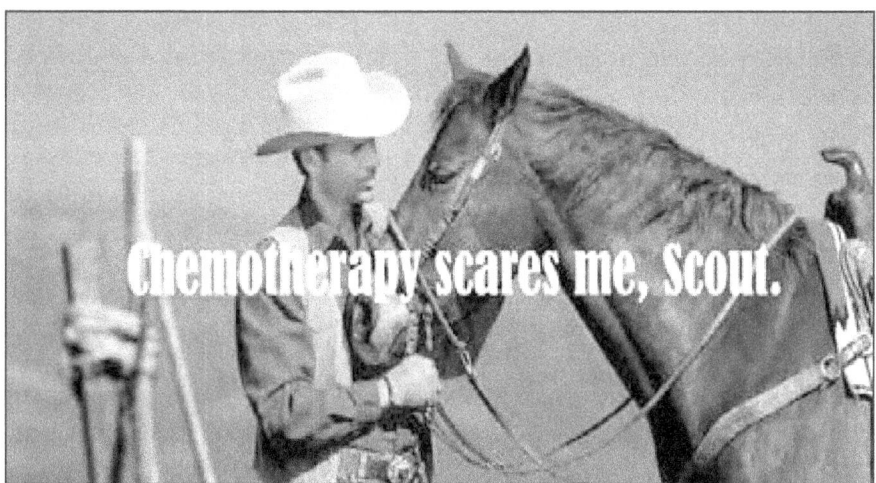

"promote," "protect," "minimize," "prevent," and "reduce" to describe objectives.

- **Measurable.** Clear objectives ("increase by 25 percent") will guide evaluation design and allow you to track progress. Also, determine how you'll measure results. Will the measurement rely on existing data or will new sources of data be needed?

- **Achievable.** Objectives should be realistic. Explore what degree of change is reasonable to expect within your program budget and your timeline for program implementation.

- **Relevant.** Objectives should be related to your program's overall goals and should be logical, based on what you plan to do.

- **Time-bound.** Determine the time frame during which you expect certain changes to take place.

An example of a SMART objective might be to increase by 20 percent the number of smokers who call the state quitline and attempt to stop smoking by the end of 2003. In addition to counter-marketing, other strategies and tobacco control activities conducted over a period of time are likely to be needed to change behaviors, policies, and social norms.

Step 4: Determine counter-marketing approaches, channels, and program strategies.

Now you can begin to develop a detailed plan. Select which counter-marketing approaches and channels you'll use; then define program strategies. Although these decisions are described here in sequence, they are interrelated. In most cases, these decisions will be made together, not sequentially.

4a. Review and select the counter-marketing approaches to use.

Five counter-marketing approaches are described here: advertising, public relations, media advocacy, grassroots marketing, and media literacy. Most of this manual is devoted to helping you to plan and implement these specific counter-marketing tactics, and each one is discussed in detail in a separate chapter. Instead of jumping to conclusions about the approaches to use, consider which are most likely to help you reach your objectives. Here's a quick look at these approaches, along with examples of what they can and can't contribute to your counter-marketing program:

- **Advertising** is a communication tactic in which messages are repeatedly delivered directly to a mass audience. Advertising permits control over the message's tone, content, and amount of exposure.

  – Advertising *can* communicate a single, simple message to many people, change attitudes, create an image for the campaign, and expose the practices of adversaries or competitors.

  – Advertising *can't* provide complex information, feedback, or services.

- **Public relations** is used to reach target audiences through "earned" media coverage—coverage of the program and issue generated through activities and relationships with reporters and other media gatekeepers.

  – Public relations *can* establish ongoing relationships with media, stakeholders, opinion leaders, and others; reach audiences with information and messages often seen as more credible than advertising; gain public support and create a positive environment for the program; expose the practices of adversaries or competitors; and provide a quick response to issues and events as they arise.

  – Public relations *can't* guarantee a story's placement, exposure, focus, slant, content, or accuracy.

- **Media advocacy** is the strategic use of media and community advocacy to create social or policy change.

  – Media advocacy *can* help communities create lasting environmental change.

  – Media advocacy *can't* guarantee individual behavior change based on new information.

- **Grassroots marketing** is used to involve people in the community as participants in a counter-marketing program.

  – Grassroots marketing *can* get people in the community involved in the issue or program, create interpersonal exposure to the message, channel feed-back, and build community support.

  – Grassroots marketing *can't* be tightly controlled or expose a broad audience to a very specific message.

- **Media literacy** helps people ask questions about what they watch, see, and read. It helps them critically assess how the mass media normalize, glamorize, and create role models for unhealthy lifestyles and behavior. Also, it includes an examination of techniques, technologies,

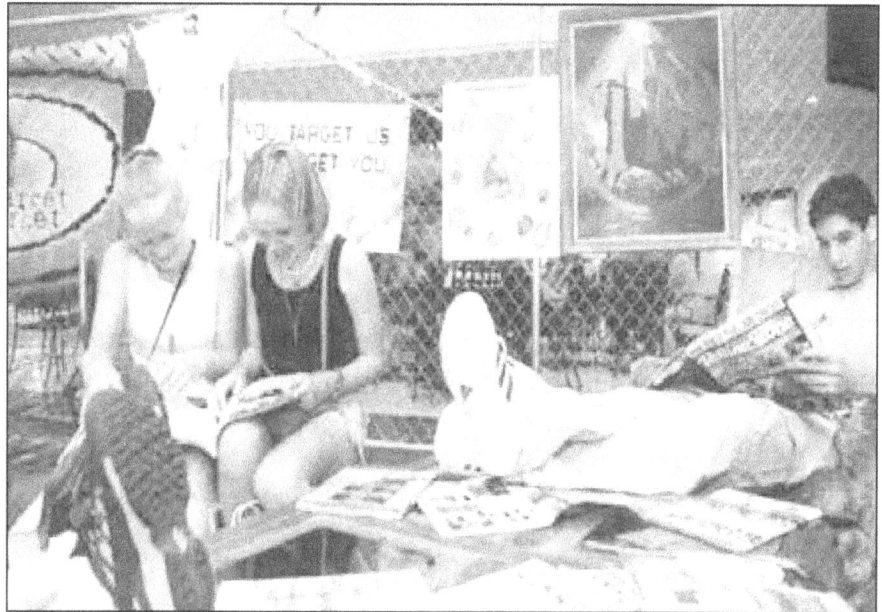

and institutions involved in media production.

- Media literacy *can* help change attitudes, teach people to recognize how messages are used to influence them, and show them how to counteract those messages by developing their own messages.

- Media literacy *can't* change industry marketing practices or replace classes or programs that explain tobacco's impact on health.

Combining several approaches is usually better than using just one. Any approach you choose must fit into your broader strategy. The best advertising or public relations work won't make up for a lack of strategy. The following questions can help you decide which approaches to use:

- Which approach or combination of approaches best addresses the problem and your program objectives?

- Which options are most appropriate for your target audience(s)?

- Which approach(es) can your organization afford and successfully implement, taking into account the available skills, budget, and experience?

- Could any of the approaches cause undesirable or unintended effects, such as public or political criticism?

4b. Review and select the channels to use.

Channels are pathways used to deliver program messages, materials, and activities to your target audience. Channels can be categorized into four broad groups: interpersonal, community and organizational, mass media, and interactive media channels.

Interpersonal channels put health messages in a familiar context. Examples of interpersonal channels to reach intended audiences are physicians, friends and family members, counselors, parents, clergy, educators, and coaches. These channels are more likely to be trusted and influential than are mass media sources. Developing relationships with and creating messages and materials for interpersonal channels may take some time, but these channels are among the most effective, especially for affecting individual attitudes, skills, and behavior/behavioral intent. Influence through interpersonal contacts may work best when the person is already familiar with the message, for example, from hearing it through the mass media. Similarly, mass media approaches are most effective at changing behavior when they're supplemented with interpersonal channels.

Community and organizational channels can reinforce and expand on other media messages and add credibility and legitimacy. Community groups and organizations can disseminate your materials, hold events, and offer instruction related to your message. Establishing links with these groups can be a shortcut to developing interpersonal channels to your audience(s). Community and organizational channels, like interpersonal channels, can offer support for action and can function in two directions. They allow discussion and clarification, encouraging motivation, and reinforcing action. Community leaders can be effective channels, because they influence other people and can influence policy. They may include physicians and other health care professionals; religious, political, and social leaders; business and union leaders; and "rule makers," who control the audience's environment (e.g., teachers, parents, policy makers, and law enforcement personnel). Community leaders can disseminate messages broadly to groups or become part of an interpersonal channel. Also, garnering the support of many organizations that work together toward a common goal can create a "critical mass" resulting in a bandwagon effect for your efforts.

Mass media channels offer many opportunities for dissemination of a message. Examples of mass media channels are radio, broadcast and cable TV, magazines, direct mail, billboards, and newspapers. The opportunities provided include mentions in news programs; entertainment programming ("entertainment education"); public affairs, "magazine," and interview shows (e.g., radio call-in programs); live remote broadcasts; editorials on TV and radio and in newspapers and magazines; health and political columns in newspapers and magazines; posters; brochures; advertising; and public service campaigns. You may decide to use a variety of formats and media channels, but you should choose the ones that are most likely to effectively reach your audience(s).

Mass media campaigns are a tried and true approach. They've been conducted on topics ranging from general health to specific diseases, from prevention to treatment. Overall, research has demonstrated that mass media approaches are effective in raising awareness, stimulating an audience to seek information and services, increasing knowledge, changing attitudes, and even achieving some change in behavioral intentions and behaviors (Snyder and Hamilton 2002). However, behavior change is usually associated with long-term, multiple-intervention campaigns, rather than with one-time, communication-only programs (Smith 2002). Mass media campaigns also can contribute to changes in social norms and to other collective changes (e.g., policy and environmental changes) (Hornik 2002).

Interactive media channels are useful now and may have even greater reach in the future. Examples include Web sites, Internet bulletin boards, newsgroups, chat rooms, CD-ROMs, and kiosks). These media channels allow delivery of highly targeted messages to and feedback from the audience. Your program can use these media to send individual messages via e-mail (electronic mail) and post-program messages, such as information about health-related campaigns on popular Web sites, to create and display ads, to survey and gather information from computer users, to exchange ideas and ready-to-use materials with peers and partners, and to rally or demonstrate support for a policy or issue. Before choosing an interactive channel, you'll need to determine whether it's accessible and whether your audience is comfortable with it.

To identify possible channels for reaching your audience, find answers to the following questions:

- Where can you reach audience members (e.g., at home, at school or work, in the car, on the bus or train, or at a community event)?

- When are they most likely to be attentive and open to your efforts?

- Where can they act on your message?

- In which places or situations will they find your messages most credible and influential?

- Which places or situations are most appropriate for the counter-marketing approaches you are considering?

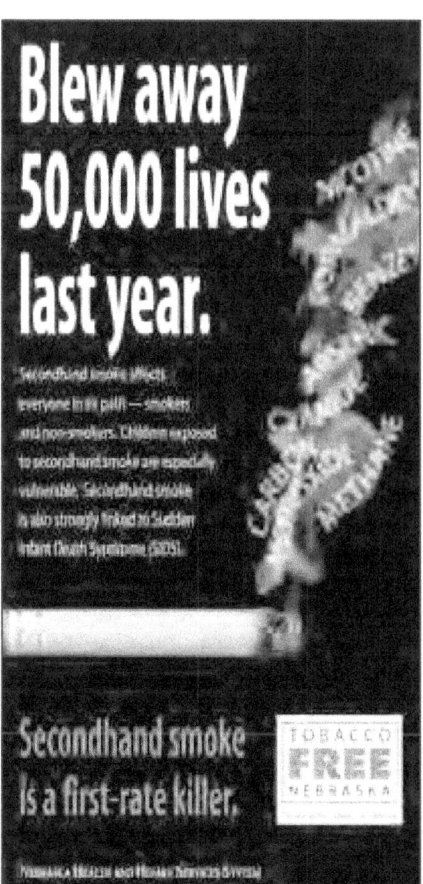

The use of several channels has been most effective in producing desired results, including behavior change (NCI 2002). Using a combination of channels not only improves your chances of reaching more members of your audience(s), it also can increase the repetition of your message, which in turn increases the chance that the audience will be exposed to it often enough to internalize and act on it. Finally, some messages may seem more legitimate when they come from several sources or channels.

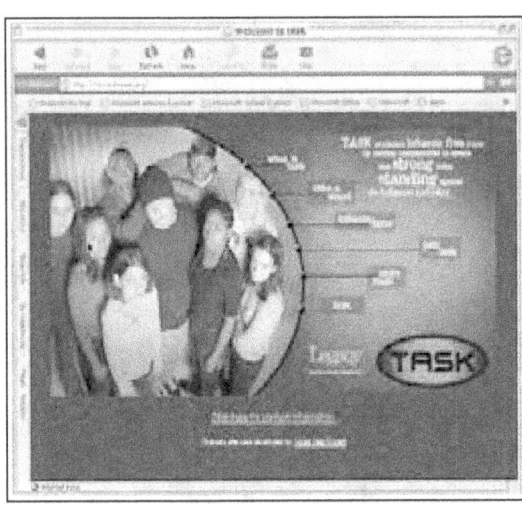

Here are some tips for selecting channels to include in your program:

- Choose channels that suit your objectives, and decide how the approaches described in this manual can be used with those channels.

- Select channels and activities that fit your budget, time constraints, and resources.

- Consider the attributes and limitations of each type of channel. For example, electronic media can reach many people quickly to inform and create awareness, but they may not be as suitable as other channels for more complicated messages and purposes. The recommendations of physicians may be persuasive to smokers but may not reach many people; TV ads may reach many people but may not be as credible as physicians' recommendations; and print ads may deliver a complex message better than TV can but may not be as engaging, because they lack action and sound. For these reasons, the best approach often is to use multiple channels to take advantage of the strengths of each channel. Table 2.2 lists some of the pros and cons of different channels.

4c. Draft program strategies.

A strategy is the approach you plan to take with a specific audience. Although you may develop many different materials and use a variety of activities, your strategies are guiding principles for all your products and activities.

The strategy includes everything you need to know to work with your audience. It defines the audience, states the action audience members should take, tells how they will benefit (from their perspective, not necessarily from a public health perspective), and explains how you can reach them. The strategy is based on knowledge

Table 2.2: Counter-Marketing Channels and Activities: Pros and Cons

Channel	Activities	Pros	Cons
Interpersonal			
• Influential adults • Health care providers • Family members • Friends	• Hotline counseling • Patient counseling • Instruction • Prompted, informal discussion	• Can be credible • Permit two-way discussion • Can be motivational, influential, supportive • Most effective for teaching and helping/caring	• Can be expensive • Can be time consuming • Can have limited reach of intended audience • Can be difficult to develop; sources need to be convinced and taught about the message themselves
Organizational and Community			
• Schools • Employers • Community groups	• Town hall and other events • Organizational meetings and conferences • Workplace campaigns • Media literacy	• May be familiar, trusted, and influential • May provide more motivation or support than media alone • Can sometimes be inexpensive • Can offer shared experiences • Can reach larger audience in one place	• Can be time consuming to establish • May not provide personalized attention • Organizational constraints may require message approval • Control of messages may be lost if they are adapted to fit organizational needs
Mass Media			
• Newspaper	• Ads (paid or public service) • News • Feature stories • Letters to the editor • Op-ed pieces	• Can reach broad audiences rapidly • Can convey health news/breakthroughs more thoroughly than TV or radio and faster than magazines • Audience has chance to clip, reread, contemplate, and pass along material • Small papers may take print public service announcements (PSAs)	• Coverage demands a newsworthy item • PSA placement virtually nonexistent • Exposure usually limited to one day

Continues

Table 2.2: Counter-Marketing Channels and Activities: Pros and Cons (cont.)

Channel	Activities	Pros	Cons
Mass Media (cont.)			
• Radio	• Ads (paid or public service) • News • Public affairs/interview shows • Dramatic programming (entertainment education)	• Range of formats available to intended audiences with known listening preferences • Opportunity for direct audience involvement (through call-in shows and remotes) • Can use ad scripts (called "live-copy ads"), which are flexible and inexpensive • Paid ads or specific programming can reach intended audience when they are most receptive • Paid ads are relatively inexpensive • Ad production costs are low relative to TV • Ads' message and execution can be controlled	• Reaches fewer people than TV • Although cheaper than TV ads, paid ads still may be too expensive • PSA placement runs infrequently and at low listening times • Feature placement requires contacts and may be time consuming • Many stations have limited formats that may not be conducive to health messages • Difficult for audiences to retain or pass on material • Stations consolidating; fewer local choices
• Televison	• Ads (paid or public service) • News • Public affairs/interview shows • Dramatic programming (entertainment education)	• Potentially the largest and widest range of audiences • Visual combined with audio good for emotional appeals and demonstrating behaviors • Can reach low-income audiences	• Ads are typically expensive to produce • Paid advertising may be too expensive • PSA placement may run infrequently and at low viewing times • Feature placement requires contacts and may be time consuming

Table 2.2: Counter-Marketing Channels and Activities: Pros and Cons (cont.)

Channel	Activities	Pros	Cons
Mass Media (cont.)			
		• Paid ads or specific programming can reach intended audience when they are most receptive • Ads' message and execution can be controlled • Opportunity for direct audience involvement (through call-in shows)	• Message may be obscured by commercial clutter • Increased channel options have fragmented audiences (some channels reach very small audiences) • Promotion can result in huge demand • Can be difficult for audiences to retain or pass on material
Interactive Media			
• Internet	• Web sites • E-mail lists • Chat rooms • News groups • Ads (paid or public service)	• Can reach large numbers of people rapidly • Information can be instantaneously updated and disseminated • Information can be controlled • Can reach specific audiences and provide personalized information • Can be interactive and engaging • Can provide health information in a graphically appealing way • Can combine the audio and/or visual benefits of TV or radio with the self-pacing benefits of print media • Can use banner ads to direct audience to your Web site	• Can be expensive • Many audiences may not have access to the Internet or skills to use it • Audience must be proactive; they must search or sign up for information • News groups and chat rooms may require monitoring • Can require maintenance over time • Thousands of health-oriented Web sites and listservs exist, so size of audience may be small • Users typically scan Web sites quickly and may not attend to health messages

This table was adapted from NCI 2002.

of the audience, guided by market research and theories and models of behavior, and tempered by the realities of organization roles, resources, and deadlines.

You'll need to develop a strategy statement that translates this information into a cohesive document articulating what you'll do, and you'll need to ensure that all key decision makers agree with it. You may be tempted to skip this step. Don't skip it. Having an approved strategy statement will save you time and effort later. Developing the statement provides a good test of whether there's enough information to begin developing messages. It offers an opportunity to convince your organization and partners to buy into your program. The statement also can serve as the guideline for all your materials and activities.

At this stage in the planning process, you should involve experts in advertising, media advocacy, marketing, or related fields, depending on the approaches you've selected. If you're working with partners, they might be a part of this program design team. Evaluation experts, if they aren't already involved, also should join the team at this point.

This stage also is a good time to do another reality check. As you develop your strategy, make sure you have the budget and other resources to include all the approaches and channels you have identified. It's better to limit your activities and do fewer things well than to stretch modest resources across many strategies and targets. Think for the long term: you may want to start with one target audience and one approach and add program components in future years. After several years, you can have a comprehensive program in place.

For each of your target audiences, write a strategy statement that includes the following elements:

- **Target audience profile.** The description will be most useful if you describe one person in the audience, rather than describing the group. The information you gathered in Step 2 should be used here.

- **Action you want the audience to take as a result of exposure to your program.** The action should be based on the objectives you drafted in Step 3.

- **Obstacles to taking action.** Common obstacles include audience beliefs, social norms, time or peer pressures, costs, ingrained habits, misinformation, and lack of access to products, services, or program activities. The additional information you gathered about the audience in Step 2 should help you identify obstacles.

- **Benefit the audience will perceive as sufficiently valuable to motivate them to take action.** Many theories and models of behavior change suggest that people take action or change their behavior because they expect to receive some benefit (e.g., have more energy, save money, live longer, or gain acceptance from peers) that outweighs the cost (e.g., time, money, or potential loss of stature among peers).

- **Reason(s) the benefit and the audience's ability to attain the benefit should be credible and important to the audience** (sometimes called the "reason to believe"). Support can be provided through hard data, peer testimonials about success or satisfaction, demonstrations of how to perform the action (if audience members doubt their ability), or statements from people or organizations the audience finds credible. Support should be tailored to the concerns of audience members about the action. For example, if they are worried that they can't act as recommended, a demonstration of the behavior may give them the confidence to act. If they question why they should take the action or whether it will have the promised health benefit, hard data or statements from credible people or organizations may be effective. If they don't believe they need to take the action, a peer testimonial may make them reconsider.

- **Channels and activities** that will reach audience members.

- **The image you plan to convey through the tone, look, and feel of messages and materials.** You should convey an image that convinces audience members that the communication is directed at them and that it's culturally appropriate. Image is conveyed largely through creative details. For example, printed

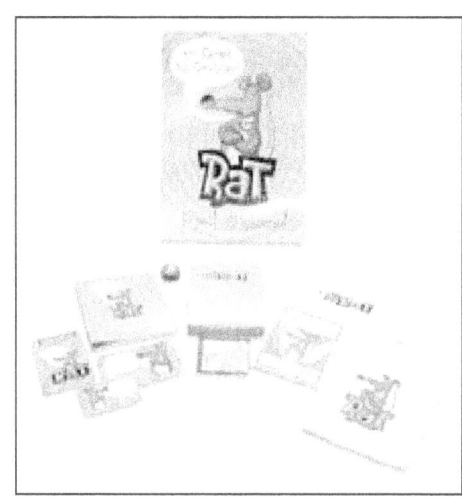

materials convey image through typeface, layout, visuals, color, language, and paper stock. Audio materials convey image through voices, language, and music. In addition, video materials convey image through visuals, the actors' characteristics (e.g., clothing and accessories), camera angles, and editing.

Developing a strategy is usually an iterative process; as you learn more about one element, other elements may need to be adjusted.

4d. Develop a logic model.

A logic model describes the sequence of events that will occur to bring about the change (objective) you have identified. This model is often designed as a flowchart (see Figure 2.1). A logic model is valuable because it accomplishes several purposes:

- Summarizes program components and outcomes at a glance

- Can display the infrastructure needed to support the program

Figure 2.1: Example of Logic Model for One Component of Youth Tobacco Use Prevention Advertising Campaign

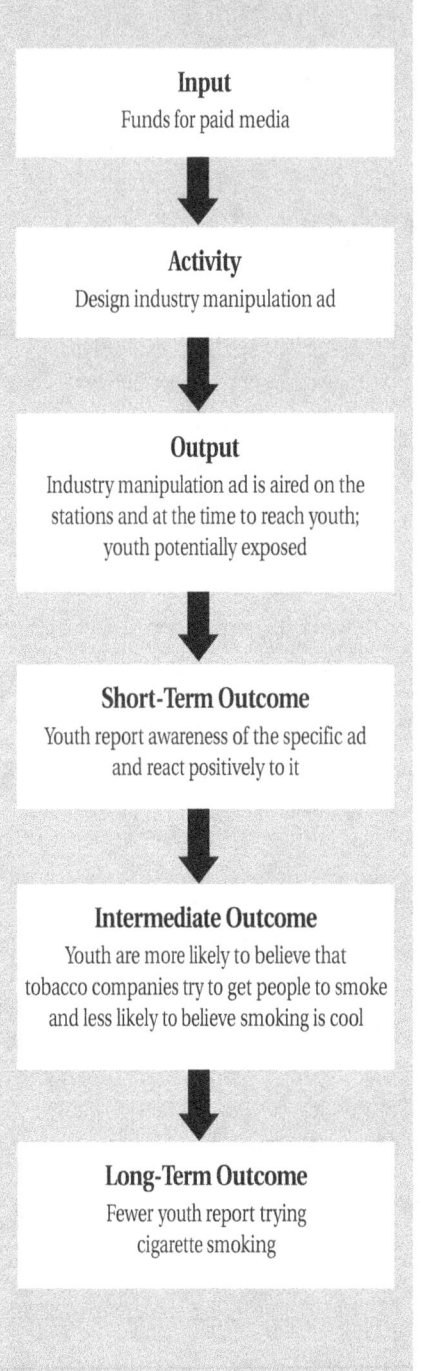

- Forces you to describe what you're planning in a simple way

- Reveals any gaps in the logic behind your plans

- Describes what will happen over the course of your program, which will be useful for working with stakeholders, partners, and evaluators

If you've identified several objectives and target audiences, you may need to develop several logic models. Chapter 5: Evaluating the Success of Your Counter-Marketing Program offers a more detailed look at logic models, but basically, your logic model(s) should include:

- **Inputs**—what is necessary to conduct the program (e.g., trained staff and materials)

- **Activities**—what you will do (e.g., provide media-literacy training or hold press conferences)

- **Outputs**—what will happen as a result of activities (e.g., messages in the media as a result of public relations initiatives)

- **Outcomes**—short-term results (e.g., changes in teens' attitudes about tobacco advertising) and long-term results (e.g., lower youth smoking initiation rates)

Step 5: Consider collaboration.

Working with other organizations can be a cost-effective way to enhance your program's credibility and reach. Many public health agencies seek partner organizations to serve as gatekeepers to reach target audiences. Think about partnerships with businesses, other government agencies, volunteer and professional organizations, schools and community groups, the mass media, or health-related institutions. These organizations can help you by providing:

- Access to a target audience

- Enhanced credibility for your message or program, because the audience considers the organizations to be a trusted source

- Additional resources, either financial or in-kind resources (e.g., volunteers, meeting space, and airtime)

- Added expertise (e.g., training capabilities)

- Cosponsorship of events

First, you'll need to weigh the pros and cons to decide whether you want to collaborate. If you decide to find partners, you'll need to consider what types of partners you want.

5a. Decide whether to collaborate.

In determining whether to recruit partners, consider these questions:

- Which organizations have similar goals and might be willing to work with you?

- Which types of partnerships would help to achieve the objectives?

- How many partners would your program need? You might want to partner with one or a few organizations for specific projects, or you may need to rally the support of many organizations.

- Will the collaboration compromise your message?

Although working with other organizations and agencies can greatly enhance what you can accomplish, be realistic about the potential disadvantages of collaboration. Working with other organizations can:

- **Be time consuming.** You'll have to identify the organizations, persuade them to work with you, gain internal approvals, and coordinate planning, training, or both.

- **Require altering the program.** Every organization has different priorities and perspectives, and partners may want to make minor or major program changes to accommodate their structure or needs.

- **Result in loss of ownership and control of the program.** Other organizations may change the schedule, functions, or even the messages and take credit for the program.

Decide in advance how much flexibility you can give partners without violating your program's integrity and direction and your own organizational procedures.

5b. Consider criteria for partner participation.

Once you've decided to partner with other organizations, you should be selective in choosing partners. Consider which organizations meet the following criteria:

- Would best reach your audience(s)

- Are likely to have the most credibility and influence with your audience(s)

- Would be easiest to persuade to work with you (e.g., organizations where you have a contact)

- Would require less support or fewer resources from you

Health care companies and other for-profit organizations may be willing to work with you even if their products or services aren't related to your program. They may view partnering with your program as a way to provide a useful public service, improve their corporate image and credibility, or attract the attention of a particular sector of the public. You must consider whether a collaboration of this type will add value or jeopardize the credibility of your program.

Step 6: Plan for process and outcome evaluation.

Evaluation is crucial for showing funding sources, partners, supporters, and critics what you've achieved. Even though most evaluation occurs later, you must plan for it at an early stage, to ensure that you have the budget and infrastructure to gather and analyze the information you'll use (CDC 1999). In addition, you'll probably want to conduct a baseline study of the target audiences' current awareness, knowledge, attitudes, and behaviors. Planning for the baseline study must be done early enough to implement the research before the campaign begins. You'll be able to determine the progress of the campaign by comparing its results with information from the baseline study.

Work with your evaluation experts on evaluation plans. If they have participated in the program planning, they will better understand what you're trying to do. Evaluation experts can help to plan an appropriate evaluation and to make decisions about data collection methods and analysis. (See Chapter 5: Evaluating the Success of Your Counter-Marketing Program for more information on planning for process and outcome evaluation.)

Your objectives and logic model for the counter-marketing program form the basis for design of the evaluation. A good evaluation plan should include both process and outcome measures:

- **Process evaluation** shows whether your program's components and flow of activities worked the way you planned. Process evaluation can help to identify any problems with implementing the program as designed.

- **Outcome evaluation** shows whether you met your program objectives.

Including both types of evaluation will provide a comprehensive "picture" of what happened and why.

As you plan for evaluation, keep these tips in mind:

- **Make sure your evaluation design is appropriate for the particular activity.** Experimental designs are the gold standard of outcome evaluation. In experimental design, a treatment group (people exposed to the program) is compared with a control group (people who aren't exposed). However, this type of design often can't be used to assess counter-marketing activities, largely because untreated control groups may not exist for statewide or community-based efforts. Even if people aren't exposed to your activities, they are likely to be exposed to some communication or other intervention on the topic. Other options include quasi-experimental, cross-sectional, and case study designs. (See Chapter 5: Evaluating the Success of Your Counter-Marketing Program for discussion of these and other types of design for evaluation.)

- **Consider how the activities are expected to work and the time frame.** Then make sure the activities are evaluated according to those expectations. For example, if you expect people to need at least five to eight exposures to your message before they'll take action, you must allow sufficient implementation time to achieve that level of exposure. If you expect people to take action immediately after exposure, then the outcome measurement should take place soon after exposure. Conversely, if you don't expect to see program effects for at least one year, outcomes shouldn't be measured until then.

- **Include process measures and milestones.** This will allow you to assess progress and to determine whether you need to make any changes in the program's implementation.

- **Determine the kind of evidence needed for the outcome evaluation.** One example is information for a report to your funding agency or partners.

- **Consider the baseline measures you have available or can collect and how you'll track changes related to desired outcomes.** Determine how you will collect data and how often.

- **Measure change against the program's specific objectives.** These objectives should be consistent with, but may not be identical to, your organization's general tobacco control goal.

- **Avoid having your program deemed a failure because it doesn't achieve sufficient reach, frequency, or duration.** Two possible causes of such a failure, real or apparent, are that activities aren't funded adequately or that they begin later than expected and aren't in place long enough before outcomes are measured. Process evaluation can track the level of intensity and the duration of exposure to the message and can help you learn why expected outcomes did or didn't occur.

6a. Write questions about the program that you want the evaluation to answer.

Planning for evaluation includes developing questions that you want the evaluation to answer about the implementation and outcomes of your program. Determine which key measures will be necessary to demonstrate to key decision makers, funding sources, other stakeholders, staff, and the public at large that the program is making progress toward its objectives. Questions may include the following:

- Did your counter-marketing program achieve the outcomes you expected (e.g., increased awareness of program messages and changes in knowledge, beliefs, and attitudes)?

- What did target audiences think of your program? Did they become involved? Did it affect them in some way?

- Did partners contribute as expected? Why or why not? How might these partners want to work with you in the future?

- Did you have an adequate level of resources? Did you schedule enough time for program development and implementation?

6b. Design the evaluation.

To decide on the appropriate evaluation design, you'll need to consider the following questions:

- Which evaluation questions are most important? (You may have to decide which ones you can realistically answer.)

- What information will you need to answer each evaluation question?

- How will you gather the information?

- How will you analyze it?

By now, you may be thinking that good evaluation is beyond your capacity. It's true that evaluation can be complex and costly, but it also can be relatively simple and inexpensive. Look at what other states have done and what might be useful in supporting future efforts. Also, examine the evaluation designs others have used and borrow what you can. Ask others what worked for them and what changes they'd make in future evaluation designs.

In addition to designing the program evaluation, you'll need to plan to pretest messages and materials. (See Chapter 3: Gaining and Using Target Audience Insights for more information.) You also may want to consider conducting a pilot test for your program. In a pilot test, you run and evaluate your program in a limited area for a limited time, then make adjustments based on the test results, before expanding the program. Consider pilot testing if your program meets the following criteria:

- Designed as a new type of program for your organization

- Intended to become a large investment

- Planned to cover many communities

- Expected to continue over several years

Step 7: Begin counter-marketing program development.

Now you're ready to start putting the pieces together. Program development and management are discussed more fully in Chapter 6: Managing and Implementing Your Counter-Marketing Program, but here are some key points:

- Develop a communication plan that includes all the elements of your planning. It should be used to explain your plans to those within your organization and to others; support and justify budget requests; provide a record of where you began; and show the program's planned evolution. Some sections of the plan, such as implementation and process evaluation, may not be as detailed as others at this point. But you can always update the plan later.

- Add a budget and a timeline that lists and assigns tasks and identifies deadlines.

- Find out more about similar programs in other states and how you may be able to use their "lessons learned" and any messages and materials they've developed.

- Conduct any market research needed to understand more about your target audience's culture, motivations, interests, and lifestyle.

- Begin to develop program activities. (See Chapter 7: Advertising, Chapter 8: Public Relations, Chapter 9: Media Advocacy, Chapter 10: Grassroots Marketing, and Chapter 11: Media Literacy for guidance.)

- Plan for testing messages, developing materials, organizing activities, negotiating partner roles, and conducting a program review for stakeholders.

The timeline should include every imaginable major task from the time you write the plan until the time you intend to complete the program. The more tasks you build into the timetable, the more likely you'll be to remember to assign the work and stay on schedule. Also, detailing the tasks will make it easier to determine who's responsible for completing tasks and what resources will be required. The timeline is a flexible management tool. You may want to review and update it regularly (e.g., once a month), so you can use it to help manage and track progress. Computer-based tools, such as project management software, can be especially useful for this task.

Points To Remember

- Effective planning will help you:
    - Better understand the tobacco control issue you're addressing
    - Identify the most appropriate approaches to bring about or support change
    - Create a counter-marketing program that supports clearly defined objectives
- Your counter-marketing program plan should complement the broader tobacco control effort and overall plan.
- Many of the planning activities in this chapter can be completed simultaneously.
- A plan is a living document. As the program progresses, review the plan to clarify and revise it as needed.
- Be prepared to evaluate what you do.

Bibliography

Backer TE, et al. *Designing Health Communication Programs: What Works?* Newbury Park, CA: Sage Publications, 1992.

Centers for Disease Control and Prevention. *CDCynergy for Tobacco Prevention and Control (CD-ROM)*. Atlanta, GA: U.S. Department of Health and Human Services, CDC, National Center for Chronic Disease Prevention and Health Promotion, Office on Smoking and Health, 2003.

CDC. Framework for program evaluation in public health. *Morbidity and Mortality Weekly Report* 1999; 1748(RR–11):1–40.

Hornik RC, editor. *Public Health Communication: Evidence for Behavior Change*. Mahwah, NJ: Lawrence Erlbaum Associates, 2002.

National Cancer Institute. *Making Health Communication Programs Work: A Planner's Guide*. Bethesda, MD: USDHHS, Public Health Service, National Institutes of Health, NCI, 2002. NIH Pub. No. T068.

NCI. *Theory at a Glance: A Guide for Health Promotion Practice*. Bethesda, MD: USDHHS, Public Health Service, National Institutes of Health, NCI, 1995. NIH Pub. No. 95-3996.

Schar E, Gutierrez K. *Smoking Cessation Media Campaigns From Around the World: Recommendations From Lessons Learned*. Atlanta, GA: Centers for Disease Control and Prevention; Copenhagen, Denmark: World Health Organization, 2001.

Smith W. From prevention vaccines to community care: new ways to look at program success. In: Hornik RC, editor. *Public Health Communication: Evidence for Behavior Change*. Mahwah, NJ: Lawrence Erlbaum Associates, 2002, pp. 327–56.

Snyder LB, Hamilton MA. A meta-analysis of U.S. health campaign effects on behavior: emphasize enforcement, exposure, and new information and beware the secular trend. In: Hornik RC, editor. *Public Health Communication: Evidence for Behavior Change*. Mahwah, NJ: Lawrence Erlbaum Associates, 2002, pp. 327–56.

Chapter 3

Gaining and Using Target Audience Insights

Understanding your target audience—its culture, lifestyle, behaviors, interests, and needs—is vital to developing an effective counter-marketing program. Market research can help you gain those insights.[1]

In This Chapter

- The Importance of Market Research
- Market Research on a Limited Budget
- Qualitative and Quantitative Research Methods
- Qualitative Research
- Quasi-Quantitative Research
- Quantitative Research
- Other Market Research Tools

Once you've determined who your target audience is, you'll need to gather relevant information about that audience. This information will help you tailor your counter-marketing messages and materials and ensure that your programs will be effective.

One way to gain insights about your target audience is through market research, which can help you understand the audience's motivations, interests, needs, culture, lifestyles, and behaviors and determine the best channel(s) for reaching the audience. Market research can help you explore ideas for activities and concepts for messages and identify and develop stronger ideas and eliminate the weaker ones. It can be used to pretest messages and materials in near-final stages, to fine-tune the process while changes can be made, and to serve as a "disaster check." Market research also can be a mechanism for pilot testing new tactics and interventions before using them more broadly. Market research for development of counter-marketing efforts is often called formative research. Other types of research for the purposes of process and outcome evaluation are discussed in Chapter 5: Evaluating the Success of Your Counter-Marketing Program.

[1] This chapter has been excerpted and adapted from the National Cancer Institute's *Making Health Communication Programs Work: A Planner's Guide* (2002).

This chapter describes market research tools commonly used to gain insights into target audiences.[2] These tools include focus groups, individual in-depth interviews, central location intercept interviews, theater-style pretests, and surveys. Diaries and activity logs, gatekeeper reviews, and readability testing are also described.

Some tools are better suited for certain purposes than others, so most programs use a combination of methods. For example, focus groups with members of your target audience can help you learn which approaches, messages, and channels are most likely to succeed with that audience. The focus groups could be augmented with individual in-depth interviews to probe more deeply into motivations, particularly if the issues are controversial or very personal or if the audience members are influenced heavily by their peers. Messages and materials might be tested through central location intercept interviews, in which respondents are recruited and interviewed at malls or other public settings, or through theater-style pretests, which use a simulated television-viewing environment to replicate a real-life viewing experience. Use of multiple tools can help confirm the validity of your findings.

Regardless of the tools you use, be sure to apply the results. Market research can provide critical data at various stages of your program, but that information won't do much good if it isn't used. Other chapters in this manual explain when and how to incorporate your results into program planning and development. (In particular, see Chapter 2: Planning Your Counter-Marketing Program, Chapter 4: Reaching Specific Populations, and Chapter 7: Advertising.)

Market research generally isn't something you can do on your own. Your program could stray off course if you use the wrong method, use the methods incorrectly, recruit the wrong type or number of participants, or misinterpret results. Unless you have the appropriate skills and experience, do-it-yourself market research can yield the same kinds of results as do-it-yourself plumbing. This chapter is designed to give you background on methods and techniques that will help you work with market research professionals. However, don't turn over complete control of the research to your ad agency or market research firm. You need to be involved in every step of the process.

The Importance of Market Research

Sometimes program managers want to eliminate market research to cut costs, especially when the budget is tight. However, spending some money on market research up front can save your program money in the long run. The initial expenditure can help ensure that the program elements are likely to

---

[2] Some of the research methods described here may require Institutional Review Board (IRB) approval. Nearly all government agencies, academic institutions, and other organizations require an assessment of the impact on human subjects involved in qualitative and quantitative research, including the protection of collected data. Some data collection efforts are exempt from IRB approval. For each research project undertaken, it is recommended that you consult the IRB expert in your organization.

be effective, rather than having no impact or, even worse, creating a backlash. If you air ineffective ads, you lose much more money in media placement funds than you would have spent on market research to determine the likelihood of success. Unfortunately, this is only one example of the many negative outcomes of insufficient market research.

Market Research on a Limited Budget

Few program managers have the luxury of conducting as much market research as they would like. When faced with a tight budget, try the following:

- Contact others in tobacco control to find out what research they've done. Can you use their findings in developing your own program? Do they have research designs and instruments you can use as models? Can you solicit advice from experienced managers on making the most of your tight budget? Can they give you advice or referrals to resources from other experts, such as those in your community with expertise in commercial marketing and advertising or in market research? Have you contacted a project officer or health communication staff member from the Centers for Disease Control and Prevention (CDC) for advice, referrals, or both?

- Be sure your program plan fully explains the need for market research and spells out a thorough market research plan. If you can't secure the funds you need this year, try to convince decision makers now that investing in research next year will pay off. Point out that market research is a core component of effective counter-marketing programs.

- Beware of too many shortcuts. You need to conduct enough market research to feel confident that the findings provide clear direction. For example, if you've tested message concepts in a few focus groups and the results are inconclusive, you probably need to conduct a few more focus groups.

- Whenever possible, consult with market research experts during planning and implementation, even if you have to cut corners elsewhere. For example, you may be able to save money by recruiting research participants through community organizations instead of paying a contractor to handle recruiting.

- Always ask prospective contractors and vendors for nonprofit rates.

- Ask professionals with market research experience if they'd be willing to donate their time.

- Use a market researcher you can trust to be objective and to not "color" results to match a program or advertising agency bias.

Qualitative and Quantitative Research Methods

Two main categories of market research can be conducted with target audiences: qualitative and quantitative research. Qualitative research seeks to gain in-depth knowledge about perceptions, motivations, and behaviors. It can answer the questions "why," "when," and "how"—questions that are critical to developing effective media campaigns. Common methods of qualitative research include focus groups and individual in-depth interviews.

Quantitative research seeks to provide estimates of knowledge, beliefs, attitudes, and behaviors in a population of interest. It can answer the questions "How many?" "How much?" and "How often?" Common methods of quantitative research include surveys using random sampling and convenience sampling. Because each approach provides a different kind of information, it's often best to use both.

Qualitative research methods should be used for the following purposes:

- To develop materials and to determine reactions to concepts or draft materials

- To explore a topic or idea

- To gain insights into a target audience's lifestyle, culture, motivations, behaviors, and preferences

- To understand the reasons behind the results from quantitative research

Qualitative research should be conducted by using the following methods:

- Select a small group of people on the basis of certain common characteristics.

- Convene a discussion through focus groups or in-depth interviews or observe individuals' behaviors in their homes, schools, malls, supermarkets, or other settings.

- Keep the discussion somewhat unstructured, so participants are free to give any response, rather than choosing from a list of possible responses.

Use a discussion or interview guide to make sure you ask questions relevant to your research purpose, but be prepared to revise the sequence of questions on the basis of participants' responses, rather than having to stick to a set order. (See Step 5 in the section on Designing and Conducting Focus Groups or Individual In-Depth Interviews, later in this chapter, for discussion of how to develop a moderator's guide.)

Qualitative research results aren't quantifiable and can't be subjected to statistical analysis or projected to the population from which respondents were drawn. The participants don't constitute a representative sample, the samples are relatively small, and not all participants are asked precisely the same questions. Even though you can collect very valuable information from qualitative research, and even if you conduct a great deal of it, you won't get findings that you can project to the target audience as a whole. For that, you need quantitative research.

Quantitative research methods should be used for the following purposes:

- To determine "how many," "how much," and "how often"

- To profile a target audience for communication planning, such as measuring which proportion of the audience thinks or behaves in certain ways

- To measure how well your program is doing (See Chapter 5: Evaluating the Success of Your Counter-Marketing Program for a more complete discussion of surveys and program evaluation.)

Quantitative research should be conducted by using the following methods:

- Select a large group of people.

- Use a structured questionnaire containing predominantly closed-ended or forced-choice questions.

Quantitative research results can be analyzed by using statistical techniques that can provide estimates of behavior or beliefs of interest for the target population. These results can be representative of the population from which respondents were drawn if they were randomly selected. In some cases, oversampling of specific population groups is necessary to provide data on those groups. In addition, the results can help in segmenting broad target populations (e.g., high school students) into more specific groups with similar characteristics.

Quasi-quantitative market research tools (e.g., central location intercept interviews and theater-style pretests) are usually used to pretest messages and materials. Although these tools are used for measurement and typically involve questionnaires with mostly forced-choice questions, the results can't be projected to the audience as a whole, because participants aren't chosen in a way that produces a representative sample.

Here's a closer look at the different research methods and tools, along with a discussion of how to conduct the research and use the results to inform your project.

Qualitative Research

Use qualitative research to:

- Learn what drives the audience's behaviors and understand what is needed to influence their awareness, knowledge, attitudes, intentions, and behaviors

- Determine whether your materials communicate the intended messages effectively and persuasively

- Understand why your program is or isn't working as expected

- Gain insights into findings on the effectiveness of the program's implementation

The most common tools used in qualitative market research are focus groups and individual in-depth interviews. Many innovative methods may also be appropriate:

- Friendship pairs, in which best friends (commonly teens or preteens) are recruited to discuss sensitive subjects

- In-home observations, in which you gain permission to spend one or two hours in someone's home to learn about their habits and practices

- Video logs, in which individuals are given video cameras or still cameras to record their environment and daily activities

Because the methods for focus groups and in-depth individual interviews are similar, they will be discussed together in this section, using instructions for focus groups as a guide.

Focus Groups

In a focus group, a skilled moderator uses a discussion guide to facilitate a one- to two-hour discussion among five to 10 participants. Typically the session is conducted in person. If that isn't possible because of distance or other factors, another option is to conduct the session by telephone or computer. The moderator keeps the session on track while participants talk freely. As new topics related to the material emerge, the moderator asks additional questions.

Focus groups are commonly used to accomplish the following purposes:

- Develop a communication strategy by:
  - Learning about feelings, motivators, and experiences related to a health topic
  - Exploring the feasibility of potential actions from the audience's viewpoint
  - Identifying barriers to those actions
  - Exploring which benefits the audience finds most compelling and believes can result from taking a particular action
  - Learning about the audience's use of settings, channels, and activities
  - Capturing the language the audience uses to discuss a health issue
  - Identifying cultural differences that may affect message delivery
- Explore reactions to message concepts (concept testing) by:
  - Identifying concepts that do or don't resonate and learning why
  - Triggering the creative thinking of communication professionals
  - Showing others what audience members think and how they talk about a health issue
- Develop hypotheses (broad questions) for quantitative research, and identify the range of responses that should be included in closed-ended questionnaires
- Provide insights into the results of quantitative research by obtaining in-depth information from audience members
- Brainstorm for possible program improvements

Pros:

- Group interaction can elicit in-depth thought and discussion.
- Group interaction can encourage brainstorming, because respondents can build on each other's ideas.

- Moderators have considerable opportunities to probe responses.

- Focus groups provide richer data about the complexities of the audience's thoughts and behaviors than surveys do.

- Groups provide feedback from a number of individuals in a relatively short time.

Cons:

- Findings can't be projected to the target audience as a whole.

- Focus groups can be labor intensive and expensive, especially when they're conducted in multiple locations.

- Group responses don't necessarily reflect individuals' opinions, because some individuals might dominate the discussion, influence others' opinions, or both. In addition, the facilitator might not be able to get everyone's reactions to every question.

- Each person is limited to about 10 to 15 minutes of talk time.

- The moderator might ask leading questions of the group or might neglect to probe for critical insights.

Individual In-Depth Interviews

The process, uses, benefits, and drawbacks of individual in-depth interviews are similar to those of focus groups, except that the interviewer speaks with one person at a time. In-person interviews can take place at a central facility or at the participant's home or place of business. As with focus groups, when individual interviews can't be conducted in person, they can be conducted by phone or computer. Although the interviews take more total time, responses usually are less biased, because each participant is interviewed alone and isn't influenced by others' responses.

Insights From Focus Groups

In a series of 24 focus groups conducted in four U.S. cities by CDC and three state tobacco control programs, youth were exposed to 10 antitobacco ads developed for youth audiences. Participants were asked to rate the ads on the basis of how likely the ads were to make them "stop and think about not using tobacco." The four ads consistently rated highest had a strong message about the negative health consequences of tobacco. Three of the four ads used real stories in a testimonial format to share the risks of using tobacco.

An important insight gleaned from the research was that youth seemed to be more affected by the thought of living with the negative consequences of tobacco use than dying from them (Teenage Research Unlimited 1999).

An Experience With One-on-One Interviews

A television and movie actor who had lost several family members to tobacco offered his time for a tobacco control ad. An advertising concept and script were developed to encourage smokers to consider quitting by having them think about how their own death from tobacco use would affect their loved ones.

Before producing the ads, the sponsoring organization conducted one-on-one interviews with adult smokers to ensure that the script and visual presentations would clearly and persuasively communicate the intended message. The smokers were shown the ad concept and asked their reactions to it through a variety of questions. Individual interviews were used instead of focus groups, because it was important for the smokers to be honest and vulnerable. The sponsoring organization was concerned that if smokers were in a focus group together, they might become defensive about the ad's message that their tobacco use could ultimately hurt their loved ones.

The approach worked. The one-on-one interviews elicited honest, heartfelt responses from the smokers. The interviews also revealed that many respondents didn't recognize the actor. As a result, the decision was made to identify him on screen at the beginning of the ad. In addition, the original script included a line noting how the actor's grandfather couldn't stop smoking even though he knew it was making him sick. Respondents didn't find that line credible. They believed the grandfather should have—and would have—quit if he knew smoking was making him sick. These respondents said they would stop as soon as they found out their smoking was causing them serious harm. Whether or not that perception was realistic, the script was changed to focus on the grandfather's suffering, which research respondents sympathized with, rather than focusing on his failure in quitting.

Designing and Conducting Focus Groups or Individual In-Depth Interviews

Here are seven major steps for conducting focus groups and individual in-depth interviews:

1. Plan the research.
2. Choose the location and format for focus groups or interviews.
3. Draft a recruitment screener.
4. Recruit participants.
5. Develop a moderator's guide.
6. Conduct the focus groups or interviews.
7. Analyze and use results.

Step 1: Plan the research.

Determine the following information:

- **What you want to learn.** Decide how you'll use the results from the focus group discussion or individual interview before you conduct the research. Prepare the questions you want answered, then make sure the moderator and interviewer guide will provide the answers. (See Step 5 for more information on developing a moderator's guide.) You'll use these questions to analyze the results of the discussions and to organize the report on the focus group discussion or individual interview.

- **When you need to have that information.** Your timing needs will determine the way you'll need to recruit and, to some extent, your costs.

- **How you'll apply what you learn.** Make sure the information you'll gain will be actionable.

- **Your budget.** The size of your budget will dictate how many groups or interviews you can conduct, in how many locations, and how much of the work you will be able to delegate to contractors.

- **Your criteria for participants.** Use the following suggestions to help you select participants.

    – Choose people who are typical of your audience. Participants should have the same behavioral, demographic, and psychographic characteristics as your audience. (Psychographics are a set of variables that describes an individual in terms of overall approach to life, including personality traits, values, beliefs, preferences, habits, and behaviors.) You may want to conduct separate groups with "doers," who already engage in the desired behavior, and "nondoers," who don't engage in the desired behavior. This strategy will help to identify what actions the doers take and why. Those actions then can be explored with the nondoers.

    – Do not select experts. Exclude market researchers and advertising professionals, because of their familiarity with the methods, and exclude those who have, or might be perceived by other group members as having, expertise in the subject matter. For example, exclude health professionals from focus groups when the topic is related to health. In addition, anyone involved in the production, distribution, or marketing of tobacco products should be excluded from focus groups related to tobacco control.

    – Match participants by gender, race, age, level of formal education, or other characteristic(s) within each group. Participants with matched characteristics are more likely to express themselves freely. If your target audience includes people with different demographic traits, consider whether you need to conduct separate sessions for each audience segment to determine whether differences between the groups are significant.

    – Select people who are relatively inexperienced with interviews. Participants' reactions should be spontaneous. This consideration will help you to avoid questioning "professional" respondents who have participated in many focus groups or individual interviews and thus may lead or monopolize the discussion. Recruitment screeners typically exclude people who have participated in qualitative research in the past six months. (See Step 3 later in this section, for further discussion of recruitment screeners.)

- **The number of focus group discussions or interviews you'll conduct.** If you're using focus groups, conduct at least two groups with each audience segment. For example, if you're conducting separate groups with men and women, you'll need at least four groups: two with men and two with women. If you're using individual interviews, conduct about 10 interviews per audience segment.

If audience perceptions vary or the audience feedback is unclear, you may want to conduct additional groups or interviews, especially if you revise the moderator/interviewer guide to further explore unresolved issues.

Step 2: Choose the location and format for focus groups or interviews.

You can conduct focus groups or interviews in several ways:

- Commercial focus group facilities can recruit participants. These facilities offer audio recording equipment, video recording equipment, or both and one-way mirrors with observation rooms. However, commercial facilities are often expensive and may not be available in small towns.

- Teleconference services can set up telephone focus groups. Most teleconference services allow observers to listen without being heard. Some have the capability to allow the moderator to see a list of participants (with a symbol next to the one currently speaking) or to see notes sent by a technician from observers listening to the call. Some teleconference services also can recruit participants.

- You can conduct focus groups or interviews in meeting rooms at office buildings, schools, places of worship, homes, or other locations. If an observation room with a one-way mirror isn't available, allow staff to listen by hooking up speakers or closed-circuit TV in a nearby room or by audio recording the session, video recording the session, or both. In some cases, you may have one or two quiet observers taking notes in the room.

Step 3: Draft a recruitment screener.

A recruitment screener is a short questionnaire that is administered to potential participants, typically by telephone, to ensure that they meet the criteria you developed in Step 1. Your contractor, if you have one, will administer this questionnaire. The screener should help you to exclude people who know one another or have expertise in the subject of the sessions. Potential participants can be told the general subject area (e.g., "a health topic"), but they shouldn't be told the specific subject. If participants know the subject in advance, they may formulate ideas or study to become more knowledgeable about the subject. Furthermore, if participants know one another, they may speak less freely. For similar reasons, they also shouldn't be told who the sponsor is.

Table 3.1: Pros and Cons of Formats for Focus Groups and Individual Interviews

Format	Pros	Cons
Face to Face		
Moderator/interviewer and participants are in one room, usually around a table; observers (members of the research team) are behind a one-way mirror.	• Body language can be assessed. • Observers can be present without distracting participants. • If the session is videotaped, it can be shared with others who couldn't attend. • Participants give undivided attention.	• Responders lose anonymity. • The session has higher travel expenses because of multiple locales. • The session may be a logistical challenge in rural areas or small towns.
Telephone		
Moderator/interviewer and participants are on a conference call; observers listen.	• The session is more convenient for participants and observers. • Participants can easily include people in rural areas or small towns, as well as the homebound. • Relative anonymity may result in more frank discussion of sensitive issues.	• Nonverbal reactions can't be assessed. • It's more difficult to get reactions to visuals. (They can be sent ahead of time, but you still have less control over exposure.) • Participants can be distracted by their surroundings. • There may be noise interference from callers' environments.
Internet Chat Sessions		
Moderator and participants "chat" while observers read.	• A complete record of session is instantly available. • Relative anonymity may result in more frank discussion of sensitive issues.	• The session is useful only for participants comfortable with this mode of communication. • The relatively slow pace limits topics that can be covered. • There's no way to assess whether participants meet recruitment criteria. • Body language or tone of voice can't be assessed. • It's more difficult to get reactions to visual presentations. (They can be sent ahead of time, but you still have less control over exposure.) • Participants can be distracted by their surroundings.

Contracting With Commercial Facilities

One way to conduct face-to-face focus groups or individual interviews is to contract with a company that specializes in this service. Before you contract with a commercial facility, prepare a specification sheet detailing all the services you need, and if you will be asking the facility to recruit participants, prepare a profile of your audience. Vendors will use this information to estimate the project's cost and to develop bids.

Use this checklist to decide which vendors to consider. Each vendor should provide these items:

- ❏ Descriptions of past projects

- ❏ Descriptions of or a list of clients (If you are unfamiliar with the vendor, check the company's references.)

- ❏ Location of the facility (Is it conveniently located? Accessible by public transportation? If not, does the vendor provide transportation assistance, such as taxi money or van service? What does this add to the cost?)

- ❏ Size of the interview room(s)

- ❏ Diagram of the table/seating arrangements (What shape is the table? How big is the table? Where does the moderator sit?)

- ❏ Size and features of the observation room(s)

- ❏ Details about audio recording and video recording arrangements and costs

- ❏ Details about food arrangements for participants and observers, including staff from your organization and ad agency

- ❏ Description of the vendor's moderator services

- ❏ Description of the vendor's method of recruitment, including the database used and the geographic area the company covers

- ❏ Recommendations for participant incentives

- ❏ Reasonable rates for vendor services (Ask for nonprofit rates.)

- ❏ Examples of focus group summaries/reports, moderator notes, screeners (short questionnaires used to recruit potential participants), and other documents produced by the vendor for other clients if you're going to ask the vendor to provide these services

The screener should guarantee the approximate mix of respondents for a group that isn't separated by certain characteristics, such as a balance of men and women in a mixed-gender group. (See Appendices 3.1 and 3.2 for sample screeners.)

Step 4: Recruit participants.

Choose appropriate participants for the focus groups or interviews, so your research is more reliable. Even if a contractor does the recruiting, make sure the screener is followed carefully so that only those who qualify will be included in the research.

Participants should be recruited by telephone one to three weeks before the sessions. How you identify potential participants depends on the type of people they are and the resources you have. Focus group facilities typically identify members of the audience through their own databases. If you do the recruiting, you might need to run an ad in a local publication, work with community organizations, purchase lists of phone numbers of individuals with certain characteristics, or identify professionals through a relevant association or mailing list service. Here are some ways to recruit:

- Hire a focus group facility or independent recruiter. Two directories of facilities are the American Marketing Association's *GreenBook: Worldwide Directory of Focus Group Companies and Services* (2003) and the Marketing Research Association's *Blue Book* (2003).

- If you have many facilities and recruiters to choose from, consider getting recommendations from local companies or organizations that conduct qualitative research.

- Enlist help from students in a university marketing research or advertising class if they are knowledgeable and experienced in focus group research.

- Work through gatekeepers such as teachers (for students); instructors for courses of English as a second language (for recent immigrants); health care systems (for patients, physicians, or nurses); and religious institutions or community organizations whose members meet your audience criteria. (A small donation may encourage an organization to recruit for you.)

Getting People to Show Up

To ensure that enough people show up, offer an incentive (usually money) and recruit more people than you need. If everyone shows up, select those who best fit your screening criteria, thank the extra participants, give them the agreed-on incentive, and ask them to leave. You also can make sure you have enough people by:

- Scheduling sessions at times convenient for your potential participants (e.g., during lunchtime or after work)

- Choosing a safe and convenient site

- Providing transportation or reimbursing participants for agreed-on transportation costs

- Arranging for child care

- Letting participants know you'll provide snacks or refreshments

Recruiting for Telephone Interviews

If you're recruiting for telephone interviews, create a spreadsheet with spaces for the following information about each potential participant: the time zone in which the person is located; the date, time, and number at which they should be called; and the result of each call (e.g., scheduled an interview, no answer, busy, or refused). This type of spreadsheet also can be helpful in planning in-person interviews and using other research methods.

Step 5: Develop a moderator's guide.

The quality of the moderator's guide is critical to the success of focus groups. The guide tells the moderator or interviewer what information you want from the sessions and helps him or her keep the discussion on track and on time. Your contractor will draft the guide for you if you need this service. Before it is drafted, you'll need to determine the following information:

- What you want to learn from the focus group or interview

- How to apply what you learn

- What tools (e.g., descriptive information, message concepts, or other draft creative work) you'll need to provide for the sessions

You should write questions for the guide that relate to the purposes you've identified. Most questions should be open-ended, so participants can provide more in-depth responses than just "yes" or "no." Also, make sure the questions aren't worded in a way that will prompt a particular response. For example, don't ask, "What problems are you having with quitting smoking?" Instead, you could phrase the question more neutrally by asking, "What problems do smokers have with quitting?" Participants will then be more likely to offer honest responses, rather than the answers they think you want. The time and depth of exploration given to each issue should reflect the issue's importance to your purposes. (See Appendices 3.3 and 3.4 for examples of moderator's guides.)

In the focus groups, don't include questions for group discussion if you need individual responses. However, you can have the moderator give each participant a self-administered questionnaire to complete *before* the session. Participants also can be asked to individually rank certain items (e.g., potential actions, benefits, or message concepts) on paper during a session to combine individual and group reactions.

Step 6: Conduct the focus groups or interviews.

Focus groups and interviews typically begin with the moderator welcoming participants and briefing them on the process (e.g., that

Working With Community Organizations (Partners) To Conduct Focus Groups

You'll need a formal or informal agreement to conduct focus groups with your partner. Working with your contact at the partner organization, develop an agreement that includes the following elements:

- A description of your organization
- A description of the material/topic to be discussed and its purpose
- Details about participants to be recruited
- An outline of activities involved
- The incentives you are offering the partner organization and/or the participants
- A detailed explanation of why the partner should *not* reveal details about the topic to participants in advance
- How you will protect participants' confidentiality
- If and how you will share the information learned

Once you have an agreement, decide how you will recruit participants. One idea is to conduct your research as part of one of the partner organization's regular meetings. Here are the pros and cons of this approach:

Pros:

- Little extra effort is required to recruit participants.
- Minimal or no incentives may be involved.
- Your partner's regular, convenient, and familiar meeting place can be used.

Cons:

- You have little control over the number of people who will come or the composition of the focus group. Respondents are likely to know one another, which will affect the focus group's dynamics and make results less reliable.
- Because a focus group may last one or two hours, it is difficult to place it on the agenda of a regular meeting.
- Scheduling the focus group for the near future may be difficult, because many organizations set their calendars months in advance.

Continues

Working With Community Organizations (Partners) To Conduct Focus Groups (cont.)

An alternative is to recruit your partner's members/constituents to come to a special meeting. This approach offers the ability to screen participants. In addition, participants may be less distracted in a meeting solely devoted to your research than in a focus group conducted as part of a regular meeting.

Scheduling the focus group immediately before or after the regular meeting may make it more convenient for participants. A person with the organization—or you, on behalf of the organization—can ask members/constituents to participate. Also, if you're providing refreshments or incentives, let participants know in advance to encourage them to attend and to stay through the entire meeting.

If you do the recruiting, you'll have more control over what people are told about the focus group and you'll be able to screen potential participants. However, recruiting takes a significant amount of time, and organization members/constituents may be more likely to participate if they are asked by someone they know.

If the member organization recruits participants, you need to provide the recruiter with detailed instructions. These instructions must include (1) a written description of the general (not specific) topic, which should be read to potential participants verbatim, and (2) a questionnaire to screen participants.

---

there are no right or wrong answers, that it's important to speak one at a time and maintain confidentiality, that observers will be present, and that the session will be recorded).[3] In focus groups, participants introduce themselves to the group, noting information relevant to the discussion (e.g., number of attempts to quit smoking and number of cigarettes smoked each day). Next, the moderator asks a few simple "icebreaker" questions to help participants get used to the process and reduce their anxiety. This step also helps the moderator develop a rapport with the participants. Again, to reduce the risk of introducing bias, the sponsor of the research should not be revealed.

The session then shifts to an in-depth investigation of participants' perspectives and issues. Following the moderator's guide, the moderator manages the session and ensures that all topics are covered without overtly directing the discussion. Participants are encouraged to express their views and even disagree with one another. The moderator doesn't simply accept what participants say but probes to learn about thoughts and attitudes. The moderator also seeks opinions from *all* participants, so everyone has a chance to speak, rather than letting a vocal few dominate the discussion.

---

[3] If the group is conducted in a language that observers don't understand, provide a translator in the observation room.

The Moderator's Role

The moderator or interviewer doesn't need to be an expert on your topic, but he or she should be briefed well enough to ask appropriate questions and must have experience in facilitating group discussions. Rehearse with the moderator any topics or concerns you want emphasized or discussed in depth. The moderator's guide is just that, a guide. Experienced moderators flow with the conversation, ask questions that are not leading or closed ended, and sequence to the next topic when appropriate or deviate from it to avoid awkward transitions or unnecessary banter between topics.

A good moderator has the following characteristics:

- The moderator understands what information you're seeking, how you need to use it, and how to probe and guide the discussion to get the information. He or she makes sure all agreed-on topics are covered sufficiently.

- The moderator builds rapport and trust, and probes without reacting to or influencing participants' opinions. He or she emphasizes to participants that there are no right or wrong answers.

- The moderator understands the process of eliciting comments, keeps the discussion on track, and finds other ways to approach a topic if necessary.

- He or she leads the discussion and isn't led by the group.

Use local advertising agencies, the American Marketing Association's *GreenBook: Worldwide Directory of Focus Group Companies and Services* (2003), or the Qualitative Research Consultants Association to find a good moderator. If your organization plans to conduct focus groups regularly by using your internal staff, consider hiring a skilled, experienced moderator to train your staff to moderate focus groups.

Near the end of a focus group, the moderator may give participants an activity or simply check with the observers to find out if they have additional questions. Notes can be discreetly given to the moderator throughout the session if the observers want other questions asked or changes made.

One advantage of the focus group/interview method is that the moderator's guide and any materials presented can be revised between sessions.

Step 7: Analyze and use results.

In many analyses of focus groups or interviews, the goal is to look for general trends and agreement on issues while noting differing opinions. In some instances, the goal is to capture a range of opinions. Keep an eye out for individual comments that raise interesting ideas or important concerns, such as lack of cultural sensitivity or difficulty in comprehension.

Reviewing transcripts is the easiest and most thorough way to analyze the sessions, although the sessions can be analyzed less thoroughly by reviewing notes taken during the discussion. Avoid counting or quantifying types of responses (e.g., "75 percent of participants preferred concept A"). Because this is qualitative research, you can't quantify the results or suggest that they represent the opinions of the audience as a whole.

Results are worthless if they aren't used. Use them to answer the questions you drafted to guide the research design—to shape the campaign strategy, message, and materials design. Also, your results help you "sell" your program as "researched and tested." Share your findings with partners and others who might benefit.

Estimated Costs of Focus Groups and Interviews

The cost estimates in Table 3.2 can help you budget for pretesting if you're using commercial research firms. *Your actual costs will vary* depending on your location, the target audience being recruited, and the amount of time contributed by staff, contractors, and participants. For example, if your staff includes a focus group expert who can analyze the results, you won't have to pay a contractor for that task. However, don't jeopardize the quality of your results with a budget that's too small.

The estimates for focus groups assume that you conduct two groups, each with 10 mem-

Table 3.2: Estimated Costs of Two Focus Groups and 10 Individual In-Depth Interviews Conducted With Participants From the General Population

Item	Costs of Two Focus Groups	Costs of 10 Individual In-Depth Interviews
Develop screener*	$800–$1,000	$800–$1,200
Develop discussion guide*	$800–$1,200	$800–$1,600
Recruit participants	$1,500–$2,000	$750–$1,500
Rent facility	$700–$1,000	$1,000–$2,000
Provide respondent incentives/refreshments	$600–$1,500	$0–$500
Hire moderator or interviewer	$1,500–$2,100	$500–$1,000
Audiotape and videotape sessions Transcribe audiotapes	$500–$800	$300–$400
Analyze research findings and write report*	$1,600–$2,400	$1,600–$2,400
Total	$8,000–$12,000	$5,750–$10,600

*One-time costs that will not be incurred for each group.

bers of the general population. This size is for cost estimates only. Most program managers prefer groups of five to eight, because doing so more easily engages all group members in conversation, but others prefer groups of eight to 12. In either case, larger numbers frequently are recruited to allow for some "no-shows." However, if more people show up than you need, you must still give them any promised incentive. Also, recruiting specific, hard-to-find target audiences may be more expensive than selecting a group from the general population.

The cost estimates also assume that each session is two hours long, conducted in English, and audiotaped. Staff travel, food for participants, and videotaping, which is useful when some of your program team can't directly observe the session, are not included.

The interview estimate shown in Table 3.2 assumes 10 half-hour interviews that are conducted in English and audiotaped.

Quasi-Quantitative Research

Quasi-quantitative tools are used most often to pretest messages and materials, as noted earlier. These tools include central location intercept interviews and theater-style pretests. If you pretest many ads using the same methodology and the same questions, you can develop a database of results that allows you to assess the relative strengths of various ads.

Central Location Intercept Interviews

In central location intercept interviews, interviewers go to a place frequented by members of the target audience and ask them to participate in a study. If they agree, they're asked specific screening questions to determine whether they fit the recruitment criteria. If they do, the interviewers take them to the interviewing station (a quiet spot at a shopping mall or other site), show them the pretest materials, and then administer the pretest questionnaire. The interview should last no longer than 15 to 20 minutes.

For intercept interviews to be effective, you must obtain results from at least 100 of each type of respondent or more if you want to break out specific subgroups (e.g., males vs. females or age groups) (NCI 2002).

Pros:

- You increase your chances of finding the right participants if you choose the right location.

- You can connect with harder-to-reach respondents and present them with a stimulus (an ad, graphics, messages, or a brochure).

- The interviews can be conducted quickly.

- The interviews are a cost-effective way to gather data in a relatively short time.

Cons:

- You must train interviewers.

- Your results aren't representative and can't be generalized.

- Intercept interviews aren't appropriate for sensitive issues or potentially threatening questions.

- Intercept interviews aren't appropriate for in-depth questions, and they don't allow you to probe for additional information easily.

- Respondents might not want to be interviewed on the spot. Although setting up prearranged appointments is time consuming and more expensive, ultimately it may save time if respondents won't cooperate in a central location.

Developing the Questionnaire

Unlike focus groups or individual interviews, the questionnaire used in central location intercept interviews is highly structured and contains primarily multiple-choice or closed-ended questions to permit quick responses. Open-ended questions, which allow free-flowing answers, should be kept to a minimum, because they take too much time for the respondent to answer and for the interviewer to record. Questions that assess the audience's comprehension and perceptions of the pretest materials form the core of the questionnaire. The interview may also include a few questions tailored to the specific item(s) being pretested (e.g., "Do you prefer this picture or this one?"). As with any research instrument, the questionnaire should be pilot tested before it's used in the field. (See Appendix 3.6 for a Sample Intercept Interview Questionnaire.)

Setting Up Interviews

A number of market research companies throughout the country conduct central location intercept interviews in shopping malls. You can also conduct these interviews in clinic waiting rooms, religious institutions, Social Security offices, schools, work sites, train stations, and other locations frequented by audience members. You must obtain permission from the site well before you want to set up interviewing stations.

If you're using a market research company to conduct the interviews, provide the company with the screening criteria and the pretest materials in appropriate formats and quantities. Some companies have offices in shopping malls, and some offices have one-way mirrors that allow you to watch the interviews.

University and college departments of marketing, communication, or health education might be able to provide interviewer training, trained student interviewers, or both. Pretesting is an excellent real-world project for a faculty member to adopt as a class project or for a

Table 3.3: Estimated Costs for Central Location Intercept Interviews Conducted With 100 Participants From the General Population

Item	Costs
Develop questionnaire	$750–$3,500
Print questionnaire Schedule facility and phones	$400–$600
Screen and conduct interviews	$2,000–$3,500
Provide respondent incentives	$600–$750
Code, enter data, and tabulate	$850–$1,300
Analyze research findings and write report	$1,500–$3,500
Total	$6,100–$13,150

master's degree student to use as a thesis project. However, this approach may mean you don't get your results as quickly, and you may compromise the quality of the research if the individuals lack the appropriate experience.

Recruiting Participants

If your organization is recruiting the participants, you'll need to develop screening criteria, a script, and training for approaching audience members. The interviewer should be familiar with the screening criteria and approach only those people who appear to fit the criteria. Whenever the people approached don't qualify, the interviewer should thank them for their time and willingness to participate. If they do qualify, the interviewer can bring them to a designated location and proceed with the interview.

Table 3.3 shows estimated costs for central location intercept interviews. These costs are based on questioning 100 respondents from the general population for 15 to 20 minutes each.

Central location intercept interviews might not be feasible if your audience is geographically dispersed or does not have easy access to a central facility. In those cases, you can use telephone interviews and send materials to participants in advance. This type of pretest typically resembles an individual interviewing project in cost and number of interviews, but more closed-ended questions may be used and the question sequence may be followed more closely.

Theater-Style Pretests

Theater-style pretests are most commonly used to assess the effectiveness of TV ads. Animated video storyboards are used to select

---

Use of Theater-Style Pretesting To Compare Ad Formats

Theater-style pretesting was used with youth and adults to compare the effectiveness of two Massachusetts ads, "Cowboy" and "Models." This method was chosen because norms had been established over time, and results of the two ad pretests could be compared with those of previous pretests. In "Cowboy," a man tells the story of his brother, a former actor in Marlboro ads who died from lung cancer at a young age. In "Models," the U.S. women's soccer team discusses the negative impact of smoking on sports performance. Both ads also include a message about how the tobacco industry manipulates and influences people. Both are black-and-white ads featuring people talking to the camera.

"Cowboy" scored better than "Models" on several key measures, including recall of the main message and how convincing and engaging it was. "Cowboy" also scored better than most ads previously pretested with the same method. The respondents' verbatim comments helped explain why. The respondents were very moved by the real story of the man losing his brother because he smoked cigarettes. They vividly recalled many more details about "Cowboy" than about "Models," and male and female respondents alike said the ad was realistic and made them cry. They also frequently commented on an image in which the former Marlboro man is in a hospital bed attached to numerous tubes.

the best concept, or a rough-cut (near-finished) ad is pretested as a "disaster check." Participants are invited to a central location to watch a pilot for a new TV program. During the program, they're exposed to several ads, including the pretest ad. After the show, participants complete a questionnaire. They first respond to questions about the show and then answer questions about the pretest materials, to determine how effectively the message was communicated and what their overall reactions were. For theater-style pretests to be effective, you must obtain results from at least 100 respondents of each type (NCI 2002).

Pros:

- You can obtain responses from a large number of respondents at the same time.

- Running the ad as part of TV programming allows you to more closely replicate participants' experiences of watching TV at home.

Con:

- Your results aren't representative and can't be generalized.

During theater-style pretests, participants are invited to a conveniently located meeting room or auditorium that is set up for screening a TV program. Participants should be told only that their reactions to a TV program are being sought, not the real purpose of the gathering.

The program can be any entertaining, non-health-related video presentation that is 15 to 30 minutes long. About halfway through the program, some commercials are shown, and your message is among them.

Table 3.4: Estimated Costs of a Theater-Style Pretest Conducted With 100 Participants From the General Population

Item	Costs
Develop questionnaire	$400–$2,400
Produce questionnaire	$400–$600
Recruit participants	$4,500–$6,000
Rent facility	$0–$$$*
Rent audiovisual equipment	$0–$2,000
Conduct theater-style pretest	$0–$800
Provide respondent incentives	$3,000–$5,000
Code, enter data, and tabulate	$800–$3,200
Analyze research findings and write report	$1,600–$3,200
Total	$10,700–$23,200+

*The cost of large facilities (e.g., hotel ballrooms) varies widely by geographic region. Check with local facilities for approximate costs.

After the program, participants receive a questionnaire designed to gauge their reactions to the program. Then they complete a section of questions focusing on the ad.

In some cases, one-half of the audience is sent home and the rest are asked to stay. The remaining group watches your ad again and answers several additional questions. The participants who were sent home are called back two to three days later and asked questions about the ad, to determine how well they recalled the ad and its main message.

In more sophisticated theater-style pretests, participants answer questions by using automated audience-response systems. They are given a small device with response keys that they push when a question is asked. The data are automatically tabulated, giving you instant access to the numbers. Questions can be instantly added or deleted from the questionnaire on the basis of the previous responses. However, an automated system is much more costly to use than a standard paper-and-pencil questionnaire.

Table 3.4 shows the estimated costs of a theater-style pretest conducted with 100 participants.

Pretesting Other Media

Theater-style pretesting also can be used to assess video presentations, such as a 10- to 15-minute video on smoking cessation that will be shown in a clinic. You should have participants view a series of videos that includes yours. Participants evaluate the videos the same way they evaluate ads, but these sessions last longer than ad pretests.

If you're using print ads, try a variation of the theater-style pretest. In this method, several ads, including yours, are inserted into a magazine. Participants are asked to read an article with the ads interspersed and are given enough time to finish the article. Then they complete a questionnaire designed to gauge their reactions to the article and ads, as well as a section containing questions focusing on the ads. Finally, your ad is displayed alone, and participants respond to several more questions.

Using a Mix of Research Methods

The World Health Organization and CDC worked with an agency to develop several advertising concepts to encourage smokers to try to quit with help. The likelihood of successful smoking cessation increases greatly if the smoker takes advantage of help (e.g., counseling, a "quitline," written materials, physician's advice, and pharmacological products). The concepts were shared with smokers in one-on-one interviews, and one ad concept was selected for production. The ad was produced, but before it was recommended to countries to air, it was pretested through a central location intercept method.

This research showed that the number of respondents who preferred calling a quitline was nearly equal to the number who preferred visiting a Web site for help in quitting. It was decided that when possible, both a toll-free phone number and a Web site should be provided on the tag at the end of the ad.

In addition, although smokers understood the message well, they didn't believe it was forceful enough. Because the audio presentation was a "voiceover" and the wording could be changed inexpensively before finishing the ad, the agency made the wording more direct and also selected a different actor who had a more confident voice.

Designing and Conducting a Theater-Style Pretest

There are six steps for designing and conducting theater-style pretests, but many ideas, particularly those in Step 2, also are useful for central location intercept interviews. The six steps are as follows:

1. Plan the pretest.
2. Develop the questionnaire.
3. Recruit participants.
4. Prepare for the pretest.
5. Conduct the pretest.
6. Analyze the pretest.

Step 1: Plan the pretest.

Determine your requirements for the following information:

- What you want to learn
- When you need the results
- What your budget is
- Which contractors are qualified to do this work
- What criteria participants should be required to meet (Your contractor can help you to determine these criteria.)
- Which facility you'll use (Your contractor will make this decision.)

The facility must be large enough to accommodate all your participants simultaneously. Several video monitors may be needed for all participants to see the program well. You can also rent space, such as a hotel ballroom, if you want to pretest materials among a large number of people. Hotels often have audiovisual equipment available for rent. You must reserve facilities and equipment well in advance of your pretest.

Some market research companies conduct theater-style pretesting. They can provide details about the process they follow in conducting this pretesting.

Step 2: Develop the questionnaire.

Work with your contractor to carefully construct the questionnaire. At a minimum, it should contain three parts:

- Recall and communication of the main idea of pretest materials
- Audience reaction to pretest materials
- Demographic characteristics of the participants

Recall and Communication of the Main Idea

The standard questions on recall and communication of the main idea are critical to the pretest. They address some of the most important measures of a message's potential effectiveness:

- Whether it attracts the audience's attention (recall)
- Whether it communicates your main point (main idea)
- What respondents thought and how they felt when they viewed the ad (e.g., potential persuasiveness and believability)

See main idea questions in Appendix 3.6: Sample Intercept Interview Questionnaire. Keep in mind that the sample questionnaire was designed for research in which the ad was shown among a group of ads, not within a pilot TV program.

Audience Reaction

Include several standard questions on audience reaction that address your specific concerns about your message. Suppose your message asks viewers to call a toll-free number for more information. You may want to ask, "What action, if any, does the message ask you to take?" or "Did the telephone number appear on the screen long enough for you to remember it?"

If possible, develop one or more questions addressing each characteristic of your message. Use the following list of characteristics commonly found in messages to determine which ones apply to your message, and develop questions that focus on these characteristics:

- Use of music (with or without lyrics)
- Use of a famous spokesperson
- Use of telephone numbers
- Use of mailing addresses
- Request for a particular action
- Instructions for performing a specific health behavior
- Presentation of technical or medical information
- Presentation of new information
- Promotion of a sponsoring organization or event
- Representation of characters intended to be typical of the target audience
- Use of a voiceover announcer
- Presentation of controversial or unpleasant information

Some theater-style pretests don't ask specific questions about characteristics of each ad; instead, they rely on the respondents to volunteer reactions about the ads. When compiled, the responses often suggest patterns indicating perceptions about elements of the ad (e.g., confusing, polarizing, persuasive, or credible). See Appendix 3.6, Sample Intercept Interview Questionnaire, for examples of open-ended questions to gauge respondents' reactions, and closed-ended questions to assess respondents' perceptions about the pretest ad. Remember that the objective of pretesting is to uncover any problems with your ad before final production or airing.

Demographics

Questions about demographics record the participants' characteristics (e.g., sex, age, level of education, and health status). This information will help you later if you need to separate and analyze the data by subgroups.

Step 3: Recruit participants.

Your contractor will recruit participants for a recruiting fee. You'll also pay an incentive to participants. (See section on Focus Groups, earlier in this chapter, for information on recruiting participants.)

Step 4: Prepare for the pretest.

Before the pretest session, your contractor should make sure that all arrangements are made. This checklist may be helpful:

- Has participant recruitment taken place as scheduled? Were participants reminded to attend? Do they have transportation and correct directions?

- Have the moderators or interviewers rehearsed?

- Is the meeting room or other facility reserved for you? Is it set up? Are enough chairs available? Are extra chairs available in case more people show up than you expect? Is the heating or air conditioning working properly? Do you know where the light switches are? If a microphone is needed, is it set up and functioning properly?

- Is the pretesting videotape ready? Are the video and audio portions of the tape clear?

- Are the videocassette recorder (VCR) and TV monitors working properly? Do you need another monitor so that everyone will be able to see the program?

- Are enough copies of the pretest questionnaire on hand? Is each questionnaire complete (no pages missing)? Are there enough pencils for participants? Will they need clipboards or pads?

Step 5: Conduct the pretest.

The following checklist is useful for conducting the pretest:

- Have everything organized and working before the session.

- Conduct a dry run to check on equipment and timing.

- Be friendly and courteous to participants from the moment they arrive until they leave. (Remember to thank them.)

- Have a backup plan in case "surprises" occur (e.g., a large number of no-shows, too many participants, equipment failure, or a disruptive individual).

The session should take no more than one hour and 15 minutes if you're organized and well prepared.

Step 6: Analyze the pretest.

Analyze the questionnaires in two steps. First, tabulate or count how many participants gave each possible response to each question, and look for patterns in the responses to both closed-ended and open-ended questions. The patterns will help you to draw conclusions about the effectiveness of your message.

Then look at the overall results, and answer these questions to determine whether your message is both effective and appropriate or whether you need to revise your message before implementation:

- What did you learn from the pretest?

- Did your message receive a favorable audience reaction?

- Did your message fulfill its communication objectives?

- What are your message's strengths? Weaknesses?

- Did answers to any particular question stand out?

- Should you revise your message? If so, how?

Quantitative Research

Quantitative research is used to:

- Determine the percentage of your target audience that has certain behaviors, behavioral intentions, attitudes, and knowledge of your subject

- Monitor the audience's use of materials and awareness of your communication program and its tactics

- Measure progress toward the program's objectives, such as changes in beliefs, knowledge, attitudes, and behavior (See Chapter 5: Evaluating the Success of Your Counter-Marketing Program for more information.)

Surveys are a primary tool in quantitative research. They're used in a program's planning and assessment stages to obtain baseline and tracking information. They also can be useful in gaining insights into a target audience and gauging reactions to potential core messages. Surveys generally involve large numbers of respondents (300 or more) and questionnaires with predominantly closed-ended questions.

Pros:

- Random sampling can be used in surveys to obtain results that can be generalized to the target population, providing better direction for planning programs and messages.

- Participants can be anonymous, which is beneficial for sensitive topics.

- Surveys can include visual material and can be used to pretest items such as prototypes.

Cons:

- Surveys limit the ability to probe answers.

- There's a risk that the people who are more willing to respond may share characteristics that don't apply to the audience as a whole, creating a potential bias in the research.

- Surveys can be costly and time consuming.

- Response rates are declining, especially for telephone and Internet surveys (Singer, et al. 2000).

Most surveys are customized to answer a specific set of research questions. Some surveys are omnibus studies, in which you add questions about your topic to an existing survey. A number of national and local public opinion polls offer this option.

Table 3.5 displays the pros and cons of different survey formats.

Designing and Conducting a Survey

To design and conduct a survey, follow the same basic steps used for the other types of research outlined earlier in this chapter:

1. Plan the research.
2. Decide how the survey participants will be selected and contacted.
3. Develop and pretest the questionnaire.
4. Collect the data.
5. Analyze the results.

Quantitative surveys involve complex topics—such as sampling size and composition, questionnaire design, and analysis of quantitative data—that are beyond the scope of this chapter. (See Chapter 5: Evaluating the Success of Your Counter-Marketing Program for more information on planning a survey.)

Other Market Research Tools

Other tools can help you gain insights into your target audience and develop effective messages and materials. These tools include diaries and activity logs, gatekeeper reviews, and readability pretesting.

Diaries and Activity Logs

Diaries and activity logs are written records of what occurred each day, week, or other time period during a program's planning or execution. These records are kept and updated by people from whom you want input and feedback about the program. They're commonly used to:

- Track program implementation
- Assess the effectiveness of program implementation
- Pilot test an intervention
- Monitor whether planned activities are on schedule and within budget
- Learn what questions program participants asked
- Determine what technical assistance program staff needed
- Track the audience's exposure to program components
- Gain insights about the audience's relevant day-to-day experiences (e.g., smokers can record each time they smoked a cigarette, and how they felt before, during, and after smoking the cigarette, providing insights into how smokers feel about smoking and how you might be able to help them quit)

If you plan to use diaries or activity logs to gauge the quality of program planning or execution, be sure the diaries and logs are started as soon as you begin program planning. Have program managers or participants

Table 3.5: Pros and Cons of Survey Formats

Format	Pros	Cons
Mail		
	• Mail can be a cost-effective way to access hard-to-reach populations (e.g., the homebound or rural residents). • Respondents can answer questions when it's most convenient for them.	• Mail is not appropriate for respondents with limited literacy skills. • Low response rate diminishes the value of results. • Expensive follow-up by mail or telephone may be necessary to increase the response rate. • Respondents may return incomplete questionnaires. • Responses can be difficult to read. • Receiving enough responses may take a long time. • Postage may be expensive if the sample is large or the questionnaire is long.
Telephone		
With interviewer using paper-and-pencil questionnaires.	• Telephone is appropriate for those with limited literacy skills. • Questionnaires can be more complete. • The sequence of questions can be controlled.	• Potential respondents without telephones can't participate. • Respondents may hang up if they believe the survey is part of a solicitation call or if they don't want to take the time to participate. • Response rates are declining, especially for telephone and Internet surveys (Singer, et al. 2000).
With interviewer using computer-assisted telephone interviewing (CATI).	• "Skip patterns" can be included, which is useful for complex questionnaires. • The need for data entry is eliminated.	• CATI software and computers are required. • Extensive interviewer training is needed. • Time is required to program questionnaire into CATI.

Continues

Table 3.5: Pros and Cons of Survey Formats (cont.)

Format	Pros	Cons
In Person		
Administered by interviewer.	• Face-to-face persuasion tactics can be used to increase response rates. • Participants with limited literacy skills can use this method. • The method is useful with hard-to-reach populations (e.g., homeless or with low literacy) or when the intended audience can't be surveyed by using other data-collection methods. • Interviewer can clarify questions for respondents. • More questionnaires are completed.	• Administration is more expensive than self-administered surveys or telephone data collection. • This method may not be appropriate for sensitive issues because respondents may not answer as truthfully in person.
Self-administered: Respondents asked to complete survey at a location frequented by the target population (e.g., during a conference, in a classroom, or after viewing an exhibit at a health fair).	• Harder-to-reach respondents can be contacted in locations convenient and comfortable for them. • The survey can be conducted quickly. • Data can be gathered cost-effectively in a relatively short time. • Selecting an appropriate location can result in an increased number of respondents from intended population.	• The ability to reach respondents in person at a central location or gathering is required. • Respondents must have complex, mature literacy skills.
Self-administered on computer: Questionnaire is displayed on a computer screen and respondents key in answers.	• "Skip patterns" can be included, which is useful for complex questionnaires. • The sequence of questions can be controlled. • Need for data entry is eliminated, and quick summary and analysis of results are provided.	• Use is not appropriate for audiences with limited literacy skills or those uncomfortable with computers. • Expensive technical equipment is required that may not be readily available or may be cumbersome in many settings. • Respondents must have access to programmed computers and be comfortable using computers.

Table 3.5: Pros and Cons of Survey Formats (cont.)

Format	Pros	Cons
Internet		
Self-administered on computer: Questionnaire displayed on respondent's computer screen through a Web site.	• "Skip patterns" can be included, which is useful for complex questionnaires. • The sequence of questions can be controlled. • The need for data entry is eliminated, and quick summary and analysis of results are provided.	• Use is not appropriate for audiences with limited literacy skills or those uncomfortable with computers. • Respondents must have Internet access and be comfortable using computers. • There's no way to confirm the validity of identifying information provided by respondents. • Response rates are declining, especially for telephone and Internet surveys (Singer, et al. 2000). • Samples are not representative.

put the diary or log information into a specific format. This information may cover issues such as the quality of program components or how your audience uses the components. (See Chapter 5: Evaluating the Success of Your Counter-Marketing Program for guidance on planning and conducting program evaluation.)

Pros:
- Diaries and logs give respondents flexibility in their answers.
- These records enable researchers to observe behavior over time, rather than only once.

Cons:
- Diaries and logs require considerable effort by respondents and may not be filled out in a timely or thorough manner. For this reason, offering incentives for completing the diaries or logs is important.
- The data may be voluminous and challenging to code and compare.
- These records can be hard to read and are thus not appropriate for respondents with low literacy or poor writing skills or penmanship. Here are the five major steps for diary or activity log research:

1. Plan the research.
2. Identify who will complete the diaries or activity logs.
3. Develop and pretest the form for collecting information.
4. Collect the data.
5. Analyze the results.

Step 1: Plan the research.

Determine the following information:

- What you want to learn
- How much information you need
- When you need the information
- How you'll apply what you learn
- What your budget is
- What your criteria are for participants

Step 2: Identify who will complete the diaries or activity logs.

The participants you select depend on the goals of your research. If you're focusing on your audience's day-to-day experiences in relation to some aspect of tobacco use, you'll want audience members to complete the diaries. For example, if you want teenagers to keep diaries documenting when they encountered tobacco among friends, family members, and others in their lives and how those encounters made them feel, recruit teenagers willing to participate. (When recruiting youth respondents, you may need parental permission.)

If you're focusing on participants' experience with a program as a pilot test, you'll want the participants to keep the diaries. You're likely to recruit participants on site. You'll probably need to provide an incentive (e.g., a gift certificate once the completed diary is received), and you also may need to remind participants to return the diaries at the end of the research period.

Step 3: Develop and pretest the form for collecting information.

Here's how to create a user-friendly document to collect the data:

- Write questions that are specific to your objectives. For example, for a pilot test of a health education program, provide a description of the module(s) used each day and include entries such as the following:
  - Date
  - Title of module used
  - Description of activities completed
  - Record of how long activities took to complete
  - Response to whether the respondent would participate in these activities again
  - Reasons the respondent would or would not participate again
- Include examples of participant feedback.
- For a log related to smoking behavior, you might include entries such as the following:
  - When the first cigarette of the day was smoked
  - What the person was doing when smoking each cigarette
  - Whom the person was with when smoking each cigarette
  - How the person was feeling when he or she most wanted a cigarette

- Pretest the draft diary or log with members of your audience.

- Revise questions people found confusing during the pretest. If a question was confusing to only one person, use your judgment about whether to change the question. If you make substantial changes to the diary or log, conduct another pretest before finalizing the form.

Step 4: Collect the data.

Produce enough diaries or logs so that each respondent has several extra forms in case they are needed. Attach detailed written instructions to each form. Deliver the diaries or logs to respondents before training, as necessary or at least one week before the research begins. If you're asking program participants to complete diaries or logs, you'll have to distribute the materials on site. Give respondents a fixed time frame to complete these records (e.g., one week or six months), and provide a way to return the data to you (e.g., an envelope and postage). If your research period is longer than one or two weeks, you may want to ask respondents to send the first week of data, so you can review the logs for accuracy and completeness and even begin to tally information. Collect the logs at several points during the research period, to ensure that participants are filling them out regularly; otherwise they may fill them out all at once at the end of the period.

Step 5: Analyze the results.

In the planning phase, you determined what you wanted to learn from the research. Now you can look through the diaries or logs to answer those questions. Diaries generally contain qualitative information. Activity logs may contain both quantitative information you can tabulate easily (e.g., how many people called a hotline each day) and qualitative information (e.g., reasons people liked or participated in an activity). Here are some suggestions for analyzing both types of information:

- To analyze qualitative information, search the data for similarities and differences among diaries or logs, for all the questions. Look for general themes or patterns. The best way to analyze these themes is to develop categories for the responses. For example, if you want to know why teachers thought their students liked or disliked a certain educational module in your program, you might group responses into categories such as "challenging," "fun," "too much work," and "boring." You may add or combine categories as you go along. You can make inferences about the diary information (e.g., "most teachers liked the module because…"), but resist the temptation to quantify this information.

- To analyze quantitative responses, create a coding sheet for each quantitative question, writing the question at the top and creating columns for each possible response. For example, for a question in an activity log about how many people picked up particular brochures, you could create these columns: 0, 1–5, 6–10, 11–15, 16–20, and >20. Then record the response from each log by making a check mark in the appropriate column. Tally the check marks in each column, and calculate the percentage of participants who gave each type of response.

Gatekeeper Reviews

Educational materials for the public and for patients often are routed to their intended audiences through health professionals or other individuals or organizations that can communicate for you. These intermediaries act as gatekeepers, controlling the distribution channels that reach your audiences. Their approval or disapproval of your materials can be a critical factor in your program's success. If they don't like a poster or don't believe it's credible or scientifically accurate, it may never reach your audience.

Gatekeeper review of rough materials should be considered part of the pretesting process, although it's no substitute for pretesting materials with audience members. It's also no substitute for obtaining clearances or expert review for technical accuracy; that should be done before pretesting. Sometimes telling the gatekeeper that technical experts have reviewed the material for accuracy will reassure them and may speed approval of your message.

How you obtain gatekeeper reviews depends on your resources, including time and budget. Two methods are common:

1. **Self-administered questionnaires.** Gatekeepers are sent the materials and the questionnaire at the same time. (See Appendix 3.5 for an example.)

2. **Interviewer-administered questionnaires.** Typically, an appointment for the interview is scheduled with the gatekeeper, and the materials are sent for review in advance.

Questionnaires should be written to ask about overall reactions to the materials, including an assessment of whether the information is appropriate and useful.

In some cases, a formal questionnaire might not be feasible, especially if you don't think the gatekeeper will take the time to fill it out. Arrange a telephone or personal conversation or a meeting to review the materials. Consider in advance which questions you want to ask, and bring a list of these questions with you. One advantage of this approach is that you can use the discussion with gatekeepers to introduce them to your program and to ask if they want to become involved.

Readability Pretesting

Readability formulas often are used to assess the reading level of materials. Reading level refers to the number of years of education required for a reader to understand a written passage. Some experts suggest aiming for a level that is two to five grades lower than the average grade your audience has achieved, to account for a probable decline in reading skills over time. Others say a third- to fifth-grade level is frequently appropriate for readers with low literacy.

When the target audience is the general population, keep publications as simple as possible to increase reader comprehension. However, if publications are meant for a more educated, professional audience, simple materials might be considered insulting.

You'll need to decide which reading level is appropriate for your materials. Then use one or more readability formulas to determine whether your text is written at that level. Fry, Flesch, FOG, and SMOG are among the most commonly used readability formulas (NCI 2002). Applying these formulas is a simple process that can be done manually or with a computer program in only a few minutes. (See the National Cancer Institute's *Making Health Communication Programs Work: A Planner's Guide* [2002] for more information on readability formulas.)

Typically, readability formulas measure the difficulty of the vocabulary used and the average sentence length. Readability software such as RightWriter and Grammatik analyze a document's grammar, style, word usage, and punctuation and then assign a reading level. Some popular software programs such as Microsoft Word include a readability-testing function. However, these formulas don't measure the reader's level of comprehension. Researchers in one study suggest three principles for the use of readability formulas (NCI 1994):

1. Use readability formulas only in concert with other means of assessing the effectiveness of the material.

2. Use a formula only when the readers for whom a text is intended are similar to those on whom the formula was validated.

3. Do not write a text with readability formulas in mind.

> ### Points To Remember
>
> - Gaining insights about the target audience is central to developing effective counter-marketing strategies, tactics, and messages.
>
> - Market research should be an integral part of your counter-marketing program.
>
> - Market research isn't a do-it-yourself effort. Not only do you need to be knowledgeable, but you also need to seek the appropriate resources to ensure that your research is successfully designed and conducted.
>
> - Many tobacco control program staff have used market research and are good sources of advice on design, instruments, analysis, and findings.
>
> - Market research findings must be used to be worthwhile. Before you conduct research, decide how you'll use the results to plan, alter, justify, support, and/or promote aspects of your program.

Bibliography

American Marketing Association, New York Chapter. *GreenBook: Worldwide Directory of Focus Group Companies and Services*. New York, NY: American Marketing Association, 2003.

American Marketing Association, New York Chapter. *GreenBook: Worldwide Directory of Marketing Research Companies and Services*. New York, NY: American Marketing Association, 2003.

Marketing Research Association. *Blue Book Research Services Directory*. White Plains, MD: Marketing Research Association, 2003.

National Cancer Institute. *Clear and Simple: Developing Effective Print Materials for Low-Literate Readers*. Bethesda, MD: National Cancer Institute, 1994. Pub. No. T936.

NCI. *Making Health Communication Programs Work: A Planner's Guide*. Bethesda, MD: U.S. Department of Health and Human Services, Public Health Service, National Institutes of Health, NCI, 2002. Pub. No. T-0638.

Singer E, et al. Experiments with incentives in telephone surveys. *Public Opinion Quarterly* 2000;64:171–88.

Teenage Research Unlimited. *Counter-Tobacco Advertising Exploratory, Summary Report, January–March 1999*. Unpublished.

Chapter 4

Reaching Specific Populations

[Cultural] competence is not just changing how somebody looks in an ad or the language. It's about understanding people as whole entities: their history, their culture, their context, and their geography.

— Robert Robinson, Office on Smoking and Health
    Centers for Disease Control and Prevention

In This Chapter

- Developing Cultural Competence
- Identifying and Describing Specific Populations
- Conducting Formative Research
- Additional Considerations in Reaching Specific Populations

Although the main emphasis of your tobacco counter-marketing campaign may be on one or more broad target audiences, you may also want to conduct efforts that focus on specific populations—groups of individuals who share unique characteristics and may be particularly affected by tobacco. These shared characteristics include racial, ethnic, cultural, geographic, age, physical, and socioeconomic traits, and level of education. Examples of specific populations include:

- Racial/ethnic minority groups
- Gay, lesbian, bisexual, and transgender populations
- Rural residents
- Groups with low socioeconomic status
- People with disabilities
- College students
- Restaurant workers
- Blue-collar workers

Developing and implementing successful counter-marketing strategies to reach these populations may be challenging. Although you'll follow the same basic processes used to design any counter-marketing campaign, reaching specific populations requires additional approaches and considerations. For example, you may need to take a closer look at your organization's operating practices to ensure that they are inclusive, culturally competent, and adequately address the needs of the specific populations in your state. You will also need to develop an understanding of the specific populations you plan to target to ensure that messages, language, imagery, and other aspects of your counter-marketing materials and interventions are appropriate and effective.

It is important to devote adequate resources to reaching the specific populations in your state. When appropriate, it can be cost-effective to design your specific population campaign to supplement your mainstream effort. Creating messages that are coordinated with your mainstream campaign can help provide specific populations with the multiple exposures needed to contribute to attitude and behavior change, as well as to build support in populations for tobacco control policies.

If your budget won't permit you to reach all audiences at once, you'll need to decide which audiences you can reach with your current funding, and which audiences you'll want to target if your funding increases. Lack of information may also constrain the breadth of your efforts and may require that some population groups not be included initially.

Developing Cultural Competence

When developing a counter-marketing effort for a specific population, the first step is to look at your organization's level of cultural competency. The main goal of building an organization's cultural competence is to be more effective in representing and serving its constituents by developing strategies and programs that reflect the needs and priorities of those served. An organizational and philosophical commitment to diversity and inclusivity provides the basis for achieving cultural competence. In essence, it reflects the commitment to understanding specific populations and taking actions to serve them. Developers of tobacco counter-marketing programs need to recognize the differences and similarities within and among groups, including how they are influenced by their particular cultures, histories, the prevailing social and economic contexts, and the geographies in which they live. Developing cultural competence may require your organization to assess its physical environment, materials and resources, policies and procedures, training, and professional development.

Developing cultural competence may also require your staff and anyone else who works on your program to reflect on their own values and attitudes, communication style, and which community or audience they are representing, so that they are prepared to relate to diverse populations and to be responsive during interactions with them. Even if an organization has individuals from a specific population on its staff, cultural competence may still need to be addressed. Because each person has

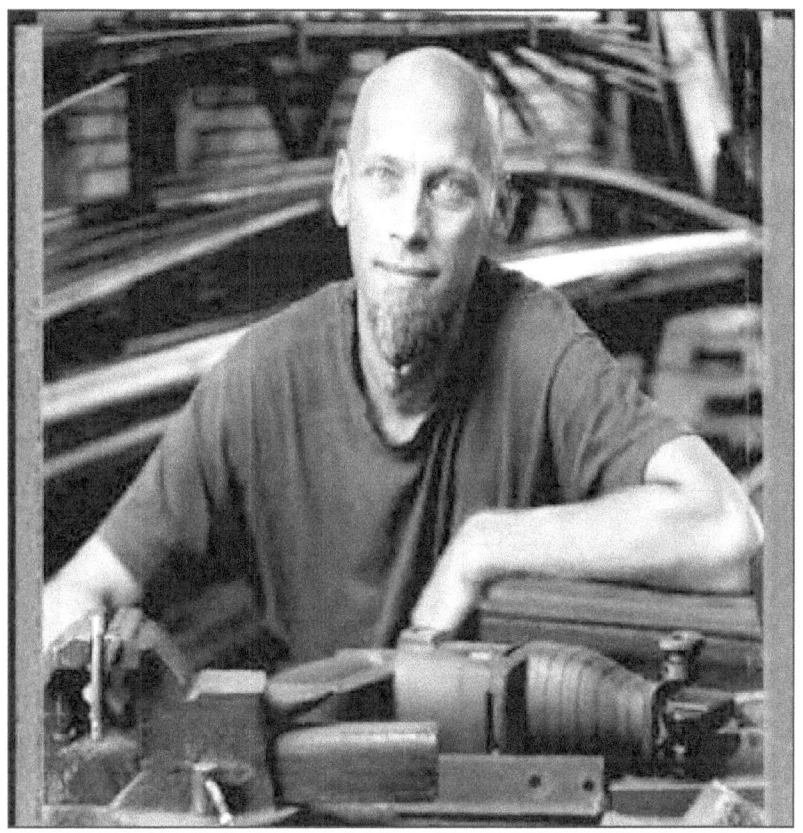

different biases and experiences, it's important for every staff member to recognize the value of being culturally competent.

Developing cultural competence within your organization should enable you to work more effectively with the communication agencies that you have hired to focus on the specific population(s) you are targeting. This will help ensure the development of culturally competent messages and materials.

Cultural competence goes beyond recognizing and incorporating the language of target audiences in your programs. For example, to make a tobacco cessation counseling program culturally competent, the program manager may need to:

- Develop an organizational commitment to cultural competence
- Employ counselors who speak languages other than English
- Develop and pretest, with each subpopulation, concepts and materials that reflect issues related to smoking in the community
- Develop and pretest materials in appropriate languages for specific communities
- Include community representatives on planning committees
- Train staff to be sensitive to cultural issues when providing tobacco cessation counseling

- Hold staff accountable for the way they interact with counseling program clients

Wisconsin's Division of Public Health provides an example of how cultural competence can be developed and promoted (National Center for Cultural Competence 1999). Its staff formulated guiding principles and strategies to promote cultural competence in the design of health programs, including the following:

- Audits of an organization's existing culture
- Clarification of the mission of diversity enhancement
- Strategic goals
- Examination of assumptions dealing with cultural competence
- Training
- Visionary leadership

The National Center for Cultural Competence, at Georgetown University Center for Child and Human Development, offers several helpful self-assessment tools that you can adapt and use to gauge cultural competence within your own organization. These checklists are available online at www.georgetown.edu/research/gucdc/nccc/products.html. You may want to consider hiring a consultant to help your organization become as culturally competent as possible or to assess your organization's cultural competence. You may even want to add a diversity specialist to your staff to help increase the staff's cultural competence.

Checklist for Developing Cultural Competence in an Organization

- ❑ Reflect an organizational commitment to developing cultural competence in all of the organization's policies, procedures, physical environments, programs, and activities.

- ❑ Promote cultural competence among your staff as a developmental process though an ongoing organizational commitment to self-assessment, professional development, training, policy development, and implementation. This process will help your organization build the capacity to understand and meet the needs of the specific population(s) it serves.

- ❑ Encourage key staff to conduct cultural self-assessments. (Sample tools are available from the Wisconsin Division of Public Health and the Georgetown University Center for Child and Human Development).

- ❑ Don't make assumptions about a population's culture. Become knowledgeable regarding aspects of the specific populations (e.g., values, attitudes, communication styles, language, literacy levels, physical environments, histories, cultures, social and economic contexts, and geographies) served by your organization.

Identifying and Describing Specific Populations

Identifying and Prioritizing Specific Populations in Your State

Specific populations traditionally have been defined by demographic characteristics such as age, race/ethnicity, income, and educational level. However, you may need to go beyond basic demographics to adequately describe the specific populations in your state. Specific populations will also be shaped by history, culture, context, and geography—factors that are only partially reflected in the sociodemographic descriptors and that can affect attitudes and preferences. Group identity can also be reinforced by particular experiences with educational institutions, religions, government, businesses, and other institutions.

Identifying different specific populations is further complicated by the diversity within respective populations. For example, the broader category of Hispanics/Latinos can be further delineated into subgroups such as Cubans, Mexicans, and Puerto Ricans, each with its unique characteristics. Similarly, the gay, lesbian, bisexual, and transgender (GLBT) community is composed of subgroups with very different characteristics. Making this issue even more complex is the overlap among groups made up of individuals who share some characteristics but also identify with other populations as well. For example, people with disabilities, members of the GLBT community, and restaurant workers who are exposed to secondhand smoke at work may also identify with specific racial or ethnic groups.

The first task in selecting and prioritizing specific populations that your tobacco counter-marketing efforts will target is to identify and describe each group affected by tobacco use in your state. Sources that might help you identify these groups include U.S. Census Bureau data, public health department reports, public school data, media outlets, national organizations, immigrant assistance or resettlement programs, and language institutes, which may show trends in demand for translators or interpreters. Although these sources can help you determine the representation of various populations in your state, they also have limitations. For example, they may underestimate the size of specific groups (e.g., Cambodians within the Asian/Pacific Islander community). These sources may also fail to identify certain groups if the appropriate questions are not asked (e.g., sexual identity questions to identify GLBTs). Depending on the quantity, quality, and types of data available from existing sources, you may need to conduct new research to gain enough information about the specific populations in your state or community to make well-informed decisions.

In determining which specific populations should be priority audiences for your counter-marketing efforts, you'll also need to study epidemiologic data, media consumption patterns, and other available qualitative data to assess whether counter-marketing is an effective intervention for a particular group. Some population groups can't be reached efficiently through mass media or other traditional counter-marketing techniques,

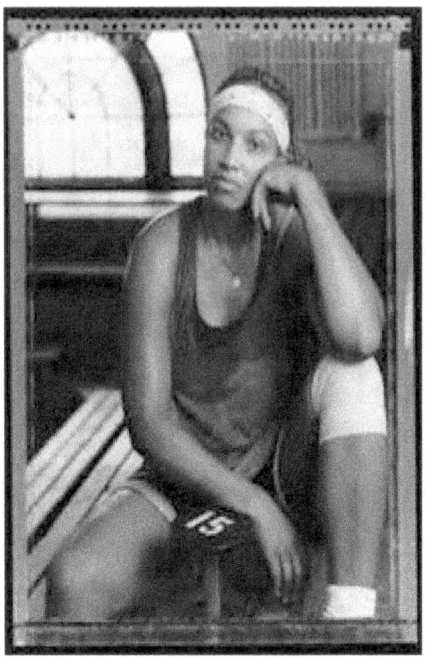

so you may want to use other program components to reach those groups.

Understanding Your Priority Audiences

Once you have chosen a specific population group as a target audience, you must learn about the characteristics shared by individuals in that group. For many populations, this means understanding such factors as their culture. Culture has been defined as "the shared values, traditions, norms, customs, arts, history, folklore, and institutions of a group of people unified by race, ethnicity, language, nationality, or religion." Culture affects how people pattern their behavior, see the world around them, and structure their environment, especially their families and communities (USDHHS 1996).

However, culture provides only one window into a community. Your tobacco counter-marketing strategies should also take into account and reflect other factors that drive any community. Geography is another way to understand how communities are differentiated. For example, African Americans who live in large urban areas will likely have different characteristics than African Americans who live in rural tobacco-growing communities, where tobacco is an important part of the economic and cultural fabric. Age, gender, and sexual orientation are other factors that impact the attitudes and behaviors of the group being targeted.

While there is heterogeneity within any group, it is important to understand that there are still likely to be common elements that bring these groups together as a broader community. It is these commonalities that allow counter-marketing programs to target such groups efficiently.

Defining Specific Populations and Targeted Segments

The challenge is to describe your target audience using the most relevant, unbiased, and data-driven characteristics possible, as well as information based on how the group describes itself and how others describe it. Formative research may reveal characteristics that provide a more accurate and appropriate description of the target group. Including more detail in the description of an audience may uncover information useful for your counter-marketing efforts. A more detailed audience profile may include media or consumer habits, lifestyle characteristics, level of acculturation, region, or place of residence (e.g., urban or rural).

You'll also want to gain an understanding of the social context of your audience by examining the social influences that may affect behavior. For example, determining the roles that family members and friends play within a specific population and identifying other supporters, such as those from whom a population's members seek advice, are parts of defining a population's social context. This kind of information can yield valuable insights into your target audience, how they interact with others, and how they interact with and are influenced by tobacco. Other contextual factors that may impact campaign development are the proportion of people of low socioeconomic status, the availability of cessation services, and the relevance of tobacco use relative to other problems confronting the target audience.

You can also target your marketing efforts more precisely if you consider subgroups within major populations. For example, recent immigrants may smoke less than members of their population who have lived in the United States longer and who have been exposed to higher levels of tobacco industry marketing. In addition, these two subgroups may consume different kinds or amounts of media. If you are focusing on a population with such subgroups, then you may want to reach recent immigrants (who have lower prevalence) with a prevention message and those who are more assimilated (who have higher prevalence) with a cessation message. There may be differences among people from the same major group based on the country of origin. For example, Asian Americans who come from China, Japan, Korea, Vietnam, or another country may have very different characteristics, attitudes, and behaviors. There also may be differences among people from the same country based on the region of origin. These differences can be understood through an assessment of particular histories, cultures, contexts, and geographies. You'll need to consider these differences when deciding what messages, tone, channels, activities, and other factors would be most appropriate for specific populations in your community or state. For example, some ads work well among all Hispanic/Latino groups, while others communicate effectively to only a few groups, based on the particular accents, vocabulary, and other ad elements chosen to reflect particular groups' lifestyles.

When your target audience has many different segments, testing messages and materials is critical to assess different potential responses among the different segments. Test messages with representatives of the target audience and other stakeholders to be sure they are understood and accepted and to avoid possible unintended negative effects. (See Chapter 3: Gaining and Using Target Audience Insights for more information on testing methods.) When evaluating messages, don't rely on the opinions of your organization's staff. Even if they are members of the target audience, they're likely to have a knowledge base about tobacco and public health that makes them atypical of the audience as a whole.

Checklist for Identifying and Defining Specific Populations

❑ Identify and describe the specific populations that are affected by tobacco use in your state.

❑ Assess whether counter-marketing is an effective intervention for the groups you have identified.

❑ Define your target group using demographics, epidemiologic data, consumer habits, lifestyle data, and other sources of information.

❑ Recognize the diversity among certain specific populations, as well as among their subpopulations.

❑ Pay close attention to the level of acculturation among immigrant groups, because the characteristics, attitudes, behaviors, and responses of recent immigrants may be very different from those of immigrants who have lived in the United States for several years.

❑ Make attempts to understand the tobacco-related social norms among the specific populations your program is targeting.

Conducting Formative Research

Findings from formative research can be used to help develop, or "form," a counter-marketing program. Formative research may consist of several parts, including environmental profiles, inventories of community resources, and audience research. As mentioned earlier in this chapter, formative research can help you understand how to separate the population into groups or segments that tend to think or act in similar ways or are affected by similar influences. It can also help you to understand the causes, or determinants, of tobacco use and other health risk behaviors, and the protective factors in target audiences. This research is also used to investigate which interventions might influence target audiences to change their behavior(s). (See Chapter 3: Gaining and Using Target Audience Insights for detailed information on research.)

Conducting an Environmental Scan

When you begin the research process, it can be extremely helpful to look at whether existing tobacco counter-marketing programs have been successful in helping to reduce tobacco use among the specific populations you've chosen to target. Look at programs that other organizations have implemented in your state, as well as those implemented by other states. Contact your representative in the Office on Smoking and Health, Centers for Disease Control and Prevention for information compiled from state efforts. Or, if you want information about a specific state's program, you can contact individuals or search Web sites within that state. If components of another state's programs appear applicable to your state, test those components—including ads and other materials—in your state before you implement them to confirm that they are likely to work in your area with your specific population. One excellent resource for accessing and using tobacco counter-advertising produced by states, organizations, and federal agencies is CDC's Media Campaign Resource Center, available online at http://www.cdc.gov/tobacco/mcrc.

You will also want to learn about organizations and individuals working with various specific populations who might be able to serve as resources to help you develop the campaign. Investigate which of these resources have the strongest expertise in developing programs, interventions, and materials for the specific populations you're targeting. Some of these organizations and individuals may be key stakeholders for your program. (See Chapter 8: Public Relations for more information on stakeholders.) Your public relations efforts will also include identifying media outlets that target your specific audiences. You need to work with these media outlets for your paid media placements and earned media coverage.

Applying Research Results to Campaign Development

To help ensure that your campaign reaches the specific populations you plan to target, you will want to follow the same guidance and processes used for general market campaigns outlined in this manual. (See Chapter 2: Planning Your Counter-Marketing Program, Chapter 3: Gaining and Using Target Audience Insights, Chapter 7: Advertising, Chapter 8: Public Relations, Chapter 9: Media Advocacy, Chapter 10: Grassroots Marketing, and Chapter 11: Media Literacy.) You'll also want to develop and implement an evaluation plan that includes evaluation of the efforts targeting specific populations. (See Chapter 5: Evaluating the Success of Your Counter-Marketing Program.)

Findings from qualitative research can be used to strategically develop materials that will reach the target audience with the intended messages. Through qualitative research, you can glean insights about your audience(s), solicit feedback on the materials and messages you are developing, and brainstorm about additional interventions that appeal to them. These findings can help you in making decisions throughout the campaign development process about aspects of the campaign, such as strategies, messages, tactics, and materials. (See Chapter 2: Planning Your Counter-Marketing Program for a more complete discussion of campaign planning steps.) It is important to remember that the findings from qualitative formative research techniques (e.g., focus groups) cannot be generalized to the population as a whole, but quantitative research techniques can provide findings that can be generalized to the entire group (see Chapter 3: Gaining and Using Target Audience Insights).

The first step is to set an overall program goal and select which specific populations you will target. For example, your overall program goal might be to increase cessation among adults, and you may have decided to supplement your general market cessation campaign with a campaign specifically targeting Hispanic/Latino men to persuade them to try to quit smoking. To accomplish your goal, you will need to develop strategies for communicating with your target audience(s). If your formative research reveals that smoking is supported by the cultural values of this audience, you might develop a strategy to communicate the cultural value of family well-being and the harm of secondhand smoke to family members. This strategy might be used to help counter the values that support smoking. Another strategy might be to show the benefits that audience members are likely to enjoy when they quit smoking or the negative consequences they might suffer if they continue to smoke.

The next step is to develop specific messages, which are the two or three key points you want to communicate to your target audience. For example, your messages to a Hispanic/Latino adult male smoker may include how much his family would suffer if he were to become ill or die from smoking, how much he would suffer physically and emotionally from the consequences of smoking, or how ill his children might become from being exposed to his second-hand smoke. These messages should be developed based on the findings of your formative research.

You'll want to develop specific tactics and activities to use in implementing your strategies. If your environmental scan identified qualified organizations and individuals in your state or community who work with the specific population(s) you have chosen, they may be able to provide valuable input to the development of tactics and activities based on their experiences and expertise. For example, one tactic would be to have people share their experiences of being harmed by smoking. Such stories can be effective because they personalize the risk of smoking. You could work with hospitals or Hispanic/Latino health organizations to identify and interview affected individuals and select the most powerful stories. This approach was used in a smoking cessation campaign in Massachusetts that featured a Hispanic/Latino man

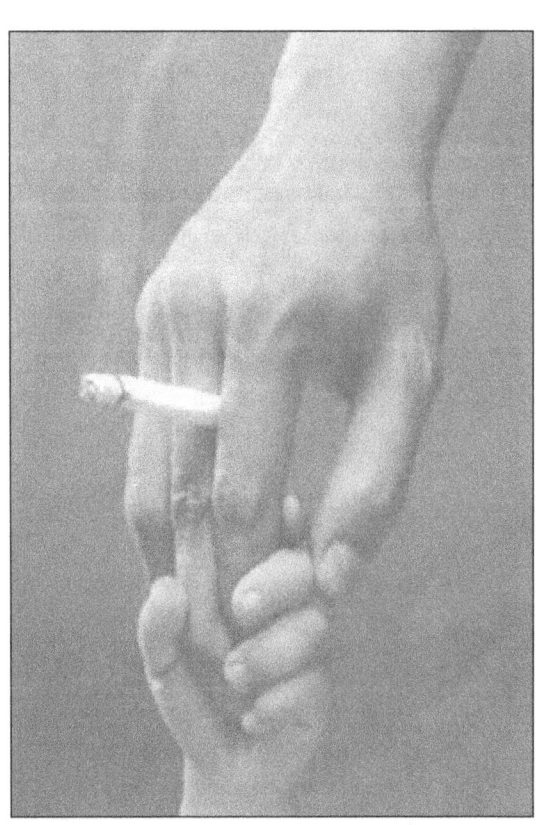

who developed emphysema early in his life from smoking. He eventually lost his voice and had to speak through an artificial-voice device. The Massachusetts Tobacco Control Program developed this story into poignant television and radio ads.

Review all your options for use of paid media to reach your audience(s), and choose ones that are cost-effective. In addition to broadcast and print media, your campaign could include billboard ads, postcards that people could send to loved ones encouraging them to quit smoking, and signs on public transit vehicles. You could also develop posters for places where people tend to meet, such as community centers.

As part of your earned media outreach efforts, you could contact reporters at the Hispanic/Latino media outlets you have identified and pitch a story about the consequences of an individual's smoking. You can put reporters in touch with the individuals featured in your ads as a way to weave your messages into a personal story.

You may want to hold a kickoff event to introduce your campaign, inviting people from your specific population, organizations that represent them, and the media. Use such an event as an opportunity to highlight your program and to give credit publicly to local individuals who helped to develop the program.

Once the campaign has started, you can begin to measure its effect. Using the same measures and indicators you used to conduct baseline research before the campaign started, conduct follow-up research after the first phase of the campaign and after the campaign ends. This evaluation will enable you to identify what worked, what progress was made, and what changes need to be made for additional campaign phases. (See Chapter 5: Evaluating the Success of Your Counter-Marketing Program for more information.) As with any counter-marketing campaign, developing campaigns to reach specific populations is an evolutionary process; you'll learn what works and what doesn't work as you go along, and you will make adjustments as necessary.

Involving Specific Populations in Research

Representatives of the targeted audience(s) should participate in the research to increase their ownership of, comfort with, level of support for, and the face validity of the counter-marketing efforts. It's important to enlist cooperation from community organizations that represent these populations. Because they are familiar with the community, they may be able to help you select contractors and facilitators who have the right skills and expertise to work with your target audience(s). You may even be able to identify and train local people to conduct the research. These members of the community—possibly social workers, community workers, religious and peer leaders, and health professionals—understand the community from the inside and have established trust with other community members. Thus, they may be able to probe more deeply into the attitudes, behaviors, and practices of the specific population you're trying to reach, and to elicit information that can more effectively guide campaign development. However, you may

> ### *Checklist for Conducting Formative Research*
>
> ❑ Choose qualified researchers who understand cultural competence.
>
> ❑ Involve specific populations at every phase of the formative research.
>
> ❑ Research specific populations' responses to the tones of different messages.
>
> ❑ Address concerns and fears expressed by the specific populations and identified in scientific literature.
>
> ❑ Share findings with the organizations that represent specific populations to keep them updated on the development of the campaign.
>
> ❑ Use research findings to help encourage specific populations to support the resulting strategies and activities of the counter-marketing program.
>
> ❑ Use research findings to help guide decisions during the development of the campaign.

run the risk of focus group participants not feeling safe with a moderator they know because of issues of confidentiality and disclosure of personal information. In addition, you must be confident that these members of the community are qualified to conduct the research. Although the process to train and develop a set of skilled moderators for specific populations may be time consuming, you may find that the audience insights you gain are a valuable long-term investment in making your campaign a success. When conducting qualitative research, you should pay close attention to ties to the tobacco industry or other potential conflicts of interest that could serve to bias results of the research.

You may need to make a special effort to address concerns that communities may have about research. These concerns could be based on negative historical experiences such as the Tuskegee Study, a research project in which treatment was secretly withheld from African-American men with syphilis. Or they could be based on the belief that the community has been overly researched and exploited by scientists more interested in publishing papers than in solving problems. Efforts may include dispelling fears, promoting involvement in the formative research at every stage, and obtaining input about how the data will be used. These efforts can help considerably to raise trust and maintain a sense of ownership of the research and its products.

Additional Considerations in Reaching Specific Populations

When developing and implementing a campaign for a specific population, you should pay close attention to the following areas:

- Involving the target population in the development process

- Using appropriate language and images in materials development

- Identifying and addressing potential barriers arising from concerns of the target audience (audience barriers)

Involving the Specific Populations in the Development Process

Tobacco counter-marketing programs should include the target audience's participation throughout the life of the program. This representation ensures that programs reflect the specific population's values, norms, behaviors, perspectives, and needs.

Each planning phase should include developing relationships and partnerships with specific populations and persons and groups that serve or have access to them. These may include professional and fraternal organizations; African-American, Asian, Hispanic/Latino, or American Indian/Alaska Native chambers of commerce; or professional media organizations, such as publishers of minority newspapers or magazines.

Give all partners the opportunity to declare conflicts of interest early in the planning process. Tobacco companies have a great deal of influence in most communities and with the media, including communities and media of specific population groups. Some ethnic media outlets receive substantial revenue from the tobacco industry and thus may not be suitable partners for developing antitobacco media strategies. Although your state may not want to partner with those outlets, you'll probably want to place antitobacco ads in the same outlets to counter the protobacco messages. In addition, because some media outlets in communities of color have depended on revenue from tobacco industry advertising, it may be strategically important to acknowledge this history when defining your relationship with those outlets. A flexible approach in the short term may make you more likely to achieve your long-term goals.

Checklist for Involving Specific Populations in the Development Process

- ❏ Assess your agency's cultural competence to avoid any bias in choosing partners.

- ❏ Include representatives of the specific population in all phases of the program, from formative research and planning through implementation and evaluation.

- ❏ Select people or groups that represent the specific population's diversity and perspectives and that are credible with the target audience.

- ❏ Include representatives who have access to large numbers of specific population members, such as media outlets (e.g., radio, TV, and magazines) and organizations (e.g., racial/ethnic, professional, religious, schools).

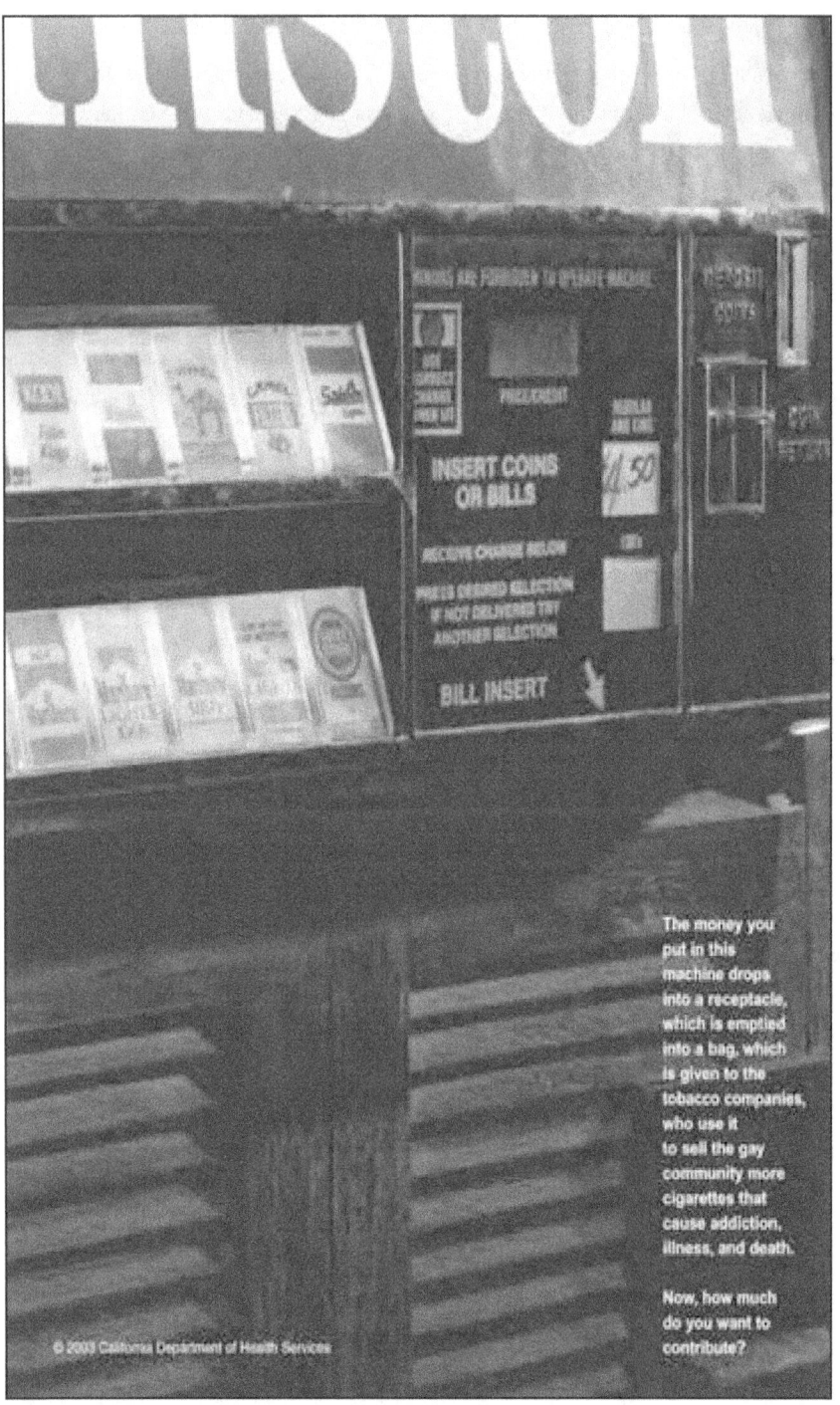

One way to gain target audiences' support for your program is to help them recognize how tobacco use harms their community and how they can help address the problem. For example, sharing with the GLBT community information about disproportionate rates of tobacco-related morbidity and mortality in their community may help members become more interested in the issue. Then, facilitating a discussion with GLBT leaders in which tobacco industry targeting of their community is highlighted may motivate them to take action against these marketing practices. When sharing information with members of a specific population, it is important to cite sources that are credible and relevant to that audience. These sources may be members of the specific population.

Using Appropriate Language and Imagery in Materials Development

Ideally, you should develop messages and materials in the language of your target audience from the start. Try to involve native speakers of the language to write and review the text, design, graphics, and images. When the language is not English, you may also want to conduct a reverse translation, in which you translate the foreign-language document into English. This serves as a quality control measure to ensure that the key messages and concepts will be communicated as intended.

If you cannot develop language-specific and culturally appropriate materials and instead must start with the original (often English) version, don't rely on a direct translation of a message. Always test the translation first. When the text is finalized, it's often helpful to have a second translator conduct a reverse translation. You should check references on translators to determine whether they have met the needs of previous clients. The following example illustrates the steps in addressing language differences:

In 1997, the CDC Prevention Marketing Initiative Nashville Demonstration Site developed an English-language radio soap opera as a mass media intervention to reach African-American teens with messages on prevention of HIV (human immunodeficiency virus) and sexually transmitted diseases. When the intervention was replicated to reach Spanish-speaking teens, focus groups and three translations of the script were needed to make the intervention appropriate for teens from the various Hispanic/Latino cultures of Central America, Mexico, Puerto Rico, and South America.

The first translation was completed by the Tennessee Foreign Language Institute, the second by a committee from the local Spanish-speaking community, and the third by a group of Hispanic/Latino teens who adapted the script to accommodate teen culture and language within the Hispanic/Latino community (CDC 1997). The final product was a consensus script that incorporated all three translations. One critical aspect of the translation was the presence of the Hispanic/Latino teens during the final translation and during the production of the soap opera. Their

¿Quiere dejar de fumar?

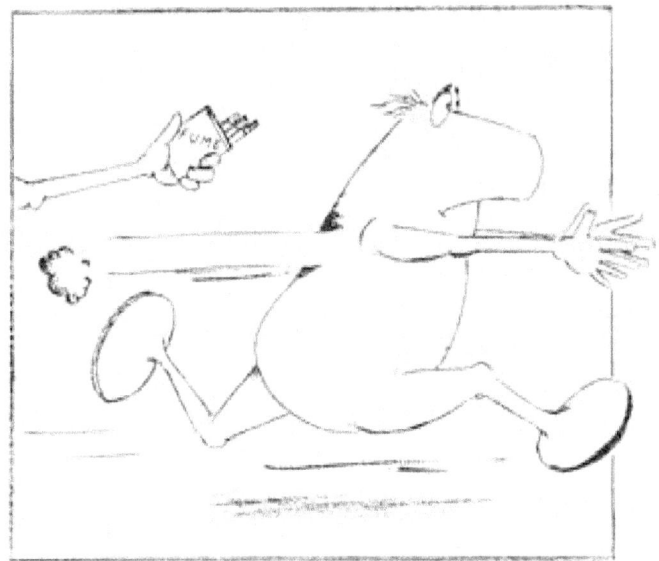

Si usted quiere dejar de fumar, recuerde la letra D.

Distancia: Ponga distancia entre usted y el tabaco. Rompa todos sus cigarros y tire sus ceniceros. Dígale a sus amistades que está dejando de fumar. Analice las situaciones en que fuma más, y si es posible, evítelas.

Tome la **Decisión:** Nadie puede hacerlo por usted. Usted se tiene que decidir por sí mismo que va a dejar de fumar.

Actúe con **Determinación:** El tabaco es adictivo y no es fácil dejarlo. No se desanime. Aunque tenga una recaída, vuelva a tratar.

Distráigase: Cuando sienta ganas de fumar, espere un minuto. Trate de hacer otra cosa: relájese, respire profundo, tome agua, háblele a sus amistades, coma frutas o verduras, salga a pasear o haga ejercicio.

Muchas personas han dejado de fumar, y usted también puede.

¡¡ SUERTE !!

> ### Checklist for Developing Appropriate Materials
>
> ❑ Use language and images that are sensitive and appropriate.
>
> ❑ Use native speakers to create foreign-language materials when possible.
>
> ❑ Ask for and check references to ensure that your translator's past work met client needs.
>
> ❑ Pretest all materials to ensure that messages and images are clear, that content is appropriate, and that language and images are not offensive to the target group or its community.
>
> ❑ Conduct a reverse translation to ensure that messages and key concepts are communicated accurately.

attendance prevented grammatical errors and ensured that a correct script was followed for each episode of the soap opera. Each step in the replication process ultimately contributed to the production of a culturally and linguistically acceptable mass media intervention for Hispanic/Latino teens.

Even if the language of the specific population is English, members of that population may have unique ways of speaking, or may use jargon or slang, so it's always important to test the materials among audience representatives to ensure that communication is as clear and effective as possible.

Materials development should also be guided by the use of appropriate and salient imagery. Positive imagery generally reflects a constructive visual of the target audience that is appropriate for the theme of the campaign. For example, an ad showing family members supporting a smoker's attempt to quit may be effective among the Hispanic/Latino community where close family ties are a priority. Salient imagery reflects visuals that are particularly important to a target audience, helping attract audience members' attention to the materials. For example, materials that integrate a rainbow image, which has been used by the GLBT community as an identifier and symbol of pride, could appeal to members of that community.

Identifying and Addressing Potential Audience Barriers

When developing your counter-marketing programs for specific populations, you may need to address existing audience barriers, such as historical mistrust of research; a resistance to targeted programs or efforts; and potentially positive perceptions of the tobacco industry, based on tobacco industry funding of

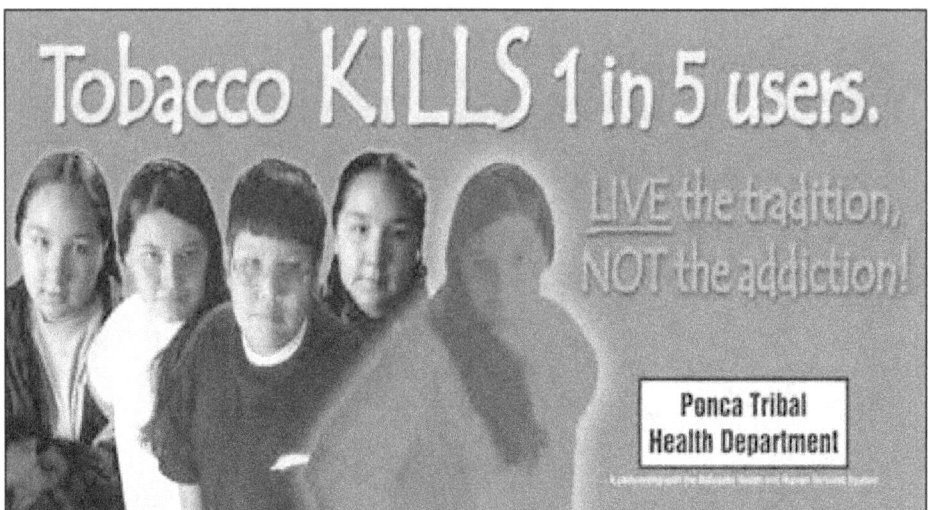

community organizations and events. In addition, some racial and ethnic communities are extremely sensitive about how their image has been portrayed in the media. For example, many African Americans are concerned about the mass media overrepresentation of African-American drug use. Such experiences of specific populations could produce negative perceptions about the integrity of targeted programs or strategies.

If you identify audience barriers in a specific population in your state, it is important that you address them. One way you can work to overcome these issues is by including the population in the campaign development process. You should work with their community leaders to communicate the value of your program. You must also be open and responsive to questions and concerns. For example, some recent immigrants may be reluctant to go to an unknown facility to participate in research or access health

Checklist for Identifying and Overcoming Audience Barriers

❑ Use formative research to identify issues, including barriers that arise from concerns of the target group.

❑ Use target group representatives and community partners to help define and address audience barriers.

❑ When possible, develop strategies for overcoming barriers, including offering benefits that have value to the specific population.

services because they fear that they could be turned in to the U.S. Immigration and Naturalization Service or because of negative experiences in their former countries. In a case like this, you might conduct research or provide health services in more familiar and comfortable locations. You could also enlist credible local spokespeople to build trust in the institutions and the facilities.

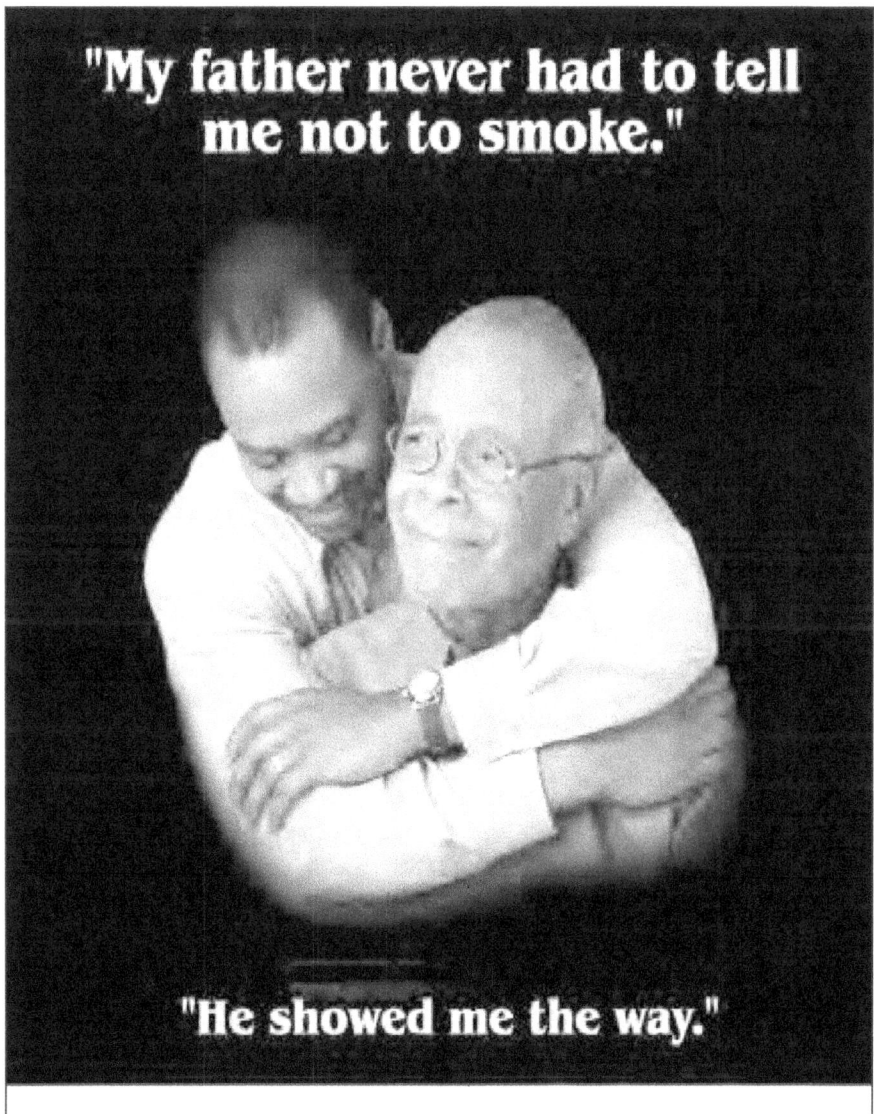

Case Study: California Smokers' Helpline (1998)

Background. The California Department of Health Services (CDHS) initiated a comprehensive tobacco control program in 1989 that was funded by revenue from an excise tax on tobacco. The main goal of the program was to reduce illness and mortality among smokers and nonsmokers caused by tobacco use. The program's strategies included exposing the truth about tobacco industry practices and products, educating Californians about the harmful effects of smoking and secondhand smoke, and providing services and support to people who wanted to quit smoking.

Developing cultural competence. The state of California has a diverse mix of residents. The CDHS tobacco control program staff needed to understand the composition of the population and why specific populations were important for reducing tobacco use. The tobacco control staff didn't simply rely on their own knowledge; they hired outside experts to teach them about the specific populations in California. They made it a priority to embrace the racial/ethnic diversity in their state. They knew that a "general population" program would not meet the needs of all groups because of language and culture differences.

Identifying and describing specific populations. Once the program staff decided to reach specific populations in California, they needed to determine some critical information:

1. The percentage of California's population that was made up of Asians/Pacific Islanders, Hispanics/Latinos, African Americans, and other major specific populations, and whether those groups were increasing in numbers

2. The major subpopulations within each of those large groups and the important differences among subgroups in areas such as language and culture

3. The absolute levels of tobacco use in each specific population and trends in tobacco use

4. How, when, and with whom tobacco was being used, and what factors were influencing each group to smoke more or to smoke less

Again, experts were hired to work with the staff to gather information in these four areas. Asians/Pacific Islanders were identified as an important specific population because of their large numbers within California and high population growth over the previous several years. The state tobacco control staff learned that Asians/Pacific Islanders included people from China, Japan, Korea, Laos, Singapore, and Vietnam, so they knew they could not communicate with all these populations in the same way. They also learned that Asian/Pacific Islander men had very high rates of smoking (up to 70 percent) and that they typically smoked in front of family members and friends when at home or socializing. The prevalence of smoking for Asian/Pacific Islander women was typically far lower (less than 10 percent), but they were an important secondary audience in terms of potential influence on their smoking husbands, brothers, or fathers. Thus, the tobacco control staff identified one primary audience (Asian/Pacific

Islander male smokers) to target for reducing smoking when around others for cessation, and one secondary audience (Asian/Pacific Islander female nonsmokers) to target for influencing the male smokers in their families. The staff also decided to communicate the main messages of the campaign in the four major Asian languages of the Asian/Pacific Islander population (Cantonese, Korean, Mandarin, and Vietnamese).

Conducting research. The first ads that were developed simply suggested that Asian/Pacific Islander smokers call the Quitline to get help from a counselor. The message was similar to the message for California's general population, but the ads for Asians/Pacific Islanders were developed using Asian talent. Awareness of, and calls to, the Quitline remained low, even though the ads and the Quitline were in the four Asian languages.

The CDHS tobacco control staff worked with its advertising agency to plan and conduct qualitative research to glean insights about why initial efforts were not working and what they could do to generate more calls to the Quitline. Research included interviews with smokers, as well as analysis of existing Quitline operations and promotions, to determine factors contributing to the low volume of calls. One important insight they uncovered was that in Asian culture, particularly among men, calling a counselor to ask for help was seen as a sign of weakness or an admission that the caller had a problem.

Developing and implementing the campaign. Based on the research findings, the Quitline was repositioned as a source for free *information* on how to quit smoking, rather than a counseling service. The new campaign included several elements. The "Jungle" campaign featured radio and print advertising that dramatized how smokers feel when they try to quit smoking: lost, trapped, hopeless, and unable to break free from their addiction to cigarettes. The ads encouraged smokers to call the toll-free number to obtain free information on ways to quit smoking.

A three-minute television ad, which was developed and aired in the four key languages, demonstrated for viewers what happens when someone calls the Quitline. The ad showed that the operator would be helpful, respectful, patient, and understanding.

In addition, an advertorial (advertisement in a format that resembles editorial content) in key print publications discussed step by step how the Quitline operates and emphasized that it was a free resource. The article featured quotes from the Asian-language Quitline staff discussing the benefits of calling. Print ads, radio ads, and advertorials were all produced in Cantonese, Korean, Mandarin, and Vietnamese and were placed in the appropriate media outlets.

Within two months of the campaign launch, the Asian-language Quitline received nearly 1,100 calls—more than all previous years combined, and a 10,000 percent increase over the previous year. Ad placements had to be suspended temporarily because the Quitline exceeded its capacity. Today, the Quitline receives a steady stream of phone calls each month because the advertising content and placement have been optimized over time.

Bibliography

Centers for Disease Control and Prevention. *Prevention Marketing Initiative Nashville Demonstration Site. "Reality Check": A Teen-Oriented Radio Soap Opera.* Nashville, TN: CDC, 1997.

National Center for Cultural Competence. *The Journey Towards Cultural Competence—The Wisconsin Story.* Washington, DC: Georgetown University Center for Child and Human Development, 1999.

Ryan H, Wortley PM, Easton A, et al. Smoking among lesbians, gays, and bisexuals: a review of the literature. *American Journal of Preventive Medicine* 2001;21:142–9.

U.S. Department of Health and Human Services. *Guidelines to Help Assess Cultural Competence in Program Design, Application, and Management.* Bethesda, MD: USDHHS, Health Resources and Services Administration, Bureau of Primary Health Care, Office on Minority and Women's Health, 1996.

Chapter 5

Evaluating the Success of Your Counter-Marketing Program

To ensure accountability and enable future improvements in tobacco control programs, state tobacco control programs must be evaluated and have explicit goals coupled to performance measures.

— National Cancer Policy Board, 2000

In This Chapter

- Evaluation and Surveillance
- Types of Evaluation
- What Evaluation Can Do
- When To Conduct an Evaluation
- Scope of the Evaluation
- How To Conduct an Evaluation

Evaluation plays a critical role in tobacco counter-marketing campaigns. Programs should be evaluated regularly to enable the program manager to build on successes, to switch to new strategies if necessary, and to be accountable to all those with an interest in the program's outcome.

Evaluation can help you to answer questions such as the following:

- What impact is the counter-marketing program having?

- Is the program being implemented as planned?

- Are the audience's attitudes or beliefs about tobacco being changed by the program?

- Is the program helping to improve the health status of the target population?

- How can the program be improved?

- Is the funding level appropriate for accomplishing the program's objectives?

Systematic collection of data for evaluation of the counter-marketing program can help to inform decisions of program managers and marketing managers, so the program can be improved and its outcomes demonstrated. However, this process doesn't take place in a vacuum. You'll need to define the purpose of the evaluation and decide which evaluation questions to ask, when evaluation should take place, how to present the questions to obtain the information needed, and how to provide this information to those who need it, in a way that facilitates its use.

An evaluation must be practical and must cover issues related to time, money, and the political context. For example, the more costly and visible the program is, the more comprehensive and rigorous the evaluation may need to be. The design of evaluation should be based on the expected use of the findings. Furthermore, it should be conducted in an ethical and high-quality manner, so results can withstand scientific scrutiny (Joint Committee on Standards for Educational Evaluation 1994; Patton 1997; CDC 2001).

Evaluation efforts should be planned during initial development of the program. Thinking about evaluation early improves both the program and the evaluation. In addition, most outcome evaluation requires a baseline study that must be conducted before any program activities take place. Evaluation should be coordinated with the program's implementation, so the results are timely and useful. If results are given to the program managers as they are generated, the managers can make adjustments to the program and share results with stakeholders.

CDC offers several resources to help you with evaluation. The Evaluation Working Group's *Framework for Program Evaluation in Public Health* (CDC 1999b) provides general evaluation guidance. The *National Tobacco Control Program: An Introduction to Program Evaluation for Comprehensive Tobacco Control Program Evaluation,* from the Office on Smoking and Health (OSH) (CDC 2001), presents an evaluation approach useful for tobacco control programs. CDC/OSH is preparing a manual that focuses on outcome evaluation specifically for paid counter-advertising campaigns. (Check http://www.cdc.gov/tobacco for availability.) States may also contact their CDC project officers for information about how to obtain resources and contact evaluation experts.

This chapter provides the basics of process and outcome evaluation for counter-marketing campaigns. It is consistent with the other CDC evaluation resources. The chapter addresses the difference between evaluation and surveillance, types of evaluation, what evaluation can do for you, and the various steps in conducting an evaluation. Additional guidance specific to each of the counter-marketing components can be found in the chapters on those topics (Chapter 7: Advertising, Chapter 8: Public Relations, Chapter 9: Media Advocacy, Chapter 10: Grassroots Marketing, and Chapter 11: Media Literacy).

Evaluation and Surveillance

The terms *evaluation* and *surveillance* are often used together, but they are distinct concepts. Program evaluation is "the systematic collection of information about the activities, characteristics, and outcomes of programs to make judgments about the program, improve program effectiveness, and/or inform decisions about future program development" (Patton 1997; CDC 2001). Surveillance is "the continuous monitoring or routine collection of data (e.g., behaviors, attitudes, deaths) over a regular interval of time" (CDC 2001). The Behavioral Risk Factor Surveillance System is an example of surveillance based on state data.

Although you may use surveillance systems and program evaluation methods to collect data on similar items, these data shouldn't be used for the same purpose. Surveillance data can be used to monitor overall trends in a population, but they can't be used to attribute observed improvements to a specific program. If a program is implemented on a sufficiently large scale and consistently across various sites, surveillance data can help to validate findings from the program evaluation. However, states should consider supplementing traditional surveillance systems that regularly monitor smoking behaviors and other tobacco-related variables with additional data collection designed to evaluate state counter-marketing programs.

Types of Evaluation

Several types of evaluation can help you to develop and assess your counter-marketing program. Three main types—formative, process, and outcome evaluation—form a continuum. Formative research and evaluation are conducted during program planning and development. (See Chapter 3: Gaining and Using Target Audience Insights and Chapter 7: Advertising for further information.) Formative research and evaluation help to answer these questions:

- How should I design my program?
- How well designed is each component of my program?

Formative research and evaluation help you to decide what to do and how to do it. Formative research is used to glean insights about the issue and your target audience(s) and to determine which messages and interventions might be effective. Formative evaluation is used to test concepts, materials, and messages, to determine whether they are communicating the intended messages and having the desired influence on your target audience.

Process and outcome evaluations, the focus of this chapter, are planned during the strategic planning stage and conducted during and after the implementation stage. Process evaluation helps you to answer these questions:

- Are we implementing the program as planned, and is it on schedule?
- What are we doing that was not in our original plan?

Process evaluation examines how your program is working while it is being implemented. It helps you to determine whether you're implementing with "fidelity"—whether you're sticking to your original program design. For an ad campaign, this evaluation might include assessments of whether the ad was aired at the times you proposed and whether your target group was exposed to the message. In addition, you might record unforeseen obstacles and potentially confounding environmental events to help you interpret findings. For public relations, process evaluation could involve documenting whether targeted key journalists were reached, the content of the pitch, and whether certain planned events took place. For a media literacy program, it might mean counting how many times the program was delivered, finding out if all the curriculum's lessons were implemented, and determining whether participants were satisfied with the content and delivery. Process evaluation enables you to report to stakeholders the plans you are implementing and the progress of your efforts.

Outcome evaluation helps you to answer the question: What effect are we having? It helps you to determine whether you're achieving the expected short-term, intermediate, and long-term outcomes. Typically, outcomes are expected changes in the audiences targeted for the counter-marketing program. For example, in an ad campaign, the outcome evaluation can show whether there's any change in the target audience's awareness and recall of the message; tobacco-related attitudes, beliefs, and other psychosocial factors; and behavior. For a grassroots marketing initiative, the outcome evaluation can show changes in the community's level of involvement in, and commitment to, the program. For a media advocacy component, the outcome evaluation can assess whether your efforts led to a change in tobacco-related policy. For public relations activities, your assessment might determine whether the target audience was aware of and understood the messages in your stories. In addition to these expected outcomes, unexpected outcomes sometimes arise, and these need to be acknowledged and included in your evaluation analysis.

Lesson Learned: Coordination

The Mistake: One state didn't establish a regular working relationship between program staff and evaluation staff. The program staff decided to stop running an ad but didn't tell the evaluation team. The evaluation team didn't check with the program staff to ensure that the ads were continuing to be aired as planned and continued to ask audience members, in subsequent waves of advertising awareness research, if they had seen the ad. Reported awareness of the ad dropped off, and the evaluation team concluded that the ad was ineffective. Fortunately, the mistake was discovered before the research report was widely disseminated.

The Lesson: Establish regular communication and coordination between the program management and evaluation teams.

What Evaluation Can Do

Program evaluation has two general purposes. First, it helps program managers to revise and improve their programs. Second, it helps them be accountable to stakeholders, demonstrate the value of the investment, and maintain or increase support and funding for program efforts. Your stakeholders range from state administrators, legislators, policy makers, and taxpayers, to tobacco control and public health decision makers, to your bosses and partners. Well-conducted evaluations can:

- Allow you to compare the program's effect among groups, particularly those most affected by tobacco's harms

- Demonstrate the role of effective counter-marketing campaigns in reducing tobacco use and exposure to second-hand smoke, thereby gaining credibility for the counter-marketing elements of the tobacco control program

- Guide administrative decisions about including counter-marketing efforts in comprehensive tobacco control programs

- Provide concrete results that can be shared with partners and the community

- Support replication, in your state or others, of counter-marketing strategies that work

- Advance the field by publishing results

If you've been working in public health for a while, evaluation won't be new to you. You evaluate your work all the time when you ask questions, consult partners, make assessments based on feedback, and then use those judgments to improve your work. Those informal processes may be sufficient for regular, ongoing assessment needs, but in a statewide tobacco counter-marketing program, the stakes are usually higher. Most tobacco counter-marketing programs affect many people and involve a good deal of time and money, so you'll need to use evaluation procedures that are more systematic, formal, visible, and justifiable.

When To Conduct an Evaluation

As noted earlier, evaluation is a continuous activity that needs to be planned along with overall program planning. Too often, evaluation is considered to be an "optional activity" rather than an integral component of counter-marketing that is included in program planning from the start.

In outcome evaluation, the timing of assessments and reports should be coordinated with the changes you expect to see in the target audience. For example, early in the campaign, you should expect changes in awareness and recall of your ads' messages. As the campaign matures, you would expect changes in attitudes and beliefs. Only after building awareness and seeing changes in underlying beliefs should you expect changes in intended behaviors and claimed behaviors. Behavior change, which is reflected by evidence such as reduction in smoking prevalence, is most likely to occur when counter-marketing is part of a more comprehensive tobacco control effort.

It's unrealistic to expect that counter-marketing efforts alone will lead to substantial changes in behavior related to tobacco use.

Some stakeholders will want the first wave of outcome evaluation results within six months of launching the program. In this case, your first wave of evaluation should concentrate on process measures and short-term and intermediate outcome measures (e.g., increases in calls to a quitline, improvements in advertising awareness, or changes in knowledge) rather than longer-term behavior changes.

Scope of the Evaluation

Every state should evaluate its counter-marketing activities as part of the overall evaluation of the tobacco control program. CDC recommends that 10 percent of a state's tobacco control funds be allocated to surveillance and evaluation (CDC 1999a). You'll need to decide the best way to allocate the funds and how rigorously to evaluate each activity.

At a minimum, good process evaluation of each counter-marketing activity will enable the program manager to monitor the scope and quality of activities and to determine whether the program is being conducted as planned. These results will help you consider the realities of conducting the program and make adjustments in its design.

Outcome evaluation is needed to determine whether your program is having the intended effects. The more rigorous an outcome evaluation is, the more expensive it is, and the more difficult it is to conduct. As a rule of thumb, you should conduct more rigorous evaluation under the following conditions:

- The program is costly, highly visible or controversial, or represents a new and untested approach.

- Sound methods for rigorous evaluation exist.

- Future funding depends on the program's success.

Because many of these characteristics apply to the counter-advertising campaign, you'll probably want to allocate a significant proportion of your evaluation resources to this component of your counter-marketing program. Counter-advertising campaigns are new to

---

Lesson Learned: Planning

The Mistake: One state didn't think about evaluation early enough and didn't do a baseline assessment before launching a paid media campaign. Consequently, the state will never know the results produced by the paid media campaign. Well-funded, paid media campaigns often produce substantial changes in awareness, attitudes, and beliefs shortly after they are run.

The Lesson: Start planning your evaluation when you start planning the program. Then you can conduct a baseline assessment before you begin to implement the program.

many states, and there is growing demand for more rigorous outcome evaluations.

The evaluation of the counter-marketing efforts should be coordinated with the evaluation of the whole tobacco control program. Counter-marketing activities are just one component of a complete tobacco control program, and evaluation can help to show whether all activities and components are working together effectively.

How To Conduct an Evaluation

To conduct a systematic evaluation of a tobacco counter-marketing program, you need to consider several steps. This detailed discussion of the steps follows the format developed by the CDC Evaluation Working Group (CDC 1999b).

Step 1: Identify stakeholders, and establish an evaluation team.

Like planning and implementation, evaluation can't be done in isolation. It involves partnerships. To identify the stakeholders, ask yourself: Who is the audience for the evaluation? What do they care about? The CDC Evaluation Working Group identified three overlapping groups that are integral to program evaluation (CDC 1999b):

- People involved in the campaign's operation, such as management, program staff, partners, the funding agency, and coalition members

Steps for Conducting an Evaluation

Step 1. Identify stakeholders, and establish an evaluation team.
Identify and involve those who will use or are affected by the evaluation.

Step 2. Describe your counter-marketing program.
Establish the need for an intervention, articulate your goals and objectives, and develop a program logic model.

Step 3. Focus the evaluation design.
Identify the purpose of the evaluation, develop and prioritize evaluation questions, and choose the evaluation study design.

Step 4. Gather credible evidence.
Develop outcome measures; identify indicators; select data-collection methods that are trustworthy, valid, and reliable; and collect the data.

Step 5. Justify conclusions.
Analyze and interpret the data, draw conclusions, and make recommendations.

Step 6. Ensure use of results and share lessons learned.
See that results are disseminated and used to inform decisions.

- People served by the campaign, such as advocacy groups and members of the target audience; elected officials; and any others who would be affected if the campaign were expanded, limited, or ended as a result of the evaluation

- The primary intended users of the evaluation or anyone in a position to make decisions about the counter-marketing efforts, such as health department decision makers, public health officials, and state legislators

In addition, if you're working with an ad agency, a public relations agency, or both, appropriate staff from these agencies should be involved in the evaluation planning.

Any serious effort to evaluate a program must consider the different values stakeholders have, ensure that their perspectives are understood, and try to respond to their unique information needs (Patton 1997). If stakeholders aren't appropriately involved, it's more likely that evaluation findings will be ignored, criticized, or resisted. If they are involved, they're likely to feel ownership and help you to gain allies who will defend the evaluation and its findings.

A Good Evaluator

To choose a good evaluator, consider whether the person:

- Has experience evaluating health promotion programs, with particular emphasis on tobacco control, marketing campaigns, or health communication programs

- Can provide references (Check all references carefully before you contract with an outside consultant.)

- Can walk you through some of his or her recent research projects, to demonstrate skill and experience

- Can work with a wide variety of people, from representatives of the target audience to high-level public officials

- Develops innovative approaches to evaluation while considering budget limitations and other realities

- Complements the in-house evaluation team and increases its evaluation capacity

- Shares all findings with the program staff regularly

- Demonstrates the ability to include cultural competency in the evaluation

You can involve stakeholders in the evaluation in various ways. The following approach has been adapted from the CDC Evaluation Working Group's *Framework for Program Evaluation in Public Health* (CDC 1999b).

1a: Establish an evaluation team.

An evaluation team should consist of the program manager, external stakeholders, and people with evaluation expertise. The program manager or someone on the counter-marketing staff should act as a liaison with the evaluation team and should be responsible for:

- Budgeting for the evaluation

- Developing and communicating program objectives and the logic model

- Managing evaluation contracts

- Coordinating evaluation activities between program staff and the evaluation team

- Incorporating evaluation findings into program planning and revision

Although the program manager should be able to understand and provide input on evaluation activities, he or she will need to find someone with the technical expertise to design and implement specific evaluation tasks.

If your health department has personnel with technical expertise, they can be part of the evaluation team, but you should also involve outside evaluation experts. Your counter-marketing program—especially the counter-advertising component—will be highly visible and possibly controversial, and the audience for the evaluation may not view the findings as credible unless they're generated and reported by outside experts. Stakeholders often see outside evaluators as being neutral and objective and without the vested interests of those inside the organization that is implementing the program. Technical expertise may be available through external partners (e.g., organizations, universities, companies, and tobacco control programs in other states) or through CDC and its Prevention Research Centers program. This national network of 24 academic research centers is committed to prevention research (CDC 2001). (Contact information is available at www.cdc.gov/prc.) States may consult with their CDC project officers for advice on finding the appropriate outside experts and working with them.

Step 2: Describe your counter-marketing program.

To effectively plan the evaluation, you'll need to have a clear description of your counter-marketing program. This description should include background information justifying the need for the program, appropriate program goals and objectives, and a logic model to help define what you hope to achieve and to guide the evaluation. Negotiating with stakeholders about a concise program description will help to gain their support and allow them to provide insights that might be useful for program planning (Patton 1997; CDC 2001).

If you followed the guidance in Chapter 2: Planning Your Counter-Marketing Program, this step will have already been completed. If you have not described your counter-marketing program, refer to the planning chapter, which offers more information on two of the program planning steps that are essential to planning an evaluation: articulating program goals and objectives and developing a logic model.

2a: Articulate program goals and objectives.

Before an evaluation can be effectively planned, you'll need to determine what your program needs to accomplish and what can be realistically accomplished within the budget and time frame. If your formative research has already been conducted, the findings can be helpful here. These results should have allowed you to identify the populations most in need and the behaviors and behavioral determinants that should be targeted for change. In addition, through pretesting of your messages and program approaches and your review of how similar approaches worked in other states, you should have gauged the amount of change to expect in your target audience.

Formative research results should be used to determine your program's goals and objectives. These goals and objectives are also critical to the evaluation, because they establish how you'll determine whether your program is being implemented as planned and how you'll measure your program's success.

A goal is the overall mission or purpose that helps to guide a program's development. In tobacco counter-marketing, as with all tobacco prevention and control components, the overall goal is to reduce tobacco-related morbidity and mortality. To fulfill this vision, CDC has identified four more specific goals, one or more of which will be relevant to your program (CDC 2001):

1. Prevent the initiation of tobacco use among young people.

2. Promote quitting among young people and adults.

3. Eliminate exposure to secondhand smoke.

4. Identify and eliminate the disparities related to tobacco use and its effects among different population groups.

Objectives are statements that describe the desired results. Tobacco control and prevention programs are complex and have multiple steps and effects. Select a limited set of objectives that will allow you to focus your evaluation on the most important results that are feasible to obtain. In addition, objectives should be conceptually linked, so that objectives at the local level are logical extensions of national and state objectives. The specific objectives outlined in *Healthy People 2010* are a good starting point for tobacco control efforts (U.S. Department of Health and Human Services 2000, available at http://www.health.gov/healthypeople/Document/HTML/Volume2/27Tobacco.htm).

Good objectives are specific and measurable (CDC 2001). Well-written and clearly defined objectives will help you to set your program priorities, aid you in monitoring progress, and serve as targets for accountability. Objectives should be SMART:

- **Specific.** The objective must identify a specific event or action that will take place.

- **Measurable.** The objective must identify the amount of change to be achieved, and there must be a way to measure the change.

- **Achievable.** The objective must be realistic and achievable.

- **Relevant.** The objective must be logical and relate to the program goal.

- **Time-bound.** The objective must provide a time by which the objective will be achieved.

One example of an objective is that, in a certain state, the proportion of restaurants with smokefree policies will increase from 40 percent to 60 percent by the end of 2005.

This objective is *specific* because it states that restaurants will have smokefree policies in place. It could be made more specific if it identified which types of restaurants and which types of smokefree policies. It's *measurable* because it identifies the current or baseline value and a level of change that is expected. It's *achievable* because it outlines a realistic amount of change, assuming a strong counter-marketing program focused on this objective. The degree to which it's achievable will depend on the context and realities within the state and the resources available. It's *relevant* because having smokefree policies will help to eliminate exposure to secondhand smoke. It's *time-bound* because a specified time frame is given.

There are two general types of objectives: process objectives and outcome objectives. Process objectives describe the scope and quality of the activities that will be implemented and the population and other entities (i.e., individuals and organizations) that will take part in these activities. A process evaluation examines how well you're achieving your process objectives or how well you're implementing your program, compared with the objectives in the original plan. If you're conducting a counter-advertising campaign in the spring to prevent initiation of smoking among youths, process objectives might be:

- By February 2003, pretest an ad countering a tobacco industry message with six focus groups of 12-to-17 year-olds.

- By March 2003, run the youth ad on TV so that 70 percent of the state's 12- to 17-year-olds are potentially exposed to the ad a minimum of three times on average per four-week period.

Outcome objectives describe the results you expect from the program. They quantify anticipated program effects by specifying "the amount of change expected for a given health problem/condition for a specified population within a given time frame" (University of Texas 1998; CDC 2001).

Outcome objectives are often divided into short-term, intermediate, and long-term outcomes (Green and Lewis 1986; Green and Kreuter 1999; Green and Ottoson 1999; CDC 2001). An example of a short-term outcome objective might be: Increase the proportion of high school youth with confirmed awareness of the youth ad campaign from 5 percent in January 2003 to 50 percent in June 2003.

An example of an intermediate outcome objective might be: Increase the proportion of high school youth who report they believe that the tobacco industry deliberately uses advertising to get young people to start smoking from 40 percent in January 2003 to 60 percent in December 2003.

Examples of long-term objectives might be:

- Decrease the proportion of high school youth who report smoking a cigarette in the past 30 days from 40 percent in 2001 to 30 percent in 2003.

- Decrease the prevalence of high school youth who report smoking five or more cigarettes a day from 25 percent in 2001 to 20 percent in 2003.

2b: Develop a logic model.

Developing a logic model of your counter-marketing program is a good way to fully explain how the program is supposed to work. (See Chapter 2: Planning Your Counter-Marketing Program for further information on developing a logic model.) A logic model is a flowchart of your program that shows the sequence of events in a chain of causation. Elements of a logic model can vary, but they generally include the following (United Way of America 1996):

- Inputs—what is invested in the program to support it

- Activities—the actual events or actions that take place

- Outputs—the immediate products of these activities

- Outcomes—the intended effects of the program, initial, intermediate, and long-term

Some examples of inputs, activities, outputs, and outcomes for various components of a counter-marketing program are shown in Appendix 5.1. The *inputs* are the monetary and human resources needed to do the work and the infrastructure required to support the program. These factors include funding, staff, technical assistance, partner organizations, contracts, equipment, materials, and a sound program design. The type of staff, amount of funding, and program design will often differ for each component of your program.

Activities are the actions the counter-marketing staff will take to carry out the program. Examples of such actions are identifying audiences, writing plans, creating and revising materials, contacting individuals and organizations, and organizing events. Program *outputs* (sometimes called process outcomes) are the immediate products of these activities; outputs include ads that are run, stories that are placed, events that are attended, and media literacy sessions that are conducted.

Figure 5.1: Logic Model for Youth Tobacco Use Prevention Advertising Campaign

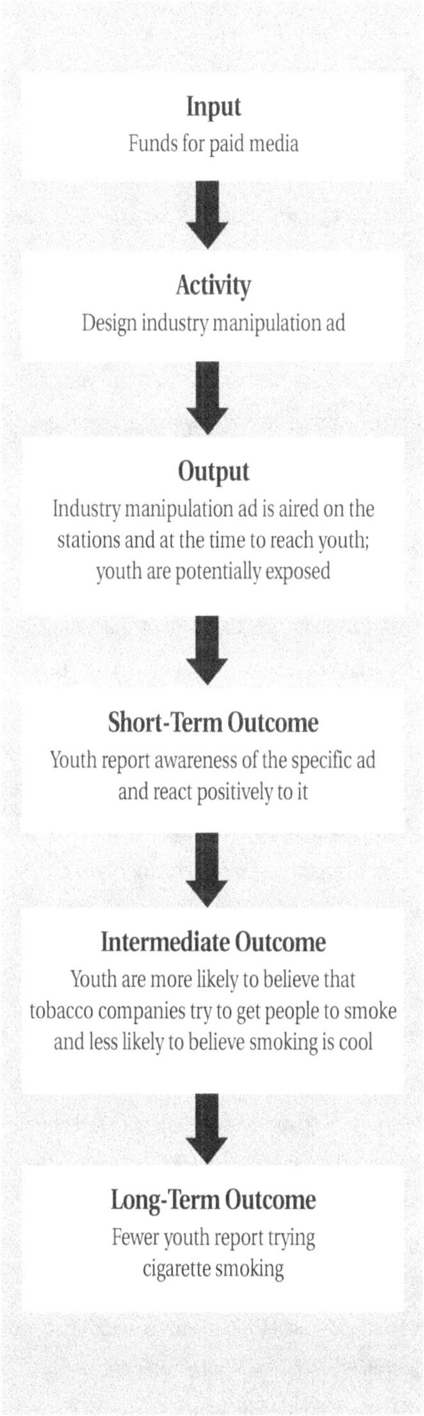

Input
Funds for paid media

⬇

Activity
Design industry manipulation ad

⬇

Output
Industry manipulation ad is aired on the stations and at the time to reach youth; youth are potentially exposed

⬇

Short-Term Outcome
Youth report awareness of the specific ad and react positively to it

⬇

Intermediate Outcome
Youth are more likely to believe that tobacco companies try to get people to smoke and less likely to believe smoking is cool

⬇

Long-Term Outcome
Fewer youth report trying cigarette smoking

Outcomes are the results you hope your efforts will achieve; they are divided into *short-term*, *intermediate*, and *long-term* (Campbell and Stanley 1963). More important than the label for the outcome, however, is the chain of causation linking one outcome logically to another. A logic model shows how you expect change to occur or how the immediate products of your activities will lead to short-term, then intermediate, then long-term outcomes.

As much as possible, the logic model should be tailored to your particular campaign, target audience, strategy for influencing behavior, and specific behavioral objective. Figure 5.1 shows an example of a logic model for a tobacco counter-advertising campaign designed to prevent youth from starting to smoke tobacco. The campaign points out that the tobacco companies try to influence young people to start smoking by convincing them that smoking is cool. Appendix 5.1 provides other examples of logic models for the components of a counter-marketing program.

Although the sample logic models list behavioral outcomes, behavior change typically results only through a combination of interventions. For example, a media literacy program would not be expected to result in a reduction in youth smoking unless other components of the counter-marketing program were also influencing these youth.

The elements of the logic model are linked in a series of if-then statements. If the ad is aired on the selected channels, then audience members who watch the channel can be aware of, comprehend, and react positively to the ad. If the audience is exposed to, aware of, and recalls the ad, then their attitudes, beliefs, and other psychosocial factors might change. (Psychosocial factors are characteristics such as attitudes, beliefs, perceived norms, and self-efficacy that, according to the major theories of behavior, are the determinants of people's behavior.) If changes in psychosocial factors occur, then one would expect changes in behavior.

This logic model is the model for one type of effort, a youth counter-advertising campaign. You could also develop a logic model for your entire counter-marketing program that shows how each component works individually and is coordinated into an integrated program. Another option is to develop a logic model for the entire state tobacco control program that shows how the various counter-marketing efforts work in combination with the other elements of the tobacco control program. Some good examples of logic models can be found in the CDC/OSH tobacco control evaluation manual, *Introduction to Program Evaluation for Comprehensive Tobacco Control Programs* (CDC 2001).

It's not uncommon for people to have different interpretations of the short-term, intermediate, and long-term outcomes for a particular program. What may be an intermediate outcome to some may be a long-term outcome to others. For example, one person may consider "quitting smoking" to be a long-term outcome for a particular smoking cessation program, while another may consider quitting smoking to be an intermediate outcome and "long-term abstinence from tobacco use" to be the long-term outcome. The logical sequence of short-term, intermediate, and long-term outcomes, based on your program's theoretical under-pinnings and the types of change that can be expected, is more important than the labels.

There are also different interpretations of how program outputs and short-term outcomes are articulated in program logic models. In a public relations effort, for example, one may consider the public relations activities of identifying and connecting with key journalists to be the program outputs and getting press coverage and audience exposure to be a short-term outcome. Others may consider the PR activities, news coverage, and audience exposure all as outputs and the target audience's actual awareness of the counter-marketing message as the short-term outcome. Here we use the latter interpretation across all counter-marketing programs, so that *program outputs* include multiple "products of activities" that allow the target audience to be exposed to counter-marketing messages and *short-term outcomes* include the target audience's increased awareness of these messages.

Step 3: Focus the evaluation design.

An evaluation can easily become too extensive and complex. In collaboration with stakeholders, the evaluation team will need to decide the evaluation's purpose and how results will be used. The evaluation plan should outline the questions you plan to answer, the process you'll follow, what will be measured, which methods will be used, who will perform various evaluation activities, what you will do with the information after it's collected, and how the results will be disseminated.

3a: Determine the purpose and questions for the evaluation.

You can help to focus the evaluation by determining the information you need and setting priorities for the evaluation questions used to get that information. Because the prioritized questions will guide the methods for gathering the information, decisions about the questions should be made *before* choosing the methods.

To prioritize the evaluation questions, the evaluation team should brainstorm with the stakeholders and intended users. You should use your process and outcome objectives to guide this discussion, so the objectives are linked to the questions you want the evaluation to answer.

Develop evaluation questions for each component of your counter-marketing campaign. One study won't effectively answer all your evaluation questions, so consider conducting several studies that will make up an evaluation portfolio. Put together a table that summarizes the objectives

Table 5.1: Sample Program Objectives and Corresponding Evaluation Questions

Objectives	Evaluation Questions
Advertising Component	
Process Objective By the end of 2003, an ad for a branded state counter-advertising campaign aimed at youth will have been aired on TV to reach 80 percent of 12- to 17-year-olds an average of six times per four-week period.	Did youth react positively to the ad in the campaign during the formative research? Based on the TV show ratings during which the ad was broadcast and its corresponding reach of the audience, were at least 80 percent of the 12- to 17-year-olds theoretically exposed to the ad at least six times? During which time periods was the ad aired?
Outcome Objective By the end of 2003, 60 percent of 12- to 17-year-olds will confirm their awareness of one or more of the TV ads in the state youth advertising campaign, and 50 percent will correctly recall the main message(s). Decrease the proportion of high school youth who report trying a cigarette from 40 percent in 2001 to 30 percent in 2003.	Among 12- to 17-year olds, were 60 percent or more aware of the ad? Were 50 percent or more able to recall the message? Were there differences in awareness and recall that were based on sex, age, or ethnic background of the youth? Did the proportion of high school youth who initiated cigarette smoking decrease from 40 percent to 30 percent? Were there differences in the decrease of initiation of cigarette smoking that were based on the sex, age, or ethnic background of youth? How does the change in youth initiation of cigarette smoking in the state compare with that in the nation? Can some of the change be confidently attributed to the advertising campaign?

Continues

Table 5.1: Sample Program Objectives and Corresponding Evaluation Questions (cont.)

Objectives	Evaluation Questions
Public Relations Component	
Process Objective By the end of 2003, representatives from the top 10 print and broadcast media outlets will have been reached with counter-marketing messages at least five times through phone, mail, and press conferences; five of these media outlets will have included these messages in their coverage and 50 percent of the target audience will have been exposed to the messages.	Were the required number of media representatives reached the designated number of times? Did the required number of media outlets cover the counter-marketing messages? How well were the messages covered (e.g., how much space and time for stories with protobacco slant and for stories with antitobacco slant)? Which outlets responded? How many target audience members were exposed to these messages?
Outcome Objective Increase the target audience's awareness of counter-marketing messages in media outlets by 25 percent from 2002 to 2003.	Did the target audience increase its awareness of counter-marketing messages by 25 percent?
Media Literacy Component	
Process Objective By December 2003, at least 1,000 middle school children will have been reached with media literacy sessions through programs offered in 10 schools and through 10 youth-serving organizations in the state.	Were media literacy sessions offered in the designated number of schools and organizations? Did these sessions reach the required number of children? What were the ages, gender, and race/ethnicity of the children reached?
Outcome Objective Increase by 50 percent the number of program participants who can competently deconstruct a tobacco industry ad and produce their own counter-marketing message.	As a result of the program, did participants increase their media literacy skills sufficiently to be able to deconstruct industry ads and develop tobacco counter-marketing messages?

and corresponding evaluation questions for each component (e.g., Table 5.1). This table will help you take the next step of determining the studies that should be in your portfolio.

3b: Select the evaluation design.

The evaluation design is the structure or plan for data collection that specifies which groups will be studied and when. The design you select influences the timing of data collection, how you analyze the data, and the types of conclusions you can draw from your findings.

Choosing the appropriate evaluation design is particularly important if you're planning an outcome evaluation. Outcome evaluation tests the effectiveness of an intervention, and the evaluation design's strength will affect your ability to attribute change to the intervention. Because you may be under considerable pressure to demonstrate the effectiveness of your program—especially the advertising component—your evaluation team needs to be familiar with various designs. This section touches briefly on various designs, but you may also need to consult other resources to help you make decisions about study design (Campbell and Stanley 1963; Spector 1981; Wimmer and Dominick 1987; Fletcher and Bowers 1988; Flay and Cook 2001; Rice and Atkins 2001; Hedrick et al. 1993; Hornik 1997; Rothman and Greenland 1998; Siegel and Doner 1998; Freimuth et al. 2001). Feasibility, scientific appropriateness, and costs must be considered in selecting a design, as well as your immediate and longer-term needs for data collection. You'll also need to know your stakeholders' standards, so you can choose a design that meets those standards.

Evaluation designs can be broadly divided into three types: experimental, quasi-experimental, and observational. As CDC (2001) notes, "*Experimental designs* use random assignment to compare the effect of an intervention in one or more groups with the effect in an otherwise equivalent group or groups that don't receive the intervention." For example, you could identify a set of schools willing to participate in an outcome evaluation of a media literacy curriculum. One-half of the schools could be randomly assigned to begin to use the curriculum immediately (test group) and one-half to use it after the study is completed (control group).

An experimental design is often unrealistic for a counter-advertising campaign, because exposure to the message is widespread and you can't control who gets it. Many times, people have ethical concerns with experimental designs, because interventions are at least temporarily withheld, during the time of the study, from those who need them. To determine whether you need an experimental design for an outcome evaluation of your counter-marketing program, consult an expert and consider issues such as scientific appropriateness and costs.

Many program managers find a *quasi-experimental design* easier to use than an experimental design, but a quasi-experimental design is not as scientifically strong. CDC (2001) comments that "this design makes comparisons between nonequivalent groups and doesn't involve random assignment to intervention or control groups." A simple example of a quasi-experimental design would be measuring the attitudes, beliefs, and behaviors of two communities, one of which chose to conduct a counter-marketing campaign and the other had no intervention. The community with no intervention would be selected for its similarity to the first community.

According to CDC (2001), "*Observational designs* include, but are not limited to, time-series analysis, cross-sectional surveys, and case studies." *Case studies* are generally descriptive and exploratory. If your program or your application is unique or you're working in an unpredictable environment, you might want to consider a case study. Case studies are often used to evaluate media advocacy projects, to provide an in-depth examination of how media coverage on a particular topic was framed and how community advocates were involved in the media advocacy initiatives (Wallack et al. 1999). *Cross-sectional surveys*, such as the Youth Tobacco Survey (YTS) and surveys performed using a time-series analysis, can be conducted with a target audience to help determine whether the desired outcomes of your counter-marketing program (e.g., reduced tobacco use) have been achieved. Cross-sectional surveys are administered to independent samples of the target population. For a *time-series analysis*, the target population is surveyed a number of times both before and during program implementation. Although this type of analysis can require considerable resources and time, the more times the target population can be surveyed and the more closely the timing of the survey can mirror the timing of your intervention (e.g., through ads in a paid media campaign) the more confident you can be that the changes in program outcomes are to some extent attributable to the program.

Step 4: Gather credible evidence.

So far, you've written measurable objectives, developed a logic model, selected the types of evaluation and the evaluation questions, and determined the study design(s) you'll use. The next step is to decide on specific outcomes to address and identify the indicators you'll use to measure progress. Once these are in place, you'll be ready to figure out which sources of data and data collection methods should be used to obtain the information you need.

4a: Develop outcomes and identify indicators.

By now, you should have decided what kind of outcome evaluation you'll conduct and which components of the counter-marketing program will be addressed in the evaluation. Make sure that the outcomes you choose reflect the evaluation's purpose(s), audience(s), and the intended uses of the results and that they're relevant to the component(s) you're studying. If your ad campaign has been running for an extended period and the legislators want to know whether youth smoking has decreased and the campaign is worthy of continued funding, then behavioral outcomes should be the evaluation's primary focus.

After you've selected the outcomes, determine which indicators you can use to show whether you've achieved these outcomes. *Indicators* are specific, observable, and measurable characteristics or changes that show the progress a program is making toward achieving a specified outcome (Campbell and Stanley 1963; CDC 1999b; CDC 2001). Indicators translate general concepts related to the program, its content, and its expected effects into specific measures that can be interpreted. For example, the percentage of high school youth who report that they've tried smoking a cigarette, even a puff or two, is an indicator that can be used to measure the long-term outcome of efforts to decrease smoking among youth. Also, the percentage of high school youth who report that tobacco companies deliberately use advertising to get them to start smoking is an indicator of the short-term outcome of efforts to increase negative beliefs about the tobacco industry.

Each outcome should have at least one indicator, and each indicator should measure an important dimension of the outcome. You must be specific about what each indicator will measure. Indicators define the criteria you'll use to judge your progress in achieving the desired outcomes. You can assess behavior in several ways. Identifying the best indicator depends on the type of behavioral outcome you're addressing. Indicators that may be useful for monitoring long-term trends in smoking prevalence (e.g., "whether a person smoked 100 cigarettes in his or her lifetime") will yield a different estimate of behavior than indicators that are appropriate for evaluating the impact of a counter-advertising campaign on a population (e.g., "on how many of the past 30 days a person smoked").

4b: Collect data.

Next, you'll need to decide which methods to use to gather data about your outcomes and indicators. Each method has advantages and disadvantages. Some methods are appropriate for process evaluation; others are appropriate for outcome evaluation. A number of common data-collection tools and methods are used for process evaluation, outcome evaluation, or both. (See Appendix 5.2: Key Data Collection Tools and Methods.)

Try to use methods that your stakeholders perceive as credible. Some stakeholders may want you to use an interview method to gather qualitative feedback from the community; others may want you to conduct an extensive population-based survey. Be prepared to explain the value of more rigorous methods to stakeholders less familiar with evaluation.

Consider conducting a custom survey.

Surveys are likely to be part of every counter-marketing evaluation. They can be roughly divided into two types: (1) primary data surveys (custom surveys), which are designed for your specific needs, and (2) secondary data surveys, which must be used as they are, because they have been developed by other individuals or organizations for particular purposes.

Primary data surveys. In most states, some form of primary data collection will be needed to evaluate the specific outcomes of the counter-marketing efforts, particularly the advertising component. Although surveys for collection of primary data can be expensive, they have many advantages. These surveys can be customized with specific items, sampling plans, and timing of administration to fit your counter-marketing campaign. You can track awareness of your specific ads and themes, the attitudes and beliefs relevant to your campaign, and behaviors in your target population. These data can be used to help you make decisions about how to improve and when to change the campaign. Many states have used custom surveys to demonstrate the effectiveness of their counter-advertising efforts.

Depending on your resources, you should consider custom surveys for each of the large components of your counter-marketing program. Alternatively, one way to integrate the outcome evaluation of several components is by conducting a customized survey to assess the full range of audience outcomes for all components of your counter-marketing (advertising, news articles and stories, grassroots events, media literacy, and media advocacy). This approach may appear to be more efficient, but it may not yield the same quality of data that could be generated from conducting an individual survey on each component.

In most cases, you should contract with an outside expert to design a customized survey for use in collecting these primary data. For assistance in finding and working with an appropriate contractor, states may consult with their CDC project officers. A good way to start work on a survey is to discuss with your evaluation expert questions associated with design, sampling and sample size, measurement, and data collection and analysis. (See Table 5.2 for sample questions.) Your survey probably will measure variables such as the target audience's awareness and recall of the counter-marketing messages and the attitudes, beliefs, intentions, and behaviors related to tobacco use. (See Appendix 5.3 for sample survey items.) Another resource is primary surveys that have been developed to evaluate other state counter-marketing campaigns.

Some research methods require Institutional Review Board (IRB) approval. Nearly all government agencies, academic institutions, and other organizations require an assessment of the impact on human subjects involved in qualitative and quantitative research, including the protection of collected data. Some data-collection efforts are exempt from IRB approval. For each research project undertaken, it is recommended that you consult the IRB expert in your organization.

Secondary data surveys and data collection systems. All states have access to secondary data, particularly on behavior. Several secondary data sets are described in CDC's *Surveillance and Evaluation Data Resources for Comprehensive Tobacco Control Programs* (Yee and Schooley 2001). These sources may include data that can be disaggregated at your state's level. Sources include the following:

- Adult Tobacco Survey
- Behavioral Risk Factor Surveillance System
- Current Population Survey Tobacco Use Supplements
- Monitoring the Future

Table 5.2: Questions To Ask in Designing a Survey To Evaluate Counter-Marketing Efforts

Design: How should I structure the study?

- How should I establish control or comparison points against which I can assess impact?
- When and how many times do I want to survey people?
- Should I survey the same or different people each time?

Sampling: Whom should I study, and how should I select the study participants?

- Whom should I survey?
- What sampling plan should I use?
- How many people should I survey?
- How large a sample do I need to make the comparisons I want to make with sufficient statistical power?

Measurement: What questions should I ask, and how should I ask them?

- What variables do I need to measure?
- How many items do I need for each variable?
- How do I ensure that my measures are reliable and valid?
- Do I create my own items, or can I use someone else's items?

Data collection: How should I collect the data?

- Should I collect custom data or use existing data?
- How should I administer my survey?
- How can I ensure a high response rate?
- What data do I need in addition to survey data?

Analysis: How should I analyze the data to answer the evaluation questions?

- Which descriptive statistics should I use to help describe and summarize the data (e.g., frequency data, raw numbers, and percentages)?
- Which inferential statistics should I use to allow generalization from my sample to a wider population and to enable me to test hypotheses that the data are consistent with research predictions?
- What analyses can I conduct to determine whether the program is effective?

- National Health Interview Survey
- National Household Survey on Drug Abuse
- Pregnancy Risk Assessment Monitoring System
- State Tobacco Activities Tracking and Evaluation System
- Youth Risk Behavior Surveillance System
- Youth Tobacco Survey

Although these secondary sources are unlikely to be ideal for evaluating your counter-marketing program, they can provide important information on trends, especially for attitudes, intentions, and behaviors. In many states, current studies can be modified to make them more relevant to the counter-marketing component. It might be possible to add items or modules, modify the sampling plan, increase the sample size of some segments, or adjust the timing. Alternatively, you could time the launch of your program to fit the timing of the routine collection of data.

Early in the planning of your evaluation, review what secondary sources are available in your state and see if they would improve your evaluation. For example, many states conduct the Youth Risk Behavior Survey (YRBS), a school-based survey of youth risk behaviors. The instrument includes several items on smoking behavior that can be used to track long-term trends and provide state-level estimates of students in grades 9 through 12. National data are available for comparison, and data from nearby states also might be available. Disadvantages of these data are that they are collected only every two years, in the spring, and that the instrument assesses only behavior. The YRBS could be and has been enhanced in many states by adding questions. Vermont, for example, has added items that help (1) to measure how easy it is for youth to get cigarettes and (2) to assess youths' opinions of their parents' attitudes toward their own cigarette use. Alabama has added an item that helps to determine whether a youth's health care provider addresses tobacco use prevention. For some states, the YRBS might prove to be a useful data source to include in portfolios.

Step 5: Justify conclusions.

Once the data are gathered, you'll need to analyze and interpret the data and formulate conclusions and recommendations. Your analysis and interpretation should be related to the evaluation questions. Essentially, analysis and interpretation are a matter of tracking what happens along each step of the logic model. (See Table 5.3 for the key evaluation questions in tobacco counter-marketing and examples of data analysis approaches for each question.)

Table 5.3: Evaluation Analysis

Evaluation Questions	Data Analysis Approach
Process Evaluation: Is the state's counter-marketing program being implemented as planned?	
Are the program activities being conducted at the planned level (quantity and quality)?	• Summary of data on the number and quality of media literacy sessions conducted
Are members of the target population exposed to the ad and participating in the program?	• Summary of ratings of TV shows during which paid counter-advertisements were aired • Summary of data on the number of participants in a youth summit
Short-Term Outcome Evaluation: Is the state's counter-marketing program having the intended effects?	
Who is aware of the ad? Who is aware of the program? Are all segments of the target population aware of the ad? Are all segments aware of the program?	• Collecting data on the percentage of the state's adult voters who recalled seeing a story or article about tobacco in a newspaper or magazine in the past month • Obtaining data on the percentage of 12- to 17-year-olds who reported seeing one of the state's counter-marketing ads in the past month • Acquiring data on the level of awareness of the campaign's brand among youth by gender, age, race/ethnicity, and community • Collecting data on the percentage of restaurant owners who reported knowing about the state's policies on secondhand smoke
Is the right message getting across?	• Obtaining data on the percentage of participants who were aware of the advertising campaign and could correctly recall the intended message • Acquiring data on the percentage of the articles on the counter-marketing theme that conveyed the intended message
How is the target population's awareness of the program changing over time? How is it changing in relation to specific counter-marketing efforts?	• Tracking data at several points over time to indicate (1) the percentage of the state's population that is aware of the counter-advertising campaign; (2) whether the percentage is higher immediately after the counter-marketing efforts; and (3) when the percentage starts to decrease, suggesting that the effects of the state's ads have peaked or that the state has reduced its media buying

Continues

Table 5.3: Evaluation Analysis (cont.)

Evaluation Questions	Data Analysis Approach
Short-Term Outcome Evaluation: Is the state's counter-marketing program having the intended effects?	
Are attitudes, beliefs, and other psychosocial factors moving in the desired direction?	• Pretest and posttest tracking of data (1) on restaurant owners' belief that secondhand smoke is harmful to health and (2) on the public's attitudes toward policies on exposure to secondhand smoke
Is behavior changing?	• Tracking data at several points over time that indicate the percentage of high school students who reported trying a cigarette or using chewing tobacco • Tracking data at several points over time that indicate the percentage of smokers who reported trying to quit smoking
Are the counter-marketing efforts contributing to the changes in attitudes, beliefs, policies, and behavior?	• Collecting data to address whether change can be attributed to the intervention: (1) the percentage of participants who believe in negative health consequences of smoking, among those who are aware of the state's ads on health consequences versus those who are not aware and (2) the percentage who understand the tactics of tobacco advertising, among those who participated in the media literacy workshop versus those who did not participate • Monitoring data on tobacco-related policies to document their stage of development, implementation, and enforcement, and comparing the timing of these stages with the timing of activities in the tobacco counter-marketing campaign
Long-Term Outcome Evaluation: Is the state counter-marketing program achieving its long-term goals?	
As part of the state's entire tobacco control program, do the state surveillance data indicate progress toward goal(s)?	• Monitoring surveillance data on the prevalence of smoking or public exposure to secondhand smoke and comparing these data with data from the tobacco control program (customized survey)

Descriptive Analyses

Analysis and interpretation of your process evaluation data will be descriptive. The data will consist of raw numbers and percentages (e.g., frequency data) that simply describe the level of activities and outputs that have taken place. As a manager, you'll want to review monthly reports on each component, to ensure that the activities are being implemented as planned. Relevant questions include the following:

- Is the public relations specialist conducting all the planned press activities?

- Have quitline operators been trained appropriately?
- Are all the media literacy sessions being held?
- Have the ads been designed, tested, and produced?
- Is the state on target in its media buying?

If the expected level of activity isn't being achieved, you need to determine what needs to be done to ensure that the necessary resources and support are available.

As another descriptive analysis, you'll want to determine whether the program is reaching enough people. Are audience members aware of the advertising campaign? Are enough articles and editorials being published? Look at the quality of the reach as well as the quantity. You'll need to know not only the column inches and placement of the ad coverage, but also its content and slant. (See Chapter 7: Advertising and Chapter 8: Public Relations for more information.) If the intended message isn't getting across, you may need to modify your materials or your approach.

Although this type of tracking of the campaign's reach is more a matter of management than evaluation, it's a critical step. If the outcomes of intervention are not ultimately achieved, it may be simply because the intervention was not implemented as planned. The regular review of these descriptive data will help you to monitor your implementation efforts.

Comparative Analyses. Beyond descriptive analyses, you'll also want to perform comparative analyses to determine whether your program is successful. In conducting comparative analyses, you'll need to use inferential statistics to determine whether the differences you observe are great enough to be statistically significant. Consider at least four types of comparisons: over segments of your target population, over time, over regions, and over levels of awareness of the counter-marketing effort.

Analyses by segments. Comparisons of levels of awareness, attitudes, beliefs, and behaviors by segments of your target population will tell you whether you're reaching a substantial proportion of each segment and how your efforts are influencing each segment. Consider analyzing the data by gender, age, and race/ethnicity. Counter-advertising programs with youth, for example, sometimes have been found to be more effective with those younger than 16 than with those 16 or older. Early analyses by race/ethnicity demonstrated to some states that they weren't influencing some segments of their target population. The media buys, media outlets, and messages needed to be adjusted.

Analyses by time. Comparisons over time will show you how the awareness, reach, and effect of your program are increasing with time, the level of your program activities, or both. Some variables should change gradually, and others should change abruptly. For example, the proportion of the population that is smoking or the percentage of youth that has tried a cigarette should decline gradually and smoothly. This result is most likely when, at the onset of the program, there is a large pool of "susceptibles" made up of individuals who have not been reached by similar interventions. Levels of exposure to the activities of your counter-marketing campaign increase as the program gradually scales up. After you run articles and ads about industry manipulation in your state, there should be sudden increases in awareness of the ads and a subsequent increase in the belief that the industry is trying to influence consumers to buy cigarettes. Examine the pattern of results with respect to time and the timing of your program activities. After the most receptive members of the population have been influenced by program messages, leaving the more resistant ones, results will show a slowdown in measurable improvement.

Analyses by region. You can also examine the pattern of awareness, beliefs, attitudes, and behaviors by region. If the different regions of your state have different amounts of program activity, this difference should show up in the findings. In Texas, for example, counter-marketing managers purposely implemented different patterns of programs in different communities, to evaluate the programs' effects. In 14 areas across the state, they implemented a mix of three levels of media activity (no campaign, low-level campaign, or high-level campaign) and five community program options (no programs, cessation programs, law enforcement programs, school-community programs, or all three programs combined). Their evaluation found a significant relative reduction in the prevalence of daily smoking in the areas where a high-level media campaign was conducted in combination with either school-community or multiple programs (Texas Tobacco Prevention Initiative 2001).

Analyses by level of awareness of the counter-marketing effort. A common approach for analysis to evaluate counter-marketing efforts, particularly counter-advertising, is to compare attitudes, beliefs, and behaviors in different groups by level of awareness of advertising. Such analysis can help you determine whether there have been more positive changes in attitudes, beliefs, and behaviors among those who are aware of the program than among those who aren't aware.

Attribution in Outcome Evaluation

Finding change is not conclusive evidence that the change is attributable to the effectiveness of your program. To demonstrate that a program is effective, you need data that show (1) a change or difference, and (2) that your program was to some extent responsible for that change or difference.

The first part is relatively simple. By conducting surveys before and after your programs, you can show increases in awareness and desirable changes in attitudes, beliefs, and behaviors over time. By comparing levels of attitudes, beliefs, and behaviors across levels of exposure to a program, you can show that people exposed to the program have better outcomes. By comparing people in regions where programs were implemented to those in regions where they weren't implemented, you can show better attitudes, beliefs, and behaviors in areas with the programs.

The second part is difficult. Methodologically sophisticated stakeholders can and do criticize each of the analyses described and claim the changes or differences observed could have resulted from factors *other than* the counter-marketing program. Critics can correctly claim that the differences or changes result from factors such as general trends in smoking, policy and pricing changes in the state, national media campaigns, or changes in the activities of the tobacco industry.

As noted earlier, it's usually not feasible to use a true experimental design with random assignment to evaluate your counter-advertising component, because it's difficult to control who is exposed to what. But there are some things you can do to avoid criticism of the evaluation. From a process perspective, you can:

- Find out early if your stakeholders want a rigorous assessment of the degree to which the counter-marketing program was responsible for changes or differences
- Allocate additional resources for that assessment
- Alert your evaluation experts, and discuss the alternative methods with them
- Find out what other states have done
- Arm yourself with high-quality studies from a variety of sources showing that strong counter-marketing efforts generally can lead to better outcomes
- Be prepared to answer questions about attribution when you present your results

From a technical or analytic perspective, your evaluation team can:

- **Conduct several types of analyses to demonstrate change.** For example, (1) show change from time A to time B; (2) show better outcomes among people who are exposed to counter-marketing activities than among those who aren't exposed; and (3) compare results for your state with those for areas of the country that have fewer or different counter-marketing programs.

- **Perform complex multivariate analyses.** For example, you can determine the effects of multiple independent variables (e.g., timing of the ads and changes in awareness, attitudes, and beliefs) on the dependent variable (e.g., change in smoking behavior), controlling for the effects of other variables (e.g., gender, age, and race/ethnicity).

- **Measure attitudes, beliefs, and behaviors that you expect to be influenced by your program, as well as those that you do not expect to be changed.** Then show that the differences for the items specific to your program are greater than the differences for the other items.

- **Conduct a longitudinal study that follows a cohort across time in order to show the causal chain of effects.** This approach allows you to conduct more complex analyses to determine whether the degree of program exposure is associated with changes in attitudes and beliefs, and whether the changes in attitudes and beliefs are associated with changes in behavior.

- **Perform a quasi-experimental study to assess the impact of different program components that have been implemented in different communities in your state.** This approach can help you determine how much different program components have changed attitudes, beliefs, and behaviors.

Step 6: Ensure use of results and share lessons learned.

The main purpose of your evaluation is to produce findings that will help to inform your decision making and help you to be accountable to stakeholders. Despite the potential usefulness of an evaluation, however, its findings, conclusions, and recommendations don't automatically translate into informed decision making and appropriate action. You must have a plan for making sure that the evaluation results are disseminated in a timely and understandable fashion and that they are used to improve programs and to help ensure support and funding for future programs. Each of the steps in the evaluation process must be executed in a way that ensures use.

6a: Develop a clear and focused evaluation plan.

The first step in using results is to have a clear evaluation plan that links the program objectives, the evaluation questions, and the methods. Linking the data source to the question not only helps you to keep your data collection pared down to the essentials, it also keeps you aware of the data's value in decision making.

6b: Consider the implications of different results.

In collaboration with your stakeholders, consider the decisions that would be made on the bases of specific patterns of results. During different stages of evaluation planning, pose various hypothetical results and discuss their implications for modifying the program. If no action would be taken, you might need to rethink the proposed evaluation plan to make sure you're asking the right questions. Consideration of the possible results also allows stakeholders to explore the positive and negative implications of those results and gives them time to develop options.

6c: Communicate with stakeholders during each step of the evaluation process.

Let all interested parties know how the evaluation is going. Involve them in the evaluation planning, in an effort to manage their expectations about what questions the evaluation will answer and when. Keep them informed, and hold periodic discussions about interim results, early interpretations, draft reports, and the final report.

6d: Follow up with stakeholders to ensure that results are used in decision making.

Efforts to make sure that results are used don't end with a final report that reaches conclusions and makes recommendations. Follow-up by the evaluation team is needed to remind stakeholders of the intended uses for the results and to help prevent results from being lost or ignored when complex, politically sensitive decisions are being made.

Tips for an Effective Evaluation Report

- Include an executive summary.
- Describe the stakeholders and how they were involved.
- Describe the essential features of the program, including the logic model.
- Outline the key evaluation questions.
- Include a description of the methods.
- List methodological strengths and weaknesses. No study is perfect; don't pretend yours has no flaws.
- Present results and conclusions.
- Put results into context. (Help readers to understand what is reasonable at this point and how the results should be interpreted.)
- Translate findings into recommendations.
- Organize the report logically.
- Minimize technical jargon.
- Provide detailed information in appendices.
- Use examples, illustrations, graphics, and stories.
- Involve stakeholders in preparation of the report.
- Consider how the findings might affect others.
- Develop additional communication products suited to a variety of audiences, for sharing the results.

6e: Use a variety of channels and approaches in disseminating results.

Dissemination is a form of communication. As with any communication, you should consider the target audience and purpose when deciding how to disseminate the results. Some people connect with numbers, some with text, some with graphs and pictures, and some with stories.

You should also think about the timing of the release of your results:

- Who should receive results first?
- When should the media be notified?
- How often should each set of stakeholders receive results?
- Who should release results to which audiences?

In addition, consider the potential criticisms that your results may receive. You may present a certain percentage decline in tobacco use as a success, but others may see that same decline as a failure. You should prepare responses to any potential criticisms you foresee and train your spokespeople to respond to attacks on your campaign. Stakeholders can be especially valuable in defending your results. For more information on preparing for and responding to media inquiries, see Chapter 9: Media Advocacy and Chapter 8: Public Relations.

A formal evaluation report shouldn't be the only product you disseminate. Work with various stakeholders to develop other products and to make sure the products' timing, style, tone, message, and format are appropriate for their audience(s). For example:

- Consider providing a briefing sheet that public health officials can use in presentations to state legislatures.
- Work with the public relations staff to develop materials for the news media.
- Consider a press conference to release results.
- Hold a community forum.
- Provide materials with more details, containing statistics and other data for technical audiences.
- Arrange to summarize key findings or complete reports and instruments on Web sites.
- Make your findings, reports, and materials available to other states and other people involved in tobacco control and prevention.

These ideas can help to ensure that your evaluation efforts don't go to waste. Again, your evaluation is useless if the results aren't understood and used to make decisions about the program.

Points To Remember

- Consider evaluation early and often. Evaluation shouldn't be left until the end of the program. Considering evaluation while the program is being planned helps to ensure that the plan is specific and clear about what the program is trying to achieve. Developing a logic model that links inputs to activities to outputs and, finally, to outcomes forces planners to articulate their assumptions about how the program will work. These assumptions can be reviewed to determine whether they're consistent with available evidence. Considering evaluation before you begin to implement your program also helps to ensure that baseline data are collected.

    Although you may be pressured to roll out your program quickly, if you don't collect baseline data, you'll never be able to clearly measure the changes caused by your intervention. Regular monitoring of activities and outputs helps the counter-marketing manager to troubleshoot and make adjustments in the program. Assessing short-term outcomes helps in modifying the program, and assessing long-term outcomes is necessary for accountability and to ensure continued funding for the program.

- Build an effective evaluation team. The evaluation team should include counter-marketing staff, evaluation expertise, and stakeholder input. At the state level, the program manager should be responsible for putting the team together. Make sure the team has sufficient expertise in technical evaluation and that it includes an external evaluator who is perceived by stakeholders as objective and capable. Many states have found it helpful to have a mix of experts from different backgrounds, such as a market researcher from the corporate sector, a public health epidemiologist, and a university-based communication researcher. Stakeholders are important to program evaluation, because their support of the process, results, and recommendations will help to ensure that the evaluation is accepted and used. Without stakeholder involvement, the evaluation may lack credibility, and the findings may be ignored.

- Develop and follow an evaluation plan that is appropriate to your state in terms of context, timing, cost, and rigor. In evaluation, one size doesn't fit all. There's no one best evaluation plan. Different states will face different marketing challenges, will have different resources, and will be working in a different context. The evaluation plan should reflect these factors. As a general rule, you should allocate 10 percent of your resources to evaluation. Evaluate as rigorously as your resources allow, and be sure to use more rigorous evaluation methods when the programs are more costly, visible, or controversial.

- Make sure findings are shared and used. Evaluation that ends as a report sitting on a shelf is wasted. Evaluation findings must be shared in such a way that they inform program decisions. Ensuring the use of results begins in the early stages of planning, as you ask what the program's objectives are, what questions need to be answered, and how the results will affect decisions. The evaluation report is a communication, so it must be appropriate for the audience.

- Build on what others have learned. In conducting outcome evaluation for your counter-marketing program, you may encounter a number of challenges. Fortunately, you're not alone. Others, such as CDC, the American Legacy Foundation, and other states, have faced the same issues and have begun to develop solutions. Talk to others, read the literature and reports, and share your experiences.

- Consult other CDC resources. This chapter provides a brief overview of what you should consider in evaluating a counter-marketing program. Consider reviewing other CDC resources and consulting your CDC project officer for specific advice. Seeking these resources and specific advice is especially important if you're conducting an outcome evaluation of a paid media campaign.

Bibliography

Campbell DT, Stanley JC. *Experimental and Quasi-Experimental Design for Research*. Boston: Houghton Mifflin, 1963.

Centers for Disease Control and Prevention. *Best Practices for Comprehensive Tobacco Control Programs—August 1999*. Atlanta, GA: CDC, National Center for Chronic Disease Prevention and Health Promotion, Office on Smoking and Health, 1999a.

Centers for Disease Control and Prevention. Framework for program evaluation in public health. *Morbidity and Mortality Weekly Report* 1999b; 48(RR-11):1–40.

Centers for Disease Control and Prevention. *Introduction to Program Evaluation for Comprehensive Tobacco Control Programs*. Atlanta, GA: CDC, 2001.

Flay BR, Cook TD. Three models of summative evaluation of prevention campaigns with a mass media component. In: Rice RE, Atkins CK, editors. *Public Communication Campaigns*, 3rd ed. (pp. 175–95). Newbury Park, CA: Sage Publications, 2001.

Fletcher AD, Bowers TA. *Fundamentals of Advertising Research*, 3rd ed. Belmont, CA: Wadsworth Publishing Co., 1988.

Freimuth V, Cole G, Kirby S. Issues in evaluating mass-media health communication campaigns. In: Rootman I *Evaluation in Health Promotion: Principles and Perspectives* (pp. 475–92), WHO Regional Publications. European Series No. 92. Copenhagen, Denmark: WHO Regional Office for Europe, 2001.

Green LW, Kreuter MW. *Health Promotion Planning: An Educational and Ecological Approach*, 3rd ed. Mountain View, CA: Mayfield Publishing Co., 1999.

Green LW, Lewis FM. *Measurement and Evaluation in Health Education and Health Promotion*. Palo Alto, CA: Mayfield Publishing Co., 1986.

Green LW, Ottoson JM. *Community and Population Health*, 8th ed. Boston, MA: WCB/McGraw-Hill, 1999.

Hedrick TE, Bickman L, Rog DJ. *Applied Research Design: A Practical Guide*. Newbury Park, CA: Sage Publications, 1993.

Hornik R. Public health education and communication as policy instruments for bringing about changes in behavior. In: Goldberg ME, Fishbein M, Middlestadt SE, editors. *Social Marketing: Theoretical and Practical Perspectives* (pp. 45–58). Mahwah, NJ: Lawrence Erlbaum Associates, 1997.

Joint Committee on Standards for Educational Evaluation. *The Program Evaluation Standards: How to Assess Evaluations of Educational Programs*, 2nd ed. Thousand Oaks, CA: Sage Publications, 1994.

Patton MQ. *Utilization-Focused Evaluation: The New Century Text*, 3rd ed. Thousand Oaks, CA: Sage Publications, 1997.

Rice RE, Atkins CK, editors. *Public Communication Campaigns*, 3rd ed. Newbury Park, CA: Sage Publications, 2001.

Rothman KJ, Greenland S. *Modern Epidemiology.* Philadelphia, PA: Lippincott-Raven Publishers, 1998.

Siegel M, Doner L. *Marketing Public Health: Strategies to Promote Social Change.* Gaithersburg, MD: Aspen Publishers, 1998.

Spector PE. *Research Designs.* Newbury Park, CA: Sage Publications, 1981.

Texas Tobacco Prevention Initiative. *Media Campaign and Community Program Effects Among Children and Adults* (2001, January). Available at http://www.tdh.state.tx.us/otpc/pilot/reports/uthsc/Rep2.pdf. Retrieved June 11, 2003.

United Way of America. *Measuring Program Outcomes: A Practical Approach.* Alexandria, VA: United Way of America, 1996.

U.S. Department of Health and Human Services. *Healthy People 2010: Understanding and Improving Health.* 2nd ed. Washington, DC: U.S. Government Printing Office, November 2000.

University of Texas Houston Health Sciences Center School of Public Health and the Texas Health Department. *Practical Evaluation of Public Health Programs.* Atlanta, GA: Centers for Disease Control and Prevention, 1998. Available at: http://www.cdc.gov/pphtn/Pract-Eval/workbook.htm. Accessed September 24, 2002.

Wallack L, Woodruff K, Dorfman L, et al. *News for a Change: An Advocate's Guide to Working With the Media.* Thousand Oaks, CA: Sage Publications, 1999.

Wimmer R, Dominick J. *Mass Media Research: An Introduction*, 2nd ed. Belmont, CA: Wadsworth Publishing Co., 1987.

Yee SL, Schooley, M. *Surveillance and Evaluation Data Resources for Comprehensive Tobacco Control Programs.* Atlanta, GA: Centers for Disease Control and Prevention, 2001.

Chapter 6

Managing and Implementing Your Counter-Marketing Program

I won't kid you; pulling all the pieces together is hard work. But it works. And when you look back and realize your efforts have impacted not only individual behavior but the culture as a whole, you'll know it was worth the effort.

— Colleen Stevens, Tobacco Control Section,
California Department of Health Services

In This Chapter

- Setting Up Your Counter-Marketing Team
- Selecting Contractors
- Developing an Annual Marketing Plan
- Reviewing Marketing Materials
- Monitoring the Counter-Marketing Budget

To have a successful counter-marketing program, you'll need to have the right team and set up the right processes to implement your program and keep it on track. Whether your budget is $100,000, $25 million, or anything in between, the steps are the same. Each step is described in detail in this chapter.

Setting Up Your Counter-Marketing Team

Finding the appropriate mix of people and expertise may be the most important thing you do. To implement your program, you'll need to establish four groups:

1. **Health department staff** to develop and monitor activities

2. **Communication agencies, communication specialists, or both,** to develop and place ads, create public relations campaigns, plan events, and conduct other activities

3. **An evaluation firm or staff** to monitor and measure the results of your efforts

4. **Community stakeholders,** whose support is critical, to provide input on various elements of the program

Health Department Staff

Staffing will vary depending on your budget and timeline, but *you need at least one person dedicated to counter-marketing activities.* Even with a small budget, you must have a skilled person to work with the news media, develop and distribute materials, and plan tobacco control events with community groups.

If your program has a large budget, you should consider several counter-marketing staff positions:

- **Marketing director**—oversees the entire counter-marketing program
- **Advertising manager**—manages the work of the ad agency
- **Press secretary**—handles press relations and works with your public relations firm
- **Manager of community relations and local programs**—works with stakeholders and health organizations throughout your state
- **Evaluator**—manages evaluation of counter-marketing activities
- **Financial manager**—reviews bills and monitors financial aspects of contracts

Some of these positions, such as the finance manager and the evaluator, may be shared within the larger tobacco control program or, in some states, within the larger chronic disease program. In your program, you may use different job titles, but the functions will be the same as the positions described here.

Each key position will need support staff if you're implementing a large program. The counter-marketing staff should have experience or credentials in health communication, advertising, marketing, journalism, or related areas. Experience with other health-related campaigns or communication programs in the state is also extremely helpful.

If you're limited in the number of staff you can hire, consider contracting with consultants. They can help you to manage separate aspects of your program. For example, you may hire an advertising expert to help you monitor the development and production of ads.

If the staff is small, typically all of the counter-marketing staff members report to the tobacco control program manager. If the staff is large like the one listed above, the advertising manager, press secretary, and others would report to the marketing director, who would report to the overall program manager.

The program manager is responsible for ensuring that the counter-marketing program and all other program elements support each other and reinforce the larger state tobacco control effort. Counter-marketing is one part of a comprehensive tobacco control program, and your communication effort must be integrated with the overall program. For example, if the state's tobacco control program focuses on prevention of smoking among youth, the counter-marketing effort should focus on messages and interventions for youth and secondary audiences that influence youth.

You'll probably also need to coordinate with other health department staff and state government staff, such as the governor's and the health department's communication teams. Appropriate political officials and their staff should be kept abreast of your program's initiatives, as well as its opposition. Some of these political officials may need to answer for the program, so you should be proactive in keeping them up to date, especially on newsworthy issues. If they support the tobacco control program, they can be strong allies. Even if they don't support the program, you need to keep them updated on what you're doing and why (i.e., how the initiatives contribute to the program's overall goals). "Keeping people in the loop can be a constant balancing act," says one state program director. "It is important to let people know what is happening with the program and to get input on various issues or ideas. However, 'too many cooks' may turn your campaign into a vanilla, politically correct, ineffective one."

Finally, your campaign should be coordinated with local program activities. Ideally the campaign should complement and reinforce programs "on the ground." Coordinate with local tobacco control programs, especially media programs. Involve them in planning, and let them know when you plan to launch various activities.

Communication Agencies

Creating a comprehensive counter-marketing program requires a variety of specialized skills. These skills include selecting, producing, and placing ads; working with the media; planning large events; and coordinating grassroots activities. To create professional-quality communications, you'll probably need to hire one or more communication firms.

For its national "truth" campaign, the American Legacy Foundation works with several media firms: two general market ad agencies, a PR agency, an events firm, and a Web design company, along with agencies that focus on specific populations, such as African Americans, Asian Americans, Hispanics/Latinos, and Native Americans; the gay, lesbian, bisexual, and transgender community; and people of low socioeconomic status. However, the budget for Legacy's media campaign is higher than the budget for any single state's tobacco control program. A state typically couldn't afford and wouldn't need the number of agencies Legacy hired. The main point is that a comprehensive counter-marketing program has many elements, and each one is very time consuming and requires the expertise that agencies and individuals specializing in communications can bring. If your program's budget is moderate to large, you may be able to hire agencies or individual consultants in several of the categories listed here, but for less of their time than the American Legacy Foundation would require.

Agencies come in all shapes and sizes. Most large communication firms offer a range of advertising and PR services. These services usually include strategic planning, market research, creative development, advertising and materials production, media planning, purchasing of media time, and tracking media placement. Other firms focus on a single area. Some firms specialize in advertising only or PR only or in advertising for specific audiences (e.g., African Americans, Asian Americans, or youth). Some firms focus on communication and marketing, others specialize in policy or advocacy, and still others specialize in planning events.

There are no hard and fast rules for what type of firm to hire. Most states contract with a lead ad agency that then subcontracts with agencies specializing in PR, planning events, or communication with specific populations. California has separate contracts for advertising and PR, so the state can work directly with its PR agency when time is limited (e.g., when a quick response is needed). If your state has a very heated political climate or you anticipate frequent attacks from the tobacco industry, consider having a separate PR contract. In a charged environment, maintaining the right dialogue on the public airwaves in a timely manner may be one of the most important things you do.

Communication firms usually perform the following functions:

- Develop creative approaches to achieve your objectives

- Recommend the type(s) of media vehicles for your messages and target audience(s)

- Identify requirements for media placement to reach your target audience(s)

- Arrange opportunities for news coverage of your messages, your program, or both

- Organize community-based activities to promote your message

- Develop relationships with community stakeholders

Running a media campaign can be intimidating for those with public health backgrounds. Don't be afraid to ask lots of questions. Agencies will always be better staffed and move faster than the health department, so be prepared to take control and slow down the process until you understand all the concepts and are comfortable with moving forward.

— Sandi Hammond, Tobacco Control Program
Massachusetts Department of Public Health

Although communication agencies bring specific expertise and create many of the campaign elements, your program staff should be closely involved and provide direction to the agencies. In general, you should work with them to develop the counter-marketing plan, then review their work to make sure it meets your objectives and stays on course. "Without ongoing direction and involvement of program staff," says one state health department manager, "even the best agencies can stray or could end up with clever creative [advertising concepts] that has little likelihood of efficacy."

Evaluation Companies and Consultants

An evaluation contractor will help you to measure your program's effectiveness. You can hire specialists who evaluate public health communications, a private company that specializes in marketing and advertising research and evaluation, a university-based group that is experienced in media evaluation, or a combination of such companies and consultants.

Duties involved in evaluation include:

- Identifying key measures on the basis of your communication objectives

- Determining the baseline, process, and outcome information needed to measure the impact of your activities

- Preparing an evaluation plan and budget for the counter-marketing effort

- Conducting appropriate research before, during, and after your program is launched

- Developing reports on the research that clearly present the data, findings, and conclusions

Don't wait until the last minute to include the evaluation team! Engage evaluators in the planning and implementation of the program from the beginning. They can help you to determine and define your program objectives, which you can measure and report to state officials and other stakeholders. Plus, they can help to ensure that baseline data are gathered before your program is launched, so you don't miss a valuable opportunity to gauge the effect of your program. (See Chapter 5: Evaluating the Success of Your Counter-Marketing Program for more information.)

Stakeholders, Gatekeepers, and Local Programs

Stakeholders are people and organizations that have an interest (stake) in your program's success. For example, local groups representing the African-American community will be interested in campaigns that target African Americans. *Gatekeepers* are individuals or organizations that can help you to reach target audiences with your program messages. Sometimes overlap exists between stakeholders and gatekeepers. *Local programs* are tobacco control efforts that focus on a specific county, city, or region of your state. State programs can't and shouldn't be developed in a vacuum, so it's essential that you address and involve these three important audiences from the start. Community organizations, voluntary organizations (e.g., the American Cancer Society, the

American Lung Association, and the American Heart Association), religious institutions, parent groups, businesses, and other groups can be instrumental in supporting your program and promoting the tobacco control messages.

Community groups and local programs can work on counter-marketing activities by:

- Carrying and publicizing the program messages to constituents
- Developing programs that tie directly into your messages
- Cosponsoring community programs
- Speaking on behalf of the program
- Supporting local legislation and policies that contribute to reducing tobacco use
- Advocating for and protecting the program and its goals

Counter-marketing programs are often highly visible and can be controversial. They can stir up negative publicity or comments from constituents in the state. Involving key stakeholders in your program's development will help you to identify controversial issues up front and gain the stakeholders' support. For example, you should solicit input from individuals representing targeted communities before, during, and after the program is launched (see Chapter 4: Reaching Specific Populations for more information).

One of the best ways to involve stakeholders is to set up an informal steering or advisory committee for your effort and include key members from stakeholder groups, as well as members of your target audience. This approach institutionalizes the involvement of stakeholders and gives you something concrete to point to as an example of your inclusiveness. Have this group review plans, concepts, and draft materials. Listen carefully to their input. You won't always be able to incorporate everyone's suggestions, but you should understand their perspectives and what is most important to them. In many states, the media campaign fuels controversy. Having stakeholders and members of the target audience on board from the beginning gives you a source of spokespeople to defend the campaign.

Keep community leaders and local programs involved in your program. Everyone likes to be involved in a successful program effort. Many programs have a newsletter, Web site, or e-mail distribution list that keeps stakeholders and gatekeepers informed of the program's progress and successes. If you're reporting results that demonstrate progress, such as survey results that show your campaign has helped reduce smoking, involve the appropriate stakeholders in the announcement of these results. If your program receives negative press, keep stakeholders and gatekeepers informed, so they won't be surprised or caught off guard; seek their help and support when needed. For example, if a state's quitline service comes under attack, the state may ask a partner who has experience with smoking cessation issues, such as the local branch of the American Cancer Society or the American Lung Association, to comment on the necessity and efficacy of the quitline.

Look for specific opportunities for stakeholders to get involved in your program. For example, you may help a local radio station develop a day of radio programming about quitting smoking. When a local company goes smoke-free, you can help the company get media attention for its effort. When there's an important tobacco control message, such as the release of a Surgeon General's report, create press materials independently or augment press materials from the Centers for Disease Control and Prevention (CDC), so the stakeholders can use them to help you publicize the information. Invite stakeholders to participate in community events, award ceremonies, and other campaign-related events. Stakeholders can advance policy issues and legislation related to tobacco control, a role not normally available for state staff. Supportive media gatekeepers can work with you or your agencies to develop special programming, newspaper inserts, or community events with media tie-ins.

Your communication agencies may think that working with stakeholders is a burden, because many of them are used to working with commercial clients who have few stakeholders. Although agencies often focus on expediency, it's important for you to explain the value of working with stakeholders and to specifically outline to your agency how stakeholders will be involved.

Steps for Selecting an Agency

To hire an agency, you need to:

- Outline the specific work you want the contractor to do. Don't be too prescriptive in the request for proposals (RFP), but do be clear about the overall goal(s) and the campaign's specific objectives. Allow the agencies to respond creatively.

- Issue an RFP for the work.

- Organize a group of knowledgeable reviewers from within and outside your organization.

- Eliminate proposals that don't meet the technical requirements specified in the RFP (e.g., deadline and format).

- Work with your review group to evaluate the proposals.

- Compare cost proposals.

- Invite and observe presentations from finalists.

- Check finalists' references.

- Select the firm that appears to be the most capable and to offer the most value for its fees.

- Inform other agencies that they didn't win the contract.

- Sign a contract.

- Begin briefing meetings with the agency.

Selecting Contractors

Once you determine the configuration of the counter-marketing team, you'll start the formal process of hiring contractors. This section provides you with guidelines for this process. (See Chapter 7: Advertising and Chapter 8: Public Relations for more information about working with contractors.)

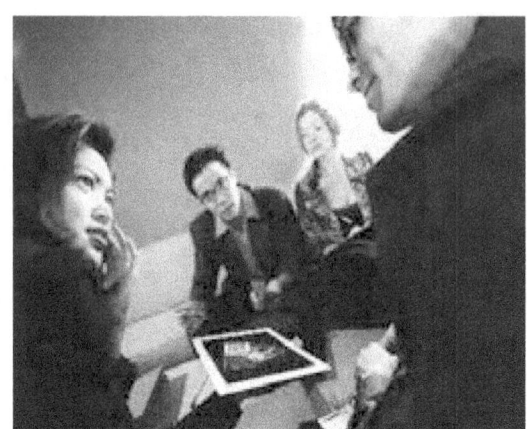

Beginning to work with a contractor is like beginning any relationship. Relationships require trust, respect, and an understanding of each participant's strengths and weaknesses. In this relationship, you bring to the table your technical expertise on content, your political acuity, and your understanding of the sometimes complex government approval process. The communication firms offer creative approaches to the message, expertise in how to develop effective communication pieces, and knowledge of the media needed to reach your audience(s). The evaluation contractor provides the technical know-how to assess how successful your messages and initiatives have been in reaching the target audiences and what the effects of those interventions have been.

The focus here is on communication and evaluation firms, but the advice can apply to hiring any private company.

Before the Bidding Process

Don't rush into issuing an RFP. Take some time to:

- **Learn what your budget can buy in your state.** Media and production costs vary in each state. Find out what it should cost to reach your audience(s) in your state. One approach is to talk to the manager of another state-funded media campaign in your state (e.g., the lottery or tourism). Your state may have a commercial campaign you can examine, too. You should also look at other states' tobacco counter-marketing efforts to see what they received for the money they spent. Find out what they spent per capita and in total, so you can make an accurate comparison with what you plan to spend.

- **Look at what has been done by other programs in your state.** Learn how other state programs selected an agency; again, the lottery and tourism programs may be a good place to start. State media campaigns can be valuable sources of government information, advice, and insights into your state's approval process.

- **Explore approaches used in other states.** Examine RFPs for media contractors in other states and the contracts awarded. The State Information Forum, a Web site operated by CDC's Office on Smoking and Health, is a source of information, resources, and other materials for state tobacco control programs. Many state RFPs are available online on the State Infor-mation Forum, at http://.ntcp.forum.cdc.gov. This Web site is password protected, so you'll need to contact CDC/OSH's Health Communications Branch to gain access if you're not a current user.

- **Learn the ins and outs of your state's contracting rules.** Find someone in your state financial or contracting office to guide you through the state's contracting procedures and to help you develop language for an RFP. A good way to start is by reviewing media RFPs from other organizations in your state. (See Appendix 6.1: Key Elements of a Request for Proposals for a Media Campaign for a description of common items included in many state tobacco control program RFPs.) Make sure that you understand the RFP and that your contracting office has reviewed the process for your RFP. You should be comfortable with the wording of the RFP and the deliverables it describes. Decide whether to ask for "speculative creative" (sample materials that a firm provides before a contract is awarded) as part of the proposal. If you make this request, you must include language in the RFP indicating that the state retains ownership of any creative materials presented during the bidding process. This language will protect you from legal action by a firm that isn't awarded the contract and may have presented creative similar to that of the winning firm.

- **Decide on the configuration of firms for your program.** Do you want one all-purpose agency that can give you a range of communication services or a set of specialized firms that work together as a team? Do you have the staff to oversee contracts with more than one firm, such as separate advertising and PR companies?

- **Avoid firms that work with tobacco companies.** Just as Coca-Cola doesn't hire firms that work for Pepsi, you shouldn't hire firms that work for the competition. This recommendation has become more complicated with the recent trend toward acquisitions and mergers. Many agencies that don't work with the tobacco industry have been bought by conglomerates that may own other firms with tobacco accounts. At a minimum, the agency you hire should have no direct connections with the tobacco industry or its affiliates (e.g., Kraft, which is owned by Altria, formerly called Philip Morris). You'll have to consider the advantages and disadvantages of hiring a firm that does no tobacco work but has sister agencies that do. *Adweek*, an advertising industry publication, publishes a directory of ad firms that lists their clients and affiliation with advertising conglomerates and holding companies. You should require that all bidding agencies disclose any connection, direct or indirect, with the tobacco industry or its partner companies, so you can consider that information in selecting an agency. If an agency you may want to use has such a connection, ask the bidder to submit a plan for providing a fire wall between your program and any potential conflicts of interest.

- **Recruit a diverse review committee.** The members of your review committee should have a wide range of expertise and backgrounds, including experience with health issues and the communication techniques you plan to use in your program (e.g., advertising, public relations, and media advocacy). Check your state's restrictions about using out-of-state reviewers.

During the Bidding Process

Most contracting rules limit your ability to com-municate directly with firms bidding on your proposal. Nonetheless, the review process gives you opportunities to learn about the firms. As you review proposals and listen to bids from each firm, keep these questions in mind:

- How strategic and thoughtful are the decisions the firm makes and the work it produces?

- How creative is the firm?

- Does the firm describe how it would approach the subject of tobacco, and, if so, do you like what you hear?

- Does the firm have experience working with community groups?

- Does the firm have experience with your target audience(s)?

- Does the firm have experience with tobacco control, social marketing, or other health-related work? If not, you don't necessarily have to rule it out; it would be much easier for you to teach the firm's staff about tobacco control than to teach them about developing and placing ads!

- Do the firm's references and samples give you insights into the quality of the work and skills of the staff assigned to your account?

- Does the firm have a track record of developing campaigns that have generated measurable results? Ask for examples.

- Has the firm bought media in every market in your state? Does it have experience in evaluating and buying a wide variety of media?

- Is the team proposed by the firm a mix of senior, midlevel, and junior staff?

- What is the experience of the primary staff to be assigned to your account?

- Are support staff in specific functional areas (e.g., market research or media buying) assigned to work on your project for a sufficient percentage of their time?

- Do you think you can work comfortably with the staff proposed for the project?

- Does the firm have the number of staff and appropriate facilities to do the work?

- Do staff of the firm have experience in negotiating for bonus airings or add-ons as part of a media buy?

(For more information on the RFP process, see Appendix 6.1: Key Elements of a Request for Proposals for a Media Campaign and Appendix 6.2: Questions and Answers on RFPs.)

Once You've Selected a Firm

Develop a team relationship with the firm that is awarded the contract. Work closely with the staff as individuals, and get to know them. Avoid thinking of them as the "suppliers" who simply deliver the goods to you; instead, think of them as an extension of your staff or as your equal partners. The better the relationship, the easier it will be to work through issues on which you may not agree.

Teach the agency what it needs to know about effective tobacco counter-marketing messages. There's a wealth of television, radio, outdoor, and print materials on tobacco control. Sharing those materials with them may help to inspire creative ideas or identify materials from other states that can be reapplied or adapted for use in your state. Although most agencies prefer to create original ads tailored specifically for the state, many states have combined new ads with available ads proven effective in other states. Ask the firm's staff to become familiar with the advertising materials

---

Tips for Selecting an Agency to Reach Specific Populations

If you decide to hire a firm to reach specific populations, choose one that offers:

- Experience in working on communication campaigns

- Examples of past communication work that an independent evaluation has shown to be successful

- References from clients for whom the firm has done similar work

- Adequate staff and facilities to do the work

- Experience in developing effective, culturally appropriate material

- Strong ties to the community

Don't pick a firm simply because its staff includes members of a specific population; choose a firm because of the merits of its work. At the same time, recognize the role that members of a specific population can play in a firm's ability to be culturally competent and culturally appropriate. (See Chapter 4: Reaching Specific Populations for more information.)

> ### *Tips for Selecting an Evaluation Contractor*
>
> Choose an evaluation contractor that demonstrates:
>
> - Experience in evaluating tobacco control programs, health communication campaigns, or both
>
> - Ability to work with a wide variety of stakeholders, including representatives of populations affected most by tobacco use
>
> - Innovative approaches to evaluation, coupled with consideration of budget limitations and other program realities
>
> - Skills that complement those of the in-house evaluation team and that increase the evaluation capacity of that team
>
> - Regular sharing of raw data, preliminary results, and full findings with the program staff
>
> - Cultural competency in conducting evaluations among various racial and ethnic groups
>
> - Expertise you need and can afford
>
> Hire your evaluation staff early in the process and involve them from the start. Don't wait until the campaign is about to be launched. The evaluation of your efforts must be seen as independent and objective, so it's important to hire a separate evaluation firm, instead of having your ad agency subcontract with one.

in CDC's Media Campaign Resource Center (MCRC), available online at http://www.cdc.gov/tobacco/mcrc. The MCRC Web site offers an online database of materials the communication firm can review. In addition, involving the agency's staff in strategic planning meetings, focus groups, community meetings, and other activities will help them to develop an in-depth understanding of the important issues. You should establish a clear process for review and approval. Mistakes can be costly to fix. Pay careful attention to the visuals and words in all communication pieces, the results of market research, and the internal and external comments about the ads.

Restrain yourself from becoming the creative director. You pay the firm to fill that role. Avoid giving prescriptive instructions about what to change. For example, don't make detailed suggestions about a proposed ad, by saying to the firm: "If you could just make this woman who stopped smoking look happier, and maybe you could have her whole family standing around her looking happy, too, and..." A better approach is to offer the agency feedback about what you'd like to change *conceptually*, and let their staff explore the specific creative alternatives. When you comment about the work the firm submits, focus on goals. For example, tell the agency: "The goal would be to make this ad focus more on the positives of quitting smoking, instead of the negatives of previous failed attempts."

Developing an Annual Marketing Plan

Once you've assembled your program staff, hired contractors, and gone through the planning process (see Chapter 2: Planning Your Counter-Marketing Program for more information on planning process), you'll need to develop a marketing plan. This plan will be the blueprint for implementing your counter-marketing tasks and activities. It should list the specific tasks, staff, time frame, and budget needs for each objective developed during the planning phase. The plan should encompass all the components you're using (e.g., advertising, PR, media advocacy, grassroots initiatives, and media literacy activities), and its timeline should allow sufficient time for technical review and approval. This marketing plan can be used to monitor program activities, and you may need to update it as you conduct the process evaluation throughout the year. (See Appendix 2.1: Counter-Marketing Planning Worksheet for guidance in developing a marketing plan.)

You may be tempted to skip the development of a marketing plan, but doing so will cause you to be reactive instead of proactive in working with your communication agencies, your target audience(s), and your management. This plan is an important tool for keeping everyone focused on how your goals will be accomplished. By developing a marketing plan, you'll ensure that your agency doesn't lead the campaign in a direction different from the one you intended. Providing a yearly marketing plan will also help the agency to know what to expect well in advance, so the staff can manage your account effectively.

Reviewing Marketing Materials

One of the key functions of the program staff will be to review the marketing materials created by the communication firm(s). You'll be responsible for reviewing these materials in three key areas: strategy, accuracy of technical content, and cultural appropriateness.

Keeping Materials on Strategy

Ad agencies pride themselves on their creativity because creative ads get noticed, are entertaining, and can influence behavior. But just because an ad is entertaining doesn't mean it's on strategy. For each key marketing piece, you and your agency should develop a creative brief. Use this creative brief to review each ad or communication piece to ensure that it's on target.

Ensuring Accurate Technical Content

Communication materials have to be on strategy, but they also have to be accurate. Any factual errors will undermine the credibility of your efforts and make your program vulnerable to criticism. Here are some ways to keep your communication work consistently accurate:

- Provide your agency with the most current tobacco-related data, and keep agency staff informed by promptly forwarding new data to them.

What Is a Creative Brief?

For almost any work with a communication agency, you'll need a creative brief (communication brief). This document spells out:

- The specific assignment—the product the agency is being asked to develop
- The goal of the communication piece(s)
- The main message(s)
- Demographic, psychographic, and other information about the audience
- Key insights about the audience that should be considered during development of the communication piece(s)
- The audience's perceived barriers to the desired behavior change
- Benefits the audience might receive from the behavior change
- Actions you want the target audience to take

The creative brief is typically drafted by the agency account team, but the health department staff can initiate it or provide input to it. It gives the agency creative team the basic message for each creative product and clarifies what the agency is being asked to do. Once the product is completed, everyone involved can refer to the creative brief to make sure the product meets the criteria in the brief. (See Appendix 6.3: Elements of a Creative Brief and Appendices 6.4, 6.5, and 6.6 for sample creative briefs.)

- Require the firm to provide documentation for all statements, facts, and figures that appear in the materials and ads it presents, even if you provided the original data. Always use the original source to substantiate data. Quotes from newspaper reports about study results may not accurately reflect the true findings.

- Maintain an easily accessible file of the ad scripts and corresponding substantiation. Program managers are often asked to back up the information in ads, sometimes months or even years after the ads were placed or aired.

- Identify technical experts within your department who can sign off on the technical content in ads and other communication materials.

- Develop a review and approval process that includes all of the key decision makers but doesn't delay ad production longer than necessary.

Producing Culturally Appropriate Materials

Communication materials must be culturally appropriate for your target audience(s). A critical step is to share the draft materials with members of the target audience early in the development process and before work on the materials is completed. You should also assess how the materials will be received by the larger community. For example, some ads designed for rebellious youth may be considered irreverent and disrespectful by adults. The state may still decide to use the ads but may choose to tightly control media placement to limit the number of adults exposed to them.

If stakeholders and members of your target community are on an advisory or steering committee for your program, you may be able to use their input to assess the cultural appropriateness of your materials. To help assess their impact on the larger community, especially if you think your messages may offend certain groups, you may need to be proactive in meeting with the community to explain the materials and your approach. This move will help to defuse potential criticism of your campaign and build relationships with stakeholders. For example, with its "Making Blacks History" campaign, the American Legacy Foundation met with the NAACP (National Association for the Advancement of Colored People), the National Urban League, the National Black Nurses Association, and other groups to explain the strategy of the campaign and get their reaction. By sharing these ads before they hit the airwaves, Legacy was reassured that the ads wouldn't be controversial because of the "Making Blacks History" phrase. (See Chapter 4: Reaching Specific Populations for more information on designing culturally appropriate materials.)

Monitoring the Counter-Marketing Budget

Managing the fiscal component of a program can be intimidating. Most people hired to manage public health communication campaigns aren't financial managers and don't have much experience with media buying, production costs, talent fees, and the range of expenses related to communication programs. These tips can help you to develop a realistic budget:

- According to CDC's *Best Practices for Comprehensive Tobacco Control Programs*, published in 1999, state tobacco control programs should allocate $1 to $3 per capita per year to counter-marketing programs. Although this amount is the minimum goal for most states, few states have been able to maintain this level of funding.

- Look at budgets for other statewide efforts, such as lottery campaigns, travel and tourism, or promotion of agricultural products (e.g., citrus fruit in Florida). These programs can give you ballpark estimates on costs for media campaigns.

- Find out what other states have spent on tobacco counter-marketing programs and determine whether any of the states have per capita and total budgets similar to yours. Learn how those funds were allocated, and ask the program managers what they would do differently if they could spend the funds again.

- Consider hiring a compensation consultant to help you negotiate your agencies' budgets. This consultant can help you to determine the appropriate profit margin for the agency and assist you in understanding how agencies bill for their work.

- Determine the amount(s) you can afford to spend and the best approach for allocating funds in your particular budget. If your budget is small, you may consider a greater mix of PR, media advocacy, media literacy, and grassroots communications rather than a paid media campaign. You can conduct innovative and effective media efforts without expensive ads.

- Conduct a media audit of your advertising media buys to ensure that you're getting your money's worth. If you have limited resources, you may want to conduct a partial audit, from a specific ad flight, to get a snapshot of the quality of your media buy. Because much of your budget may go to paid media, you need to ensure that the funds are spent appropriately.

Variables that affect a communication budget include the following:

- Cost of buying media in your state
- Amount and level of ad production (e.g., number of ads produced or reapplied and complexity of ads produced)
- Number and choice of media outlets
- Intensity and duration of campaign
- Use of existing versus original advertising
- Single focus versus multiple focuses (e.g., number of overall goals and number of target audiences)
- Number of events and activities (e.g., PR, grassroots and media advocacy)
- Communication in English only, other language, or both

Here are some rules of thumb for managing the budget of a counter-marketing program:

- Regardless of the size of the budget, remember that you're spending taxpayers' money. Be sure that your spending decisions are well informed and that every initiative is focused on the program's goals and objectives. Select initiatives that are most likely to contribute to your program's progress in a cost-effective way.

- Obtain estimates, so you know how much a project will cost before you start.

- Approve all costs before any work begins and money is spent.

- Review monthly expenditures carefully. Track expenses for each product, as well as the overall counter-marketing budget. A number of financial tracking systems are available to help you monitor expenses and project monthly expenditures. You may want to ask managers of other state campaigns (e.g., the lottery or tourism) about the procedures and tracking systems they use.

- If any products must be changed, tell staff and consultants that you must discuss and approve any additional costs in advance.

- Hold monthly budget meetings with contractors and staff to keep your expenses on track.

- Include evaluation costs in the overall campaign budget, unless they are included in another part of the tobacco control budget.

- Buy the rights to creative materials (e.g., photos and ads), whenever possible, so they can be reused by you or others.

- Ask questions at each step to better understand what you're buying and what your options are. Keep asking questions until you understand all aspects of media production and placement.

Points To Remember

- Don't skip the development of the marketing plan. Creating this blueprint will force you and your contractors to outline the specific tasks needed to reach your goals and objectives and to have all key decision makers agree. It will be a valuable tool in tracking your progress and monitoring the performance of your team and contractors. An approved marketing plan will also help you to stay on track when outside groups try to influence the direction of your program.

- Track every penny spent. You should be able to report to government officials and other funders what your specific activities cost and what you delivered for those costs. Closely monitoring the budget will help you to determine which activities were cost-effective and which were not. It will also provide you with benchmark costs for your program in future years.

- Never let anything go out the door without reviewing it. Because of the multiple reviews during the development process, you may be tempted to simply scan a product before it's finalized, but make sure you give it one last, thorough review. You need to be certain that the material is on strategy, has no technical errors, is culturally competent, and reflects the program's position. Determine your review process up front for each type of product (e.g., ads and press releases), and follow it to the letter.

- Make stakeholders and local programs your partners. Involving stakeholders in the development of your campaign is vital. This move will develop strong relationships with stakeholders, will build support for your program, and may help you to identify potential criticisms of your program and be prepared to address them proactively. On the other hand, don't feel that you have to incorporate every comment by every stakeholder. Consider all comments and feedback, but keep your campaign on target.

- Keep your eye on your goal at all times. Implementing an integrated, multifaceted program isn't easy. You may be getting input from the governor's staff, stakeholders, various contractors, and your own staff. There's a lot to consider and sort through, but no matter how exciting an ad or activity may seem or how much a key person or group pushes for something, if it doesn't support your overall goal, don't pursue it.

Bibliography

Bjornson W, Moore JM. Designing an effective counteradvertising campaign—Oregon. *Cancer* 1998;83 (12 Suppl):2752–4.

Centers for Disease Control and Prevention. *Best Practices for Comprehensive Tobacco Control Programs—August 1999.* Atlanta, GA: CDC, National Center for Chronic Disease Prevention and Health Promotion, Office on Smoking and Health, 1999.

Miller A. Designing an effective counteradvertising campaign—Massachusetts. *Cancer* 1998;83 (12 Suppl):2742–5.

Reister T, Linton M. Designing an effective counteradvertising campaign—Arizona. *Cancer* 1998;83 (12 Suppl):2746–51.

Stevens C. Designing an effective counteradvertising campaign—California. *Cancer* 1998;83 (12 Suppl):2736–41.

Chapter 7

Advertising

The (advertising) campaign is a tool to frame the debate. It can introduce an issue and create 'noise.' This not only sparks dialogue but can itself become the environment.

— Anne Miller, Arnold Worldwide
  Massachusetts Tobacco Control Program

In This Chapter

- Logistics: Hiring and Managing Advertising Contractors
- Strategy: Developing Effective Messages
- Creative: Breaking Through the Clutter
- Exposure: Show the Message Enough for It to Sink In
- Choosing a Media Approach: Paid Media, Public Service Announcements, and Earned Media
- Evaluating Advertising Efforts

Advertising is a way to speak to your audience. It's a communication tactic. For example, if you want people who use tobacco to quit, you need to give them a reason to do—so, something in exchange for giving up their perceived benefits of smoking—the nicotine high or the feeling of independence. Advertising is one way to present, in a clear and persuasive manner, the benefits of quitting tobacco use.

If you think of a tobacco counter-marketing campaign as a conversation, advertising, like public relations, is about how you do the talking. In public relations, the message is delivered through an intermediary, such as the press. In advertising, the message is delivered directly to a mass audience. With public relations, the message may change, depending on who relays it. In advertising, the audience is exposed repeatedly to the same ad. In public relations, you gain the credibility of an intermediary, but you give up a lot of control. In advertising, you don't benefit from an intermediary's credibility, but you can more tightly craft the tone and content of your message, as well as when, where, and how often people hear it. You pay a premium for this control, however, when you produce an ad or make a media buy.

Effective advertising can increase knowledge, correct myths, change attitudes, and even help to influence behavior. For example, Florida launched a major teen-oriented mass media campaign aimed at revealing the manipulative

What Advertising Can and Can't Do	
Can	*Can't*
▪ Communicate a message	▪ Substitute for strategy
▪ Reach many people	▪ Present complicated information
▪ Change attitudes	▪ Provide feedback
▪ Create an image for the campaign	▪ Provide services

and deceptive tactics of the tobacco industry. After six months, more teens felt strongly that the tobacco industry wanted them to begin smoking to replace dying smokers. A year into the campaign, tobacco use by middle school and high school students in the state declined considerably, in part because advertising had changed their attitudes about cigarettes and tobacco companies.

For advertising to work, however, it must meet the following minimal criteria:

- Offer members of the target audience a benefit they value, thus influencing them to change their beliefs, attitudes, and behaviors
- Reach the target audience enough times that the message is understood and internalized
- Engage audience members in a way that they can understand and that makes them feel understood

Although most effective advertising is created by advertising agencies—firms that specialize in analyzing audiences and finding creative ways to reach them—the counter-marketing program manager doesn't simply pay the bills and sign off on what the agency does. As with any program approach, the manager must ensure that the ads are more than just entertaining or informative. The program manager must make sure that the ads further the program's overall objectives and that the three minimal criteria are met. Furthermore, the manager must make sure these efforts are accomplished within a set budget and time frame. This chapter takes you step by step through the four key aspects of managing a successful advertising campaign: logistics, strategy, creative (advertising concepts), and exposure.

Logistics: Hiring and Managing Advertising Contractors

Campaigns that rely solely on public service announcements are unlikely to reach a target audience with sufficient regularity to make an impact because they air during time slots donated by the TV or radio stations, so most states hire contractors to create new advertising, to buy the media needed to place the ads, or to perform both tasks. Some state tobacco control programs with limited emphasis on paid advertising may not need to hire an ad agency, social marketing firm, or media buyer, but states that plan to make advertising a significant part of their overall tobacco control program probably do. Even states planning to use creative materials produced by others will need to make a media buy, and they're likely to get a better price and more effective placements if they hire professionals to do the buying.

Once a contractor is hired, the challenges are far from over. A counter-marketing manager and the creative agency should set up guidelines for everything from schedules for payment to the process for approving creative materials. Then, during the day-to-day management of the campaign, the counter-marketing manager and the agency must balance the agency's need for creative freedom with the marketing manager's need for strategic control. It's no easy task.

Selecting Marketing Contractors

Hiring an agency, media buyer, or social marketing firm is often the first challenge a counter-marketing manager must face. The typical first step is writing a request for proposals (RFP) or a similar document. The rules about writing RFPs vary by state, but one simple way to start is to look at what others have done. People who write RFPs usually review previous RFPs for government-run marketing campaigns in their state (e.g., a lottery or tourism effort) and for counter-marketing campaigns in other states. (See the State Information Forum Web site of the Centers for Disease Control and Prevention at http://ntcp.forum.cdc.gov for sample RFPs.) Take the language that is most relevant to the challenges you face, and refine it to fit your situation. The RFP should provide potential bidders with specific objectives, a description of the behavior you want to change, a list that ranks the target audiences, and a statement of your potential budget.

Most counter-marketing programs use selection committees to choose firms for creative services. A state agency can be protected from the appearance of favoritism by asking a multidisciplinary group of highly respected experts to make a recommendation or to select the marketing contractor on the basis of a thorough review of the proposals submitted and oral presentations. This approach also adds a degree of buy-in from the committee members and brings needed expertise to the decision-making process. There's no perfect recipe for a selection committee, but most states include marketing and advertising experts, grassroots tobacco control activists, policy makers, health professionals, an evaluation expert, and representatives from the organization managing the campaign. (See Chapter 6: Managing and Implementing Your Counter-Marketing Program for more information on the RFP process.)

Ultimately, the process should help ensure hiring of a firm that can understand your target audience, be responsive to your program's needs, offer breakthrough creative ideas, maximize exposure to the message, and be accountable for its use of government funds. Try to stay focused on these goals throughout the selection process. Firms that provide creative services are in the business of making things appealing. Part of your job is to make sure that an advertising approach—no matter how funny or interesting it may be—offers a logical, research-based strategy that fits within the approach of your overall program.

Ask three key questions about firms making a pitch:

1. **Are they strategic?** Do they have a clear idea about how their plan will help to encourage changes in attitudes and behaviors, not just build awareness or interest people in the topic? Do their examples of previous work reflect sound strategic thinking and positive, data-based outcomes?

2. **Are they capable?** Do they and their partners have the ability to produce breakthrough, memorable ads that can help to change beliefs and attitudes and to encourage changes in behavior? Can they manage the media buys you might want? Can they handle the financial responsibilities required by the state? Do they have sufficient staff to service your needs?

3. **Are they listening to you, to the audience, to the research?** Will they be responsive and incorporate data and expert perspectives into their plans?

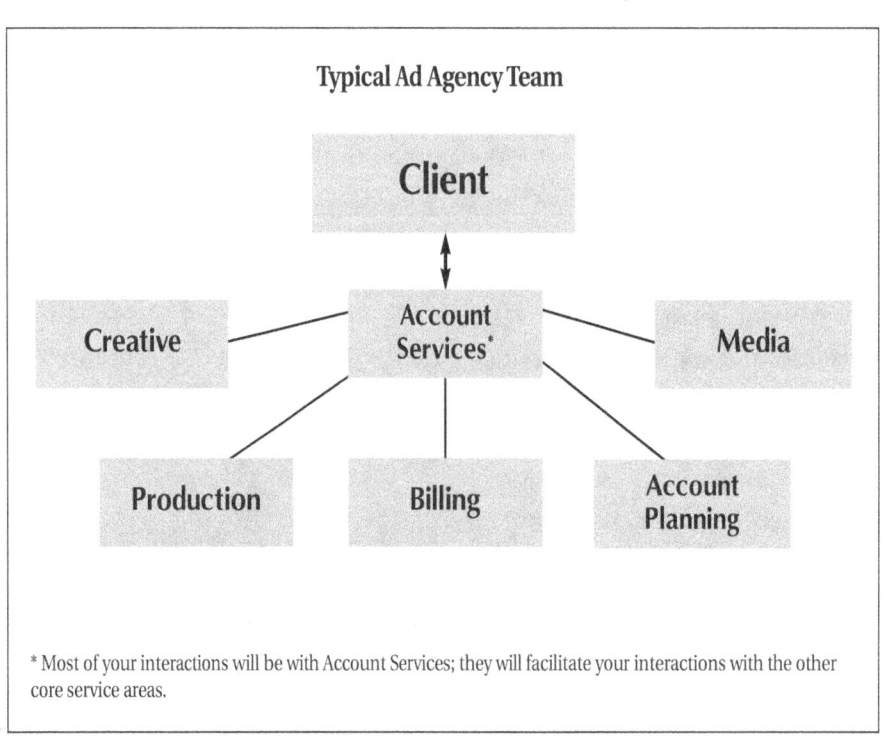

Typical Ad Agency Team

* Most of your interactions will be with Account Services; they will facilitate your interactions with the other core service areas.

Managing a Marketing Contractor

To manage an advertising agency, it's helpful to understand how agencies make money and how they handle the work you request. Most ad agencies offer these core services:

- **Account service (also known as client service).** All ad agencies have specialists who are responsible for responding to your needs and managing the work the agency is doing for you. The account service staff are your day-to-day link to the agency.

- **Creative.** An agency's creative services staff develop a range of advertising products, from TV spots to logos to billboards. Advertising concepts, typically called "creative," are developed by a copywriter and an art director. The staff, called "creatives," work on many accounts and are assigned to your projects by the account staff, as needed.

- **Account planning.** Most ad agencies have in-house experts who conduct and analyze market research, then help to develop an overall strategy. Account planners are experts on the consumer, and they provide the creatives with insights to help in development of advertising ideas. Some agencies do not have an account planning department, but have a market research department that focuses on conducting and analyzing research.

- **Media.** Agencies can buy media time or space for you, either in-house or through a subcontract with a media buyer. They keep abreast of current rates and negotiate for TV and radio time, newspaper and magazine space, outdoor advertising, and other opportunities to place your message before the audience. They offer expertise in finding cost-effective ways to reach specific audiences by selecting the best places to run your advertising and negotiating the best rates for these media placements. Some agencies hire another firm that specializes in media buying to handle this work.

- **Production.** Agencies often have in-house staff who produce materials, manage outside vendors, and help them to produce broadcast spots and other advertising.

When you contract directly with an ad agency, you hire a firm whose core business is to create and disseminate advertising products, typically print ads, billboards, and broadcast spots, based on a strategy the agency develops or helps to develop. The agency makes money by charging for creating the product, buying the media time, or both. Most agencies are paid through one or more of the following arrangements:

- **Commission.** A percentage of the media buy and, in some cases, production costs

- **Project fee.** A straight fee paid for a specific set of deliverables (Partial payments may be made as deliverables are completed.)

- **Retainer.** A fee, typically paid monthly, for a specified scope of work (Sometimes there's a guaranteed retainer and the possibility of additional charges based on the workload for a particular month.)

- **Time and materials.** A payment system consisting of an hourly rate for labor; a number by which the hourly rates are multiplied ("multiplier") to underwrite overhead; and direct reimbursement of other expenses (e.g., production costs and the media buy)

- **Performance based.** Compensation related to outcomes (For example, a portion of the payment may be based on the level of confirmed audience awareness of the advertising.)

The government rarely compensates agencies on the basis of results. However, such compensation is becoming more common in the private sector and some states are using performance-based compensation for tobacco control efforts. Florida, for example, hired a compensation consultant to help link the ad agency's multiplier to awareness, attitude, and behavior measures selected by the state's Tobacco Pilot Program. In Florida, Minnesota, and other states, the agencies have been guaranteed a base multiplier and growth of the multiplier that is contingent on achievement of certain targets.

Responses to the RFP often recommend the reimbursement arrangement as part of a cost proposal. In some states, an ad agency is selected and then the arrangement for reimbursement is negotiated from scratch, according to applicable state policies. Whatever your state's policy is, the best approach is to create an arrangement that allows the agency to make a reasonable profit by creating and placing strategically sound, memorable, insightful communication products for your target audience. The ad firm should be rewarded in particular for contributing to desired changes in the audience's awareness, knowledge, attitudes, intentions, and behaviors.

A good marketing manager should support the agency in ways that will help its creative staff develop the most effective communication products possible, while maintaining appropriate financial and creative control. How can you do that?

- Establish guidelines early.
- Designate a primary contact.
- Trust the creative expertise you hire.
- Tap expertise, not just opinions.
- Protect the agency from politics.
- Agree to brief, written copy strategies.

Establish guidelines early. If both the program manager and the ad agency know what to expect, management is always easier. States have established all types of guidelines to ensure that expectations are clear. Two of the most important guidelines relate to approval of creative materials and media buys. You should decide with the contractor how long these approvals will take, who will be involved, and how revisions will be handled. Make these decisions in advance of the first recommendations from the ad agency, not as the ad development process takes place. Then you need to hold up your end of the bargain: Don't promise five-day approvals if you can't deliver. Also, you should think in terms of the entire process. If you plan to require pretesting, schedule it. In addition, consider developing guidelines for media buying and billing. Media-buying guidelines set rules for what types of media and what kind of exposure the firm should buy. Billing guidelines create deadlines and other restrictions for prompt and accurate billing and payment. You also may want to consider placing limits on the agency's scope of work. For example, you may want to restrict a firm hired at the state level from soliciting additional tobacco control business—and more money—from your partners at the local level.

Designate a primary contact. Just as an ad agency assigns specific account staff to your program, the state must assign a primary contact for the agency. This person should coordinate everything the ad agency is asked to do, so the agency isn't pulled in several directions at once. This state staff person should have the ability to make decisions and represent the needs of the overall program.

Trust the creative expertise you hire. Outstanding advertising is rarely the result of endless tinkering or a lengthy approval process. Instead, it results from strong strategic planning that uses audience insights, creativity, and judgment. Once a creative agency is carefully selected and hired, marketing managers need to place some trust in the agency. If an agency is hired for its ability to connect with "hip" teens, for example, a middle-aged health department official probably shouldn't question the choice of colors for a youth-targeted flier. On the other hand, don't hesitate to question whether an ad concept will be understood, will be perceived as relevant, will seem credible, or is consistent with your program's goals. These are questions you may want to test with audience research. Using qualitative research, you can expose your target audience to a concept and analyze their reaction. (See Chapter 3: Gaining and Using Target Audience Insights for more information on performing qualitative research.)

Tap expertise, not just opinions. Your advertising doesn't need to work for everyone reviewing the ad; it needs to work only for the target audience. As you share a product with your peers and superiors, try to tap their expertise, not their taste. For example, ask the disease expert if the disease references are accurate, not whether he or she "liked" the ad. Consider allowing as many final decisions as possible to be made by the marketing manager, not a more senior political appointee. Some states have allowed a properly tested TV spot to air on the sole basis of a marketing director's approval. You must balance issues of control and accountability with an agency's ability to create something new, insightful, interesting, and effective.

Protect the agency from politics. Policy makers are very important in tobacco control, but they may not always be the best marketers. As much as possible, avoid pressuring your agency to make advertising decisions based on a politician's preferences. Many creative firms are very client oriented and may respond to political pressures that could be better handled by the secretary of health or another ally. Your ad agency should never be asked to lobby the legislature for funding, nor should a legislator lobby the ad agency to, for example, select for the campaign a certain celebrity who may not appeal to the audience. Many program managers inform policy makers that key marketing decisions should be made by the marketing staff because they are closest to the audience research and are skilled at interpreting it. The marketing manager has a responsibility to ensure that advertising decisions are not based on politics but on marketing information—insights about what might influence the audience and get results. On the other hand, the marketing manager should communicate regularly with state officials who make funding decisions, so they understand the campaign and will not be alienated, surprised, or offended by the ads they see, hear, or read.

Agree to brief, written copy strategies. Keeping on strategy is one of the greatest challenges of any advertising campaign. Advertising is full of creative people eager to break through the media clutter with something new and exciting. Your job, however, is to change behavior and build support for policies, not to win advertising awards or please everyone. You and the agency need to agree—in writing—on what kinds of messages will affect attitudes in a way that will lead to behavior change. Write a brief copy strategy that clearly and simply states what you're trying to do, and check everything you do against this written agreement. For each new advertising assignment, you and the agency will develop a "creative brief" that describes in detail what you are trying to achieve with each ad or campaign. This brief should include your copy strategy and more details. (See Appendix 6.3: Elements of a Creative Brief and Appendices 6.4, 6.5, and 6.6 for sample creative briefs.) By requiring all your advertising to fall under a copy strategy, you may decide not to produce some very entertaining ads, but what you do produce will be more effective.

The bottom line in logistics is to make it as easy as possible for your creative agency to develop effective advertising. As a marketing manager, you're not only an agency's client—you and the agency are partners.

Strategy: Developing Effective Messages

Just as your program must have an underlying logic to it, so must your advertising. As with your entire program, your advertising strategy should be based partly on a situational analysis—an understanding of the environment in which you operate. Who is your competition? What are they doing? How is your product—the behavior you're seeking—viewed in the marketplace? One simple type of situational analysis marketers use is a list of the strengths, weaknesses, opportunities, and threats (SWOTs) surrounding the campaign's goals. This analysis should help you to understand the current situation, so you have a clearer idea about what must change.

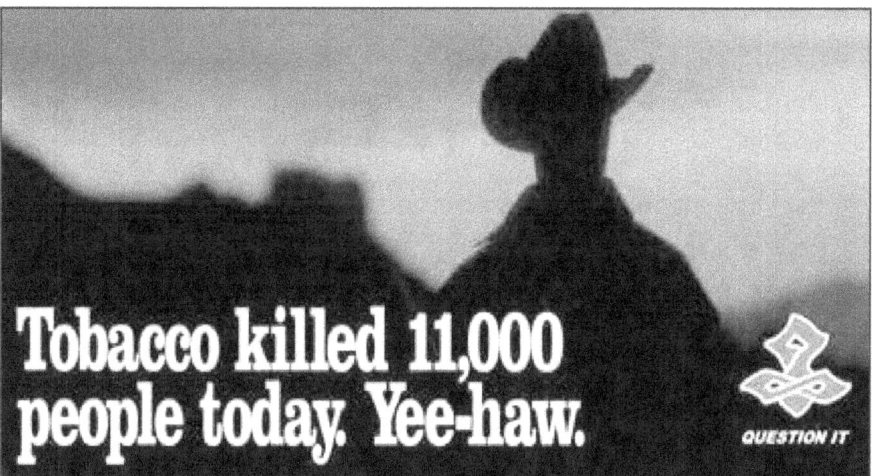

In *Principles of Marketing*, Kotler and Armstrong (2001) discuss two elements of advertising strategy: messages and media. A message should be designed to change an attitude or tell people something they don't already know. Media—TV, radio, newspapers, billboards, or some other outlet—are the channels used to expose people to the message. (See the Creative and Exposure sections later in this chapter for information about choosing media.)

The Message

What makes a tobacco control message effective? This is a hot topic debated among the tobacco control community. No single message can claim to be the silver bullet for every audience in every state. Perhaps the most effective messages have yet to be developed, but some messages have already shown promise with at least one type of audience. Several message strategies are commonly used in tobacco control. You should test messages with your audiences before you decide whether your assumptions about what might work are correct. The brief descriptions here may help you to decide on the messages that are worth testing with the audiences you select for your state program.

Health effects. The oldest and most obvious appeal in tobacco control is the argument that tobacco is bad for your health. It's the message the Surgeon General's warning carries on every pack of cigarettes. Messages range in intensity: some emphasize death, and others focus on sickness. The message can come as statistics, graphics, pictures, personal testimonials, or a combination of these forms. What makes the messages similar is the underlying logic: Health effect messages try to communicate, and often dramatize, the health risks of smoking or chewing tobacco. Some messages on health effects focus on the long term (having a shorter life or an agonizing death) while others focus on the short term (health effects suffered while one is young). Although their logic may seem counterintuitive, some researchers argue that for many smokers, especially teens and young adults, the idea of living with the effects of smoking is more frightening than the thought of dying from them.

The approach that emphasizes health effects is criticized by some people as ineffective. They argue that even though most people today know tobacco is unsafe, many still smoke. However, health concerns are probably what led to the substantial drop in cigarette use after the first Surgeon General's report on smoking and health, in 1964. Health concerns also probably led to the subsequent decline in smoking after the "Fairness Doctrine"[1] advertising from 1967 through 1970, which broadly communicated tobacco's health effects for the first time (USDHHS 1989). Today it's important to present health-risk information that is new or that comes from a novel, insightful perspective. One example of this approach is California's recent campaign linking tobacco use to impotence. The new information in this campaign alarmed some men and caused them to think about their tobacco use differently. Another example is the "Every Cigarette Is Doing You Damage" campaign from Australia. The campaign was aired in six countries, and data from follow-up research supported the effectiveness of the campaign in at least five of those countries. In this campaign, graphic visuals of a rotting lung, a brain with a blood clot, a clogged artery, and a developing tumor were coupled with the news that every cigarette smoked can contribute to similar damage. Other examples of the health effects approach are the testimonial ads developed and aired by many states and other countries. These ads poignantly describe the physical and emotional tolls that tobacco has taken on real-life smokers and their families, in the words of those individuals. The ads personalize the health effects and make them relevant to smokers and their friends and families. One caveat when using the health effects approach is that people sometimes don't believe dramatizations that are overexaggerated or are too removed from what they see every day or what they can imagine.

Secondhand smoke. Perhaps the most widely used strategy today focuses on the dangers of

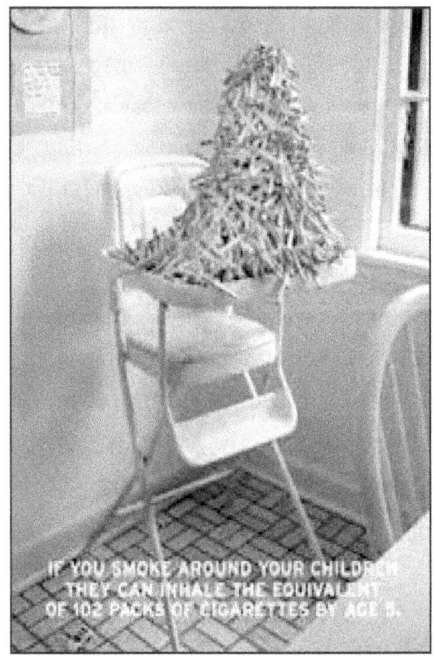

---

[1] The Fairness Doctrine was an agreement within the broadcast industry to air one antitobacco message for every three protobacco advertisements aired. As a result, significant levels of media presence for tobacco counter-advertising messages were reached for the first time for long enough to achieve a high level of awareness.

exposure to secondhand smoke. For more than a decade, counter-marketing programs across the country have communicated and dramatized the health effects of secondhand smoke on nonsmokers—to encourage smokers to protect their loved ones, discourage smoking in public places, and support policy initiatives, such as smokefree workplaces. California relied heavily on these types of messages in its successful push to support some of the nation's strongest statewide tobacco control policies, such as smokefree bars and restaurants. These messages encourage nonsmokers to question a behavior that decades of tobacco advertising have tried to frame as a norm. Secondhand smoke messages also have been found to encourage smoking cessation because smokers have fewer places to smoke, fewer people will permit a smoker to light up around them, and fewer smokers want to smoke around friends and family. The strategy also counters the tobacco industry's claim that smoking is an "individual choice."

Industry manipulation. This strategy aims to reveal to potential and current smokers how the tobacco industry uses manipulative and deceptive practices to win new customers and maintain current ones, regardless of the health consequences. These messages often talk about the industry's advertising tactics, profit motives, history of targeting children, and efforts to downplay or simply deny the health dangers of smoking. One common message is that the industry targets teens as "replacement smokers" to take the place of smokers who have died. An early California ad using this approach is one of the most memorable TV spots the state tobacco control program has ever produced.

Repositioning. Aimed at teens, this approach is a close cousin of industry manipulation, but its messages are part of a larger strategy that not only repositions the tobacco industry as a manipulative adult institution, but also gives tobacco control advocates an opportunity to take on the role of hip rebels. The goal is to undermine two benefits offered by cigarette brands popular with teens—rebellion and independence—and to offer those benefits to nonsmokers. Florida took this approach by creating and branding an edgy, rebellious anti-tobacco effort called "truth." Although teens actually played a large role in directing the campaign, much of the work and development needed to be performed by the health department and its contractors. By making the campaign appear to be organized entirely by hip teens, however, this effort repositioned the "truth" movement, and thus nonsmoking, as young and hip, while making smoking seem old and corporate. This strategy is now the basis of the national "truth" campaign funded by the American Legacy Foundation.

Defining the norm. Because most people don't smoke, some programs use the "follow-the-crowd" approach to let people know that smokers are in the minority. One TV spot, for example, informed teens that three of four teenagers don't smoke. The theory is that teens sometimes consider smoking because they think everyone is doing it. They're conforming to a perceived social norm. These messages

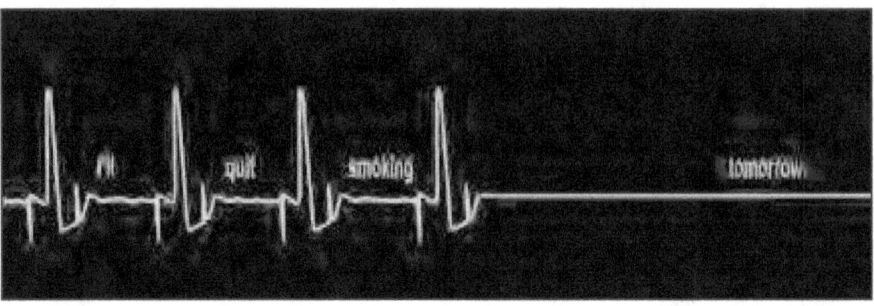

simply deflate the myth that "everyone is doing it." In addition, showing that nonsmokers are the majority may empower them to speak up about secondhand smoke. On the other hand, critics of this approach worry that some independent and more rebellious teens might be attracted to smoking, because most people don't do it.

Social consequences. Messages on social consequences consider how tobacco use might affect a person's social standing, dating opportunities, and other situations. Although teens are concerned with social consequences, messages from state health departments about social consequences in the teen culture face the same credibility challenges that parents of teens often face. One tactic to address this challenge is featuring older and seemingly hip teens as spokespeople, which gives them an authentic voice. Some states are also beginning to look at the social consequences in a global sense, considering tobacco's impact on issues such as child labor, the environment, and poverty in the developing world.

Chemical disclosure. Another strategy is to tell people about the chemicals in cigarette smoke or about the hundreds of chemical additives in cigarettes. This advertising typically tries to dramatize the implications of being exposed to the deadly chemicals known to be associated with smoking. One TV spot showed a family drinking these chemicals from beakers. Another ad interviewed professionals who worked with toxic chemicals and used protective clothing to shield themselves from those chemicals. The message highlighted their shock that the same chemicals were found in secondhand smoke inhaled every day by many people, who are unprotected from its effects.

Addiction. Several programs have attempted to illustrate the power of nicotine addiction: Once someone decides to smoke, that decision isn't always easy to reverse. One difficulty with this strategy is the message it sends to current smokers. After hearing these messages, some smokers may believe cessation attempts are hopeless. Making the addiction claim convincing for youth also has been a challenge. In focus groups, even teens who acknowledge that nicotine is addictive don't always seem to understand what that means. "Once I feel I'm getting addicted," one teen said, "I'll quit." An addiction message may be better used to supplement another message. For example, addiction has been mentioned in industry manipulation to emphasize how tobacco companies recruit "customers for life." The power of addiction also is noted often in smoking cessation messages.

Heroes and celebrities. Many tobacco control ads use famous actors, musicians, models, and athletes in the same way that commercial brands use these celebrities: to associate the product (i.e., the behavior of not smoking) with someone who is loved and admired. These heroes and celebrities have included supermodel Christy Turlington, actor Esai Morales, the musical group Boyz II Men, and the national women's soccer team. Celebrities can also attract news media. However, it's important to carefully select the heroes and celebrities to use as spokespeople, because working with them can have downsides. They can quickly fall from popularity, may suddenly become bad role models by adopting the behaviors you're trying to change in the target audience, may command significant fees, and often demand a lot of creative control.

Role models. Another strategy focuses on how adults and older teens are role models themselves, most commonly to their children and younger siblings, respectively. The essential message is that if you decide to smoke, others will follow. One ad shows a couple peering into their bedroom, where their children are playing dress up and are pretending to be adults. The couple is aghast when they see the children pretend to smoke, copying their behavior. This approach has been used with populations such as African Americans, Asians, and Hispanics/Latinos in which family connections are often very important. Counter-marketing programs have also used the role model theme to promote tobacco control advocacy. The "truth" campaign, both in Florida and nationally, under the American Legacy Foundation, showed teens taking a stand against tobacco advertising. One Florida ad featured teens ripping tobacco ads from magazines. Another ad, developed by Massachusetts, told the story of a group of teens who pressured a mall to go smokefree.

Cosmetic effects. Like messages about social consequences, messages about the effects of tobacco use are more about appearance than health. Put simply, tobacco use can be disgusting. Messages about cosmetic effects rely on people's concern about their appearance. By dramatizing consequences such as yellow teeth or cigarette breath, such messages tell an audience that tobacco makes them less appealing. Some messages emphasize the results of these effects: A Massachusetts ad shows an attractive teenage girl talking about how smokers turn her off. However, experts debate the efficacy of this approach. In focus groups, teens often say they can mask these effects of cigarettes with perfume, with breath mints, or in some other way.

Refusal skills or individual choice. Campaigns centered on refusal skills or individual choice, which nearly always target youth, typically show a teenager or group of teenagers discussing their own decisions not to smoke. These ads try to build credibility by appearing to respect a teen's ability to make an individual choice about tobacco use. Philip Morris (now renamed as Altria), the maker of the nation's most popular cigarette, Marlboro, created the largest and best known individual choice campaign, which carried the tag line: "Think. Don't Smoke." Qualitative and quantitative research on ads from that campaign showed that those ads didn't perform as well as ads from tobacco control campaigns using other approaches. Qualitative research demonstrated that individual choice ads developed by state programs did not perform well either. Survey respondents thought that giving youth the choice to smoke without giving them good rationale for not smoking (e.g., information on health effects) was not a strong or helpful message and would cause some youth to choose to smoke. (More information about the quantitative research is available from the American Legacy Foundation's First Look Report 9, *Getting to the Truth: Assessing Youths' Reactions to the "truth" and "Think. Don't Smoke" Tobacco Countermarketing Campaigns* (2002).

Smoking cessation. A number of messages have been used to encourage people to quit smoking or call a hotline to help them quit. Many use the messages described earlier with a twist that will appeal to certain smokers, such as telling parents about the dangers to their children of secondhand smoke or graphically exposing for pack-a-day smokers the health effects of their smoking. In some cases, ads to promote smoking cessation emphasize the health benefits of quitting as opposed to the dangers of continued use of tobacco. Also, cessation ads sometimes focus on efficacy, recognizing that it is difficult but very possible to stop smoking. Occasionally, these ads offer tips on how to quit. The most successful cessation ads nearly always include an easy-to-remember number for quitline services that are supported by well-qualified staff.

By jointly agreeing to a copy strategy with your creative agency, you have logic against which to judge particular advertising products. One way to do this is to determine which strategies are likely to work best, test them with your audience, and then select the strategy that seems the most powerful. Try to capture the approach in a short and simple statement, perhaps a single sentence. For example, a statement that sets direction for a secondhand smoke ad could say:

> To increase support from nonsmokers for restrictions on tobacco use in homes and public places, we will show nonsmokers how secondhand smoke endangers them.

An ad focused solely on the health dangers to smokers, as opposed to nonsmokers, would be off strategy when it comes to this objective. It might be interesting and even frightening to nonsmokers, but a message that smoking is dangerous for smokers isn't based on the logic of the message strategy on secondhand smoke. If you don't stick to your strategy, you're not giving the strategy you developed a chance to work.

You may have several copy strategies aimed at different audiences, but try not to create too many for each audience. Too many messages aimed at the same audience can have the result that no single message reaches the audience

Designing and Implementing an Effective Tobacco Counter-Marketing Campaign

enough times to make a difference. Attitudes are changed only after people are repeatedly exposed to the same basic message. To stick to the strategy without wearing out a particular ad or message, you'll probably want to illustrate the same message in different ways. You can produce or reuse different creative executions that carry the same basic message. You may want to use various media vehicles (communication channels), knowing they'll work synergistically to strengthen the message's impact. A vehicle is a route or method used to reach a target audience with a message. Examples of media vehicles are TV, radio, the Internet, bus signs, billboards, brochures, and notepads in physicians' offices.

Context of the Message

You should also consider the context of your message. You're not the only one talking to your audience. Your target audiences are being exposed to hundreds of messages every

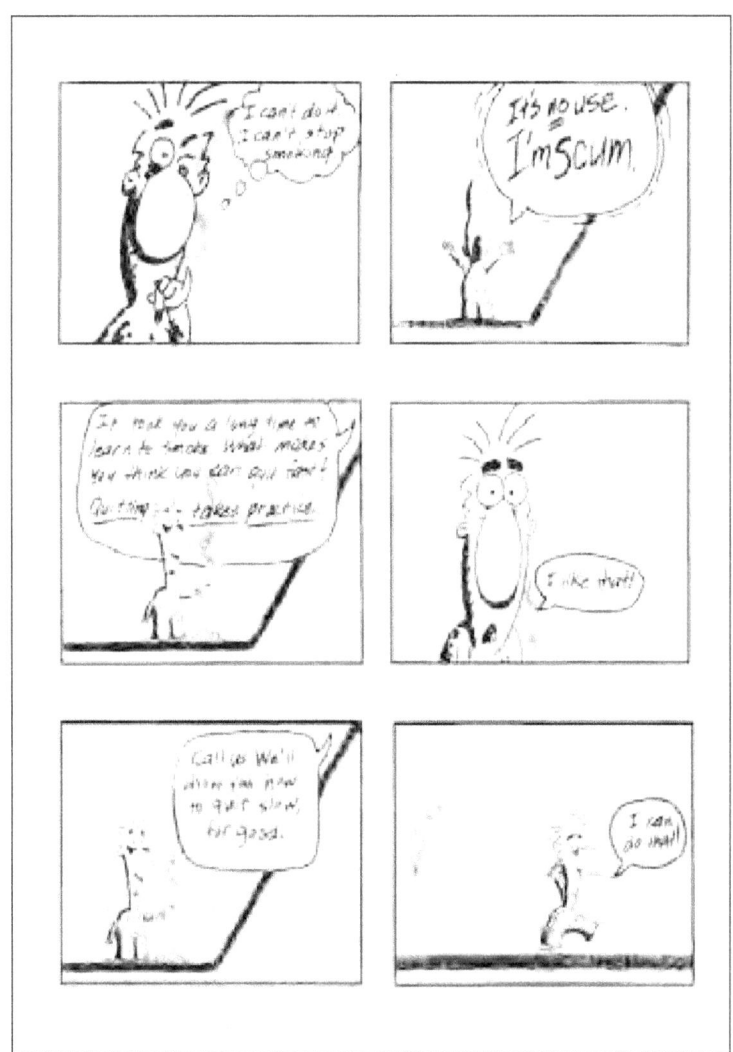

day. Some may directly pertain to tobacco. Others may not mention tobacco, but still may influence what your audience thinks is right, fashionable, or simply believable. These other messages will affect how the audience receives your message.

People consider information from many sources when they form opinions. Your audience may already be hearing from the tobacco industry, voluntary health organizations (e.g., the American Cancer Society), and the American Legacy Foundation, which is the antitobacco foundation created by the national settlement with the tobacco industry. Each campaign may have a different message, and your target audience may not recall who is saying what. For example, your audience may think the state health department's antitobacco program and the Philip Morris youth smoking prevention effort are the same campaign.

You can't coordinate everyone's messages, but you can consider how your effort might fit. For example, Legacy's "truth" campaign is spending heavily to reach teens and young adults with industry manipulation and repositioning messages. Instead of competing for teens' attention, you could choose to support this strategy, not with additional ads but with on-the-ground marketing efforts, such as the creation of youth antitobacco groups or "collateral materials" (promotional and other items such as T-shirts, posters, and fliers) to be used by interested teens. (See Chapter 10: Grassroots Marketing for more about promoting youth activism.) Or you may choose to target adults with messages that focus on changing norms around secondhand smoke or on cessation, both of which are likely to contribute to lower youth tobacco use over time.

Creative: Breaking Through the Clutter

Once you've explored various message strategies for the target audience and determined the one you believe has the most potential to influence the audience as desired, you'll begin working toward creative development of ads. Instead of developing ads, you may decide to save time and resources and reapply previously produced ads from other states, organizations, or countries. Although some parts of this section are relevant both to ad reapplication and developing new ads (for example, the process you will go through in critiquing ads), this section focuses mainly on topics relevant ONLY to developing new advertising. It's not an easy task to effectively translate your chosen message strategy into creative concepts and then to produce ads based on those concepts. This task requires a high level of strategic discipline and teamwork between you and the ad agency, with all parties contributing their talents to the effort.

In advertising, details matter as much as message strategy. Two TV spots might share the same message strategy and even the same script but may be executed very differently. Who is talking and how they present themselves will affect the impact of the final ad. Is this a message from the band 98 Degrees or from the governor? One might be more credible defining what's cool to teens; the other might be more credible with parents. Even

Table 7.1: Pros and Cons of Advertising Media

Format	Pros	Cons
TV Spots		
TV spots are usually 15, 30, or 60 seconds long. Most run 30 seconds. The longer spots are more expensive to air.	• Reach a broad audience • Deliver audiovisual impact • Have a flexible format	• Expensive to air • Fleeting exposure • Insufficient time for complex explanations • Typically expensive to produce new ads
Radio Spots		
Paid radio spots are typically 60 seconds long; public service announcements tend to be 30 seconds long. You can also use live announcer scripts ("live copy ads").	• Are cheaper than TV spots • Can typically have a narrower target than TV spots • Can be produced quickly • Are typically longer than TV spots, allowing more complex messages	• Audio impact only • Narrow reach per station
Print Ads		
Print ads run in newspapers, magazines, and student publications and can be one-quarter or one-half page or a full page.	• Reach a specific audience, often including opinion leaders • Have short lead time (newspapers) and immediate impact	• Very short life span • Compete in cluttered advertising environment • Youth and people of lower economic status often missed • Long lead time (magazines)
Outdoor Ads		
Ads include billboards and signs on storefronts, buses, trains, and benches.	• Can reinforce messages placed elsewhere (e.g., TV or radio) • Can repeatedly expose commuters to message • Can be inexpensive (e.g., transit space) • Can give high exposure	• Limited message space • Damage from weather and graffiti • Difficult to target narrowly (Everyone will see it.)

Continues

Table 7.1: Pros and Cons of Advertising Media (cont.)

Format	Pros	Cons
Point-of-Purchase Ads		
Ads are placed in stores where tobacco is sold.	• Can counter tobacco advertising where the product is bought	• Difficult to place (Tobacco industry is major point-of-purchase advertiser.)
Movie Trailers and Slides		
Ads appear in video or still photos shown before a movie begins.	• Target frequent moviegoers (e.g., teens) • Can have high impact and may serve to "inoculate" viewers against images of people smoking in movies	• Production and placement of trailers can be expensive (Production costs can be saved by using an existing TV spot.) • Targeting of specific kinds of movies not usually allowed by theaters • Ad trailers not allowed by some film distributors
Print Materials		
Many programs use informational brochures; some aim materials at a specific market.	• Can be inexpensive to produce • Have longer life • Allow large amount of message space	• Not an "interruption" medium. (Target audiences must want to read materials.) • Dissemination required • Possibility of duplicates to the same individuals
Web Banners		
"Click-through" banners can link commercial and partner Web sites to a program.	• Broaden exposure on new media • Can be inexpensive	• "Click-through" rates typically low • Pop-up ads considered annoying distractions by most people • Small message space
Web Sites		
Many programs build Web sites; some sites are aimed at specific audiences.	• Can be relatively inexpensive • Are constantly present • Have unlimited message area • Can be updated quickly	• Need to drive traffic to Web sites • Compete with a large number of other sites • Maintenance and monitoring often required

Table 7.1: Pros and Cons of Advertising Media (cont.)

Format	Pros	Cons
Sponsorships		
Payments are made in return for promotion as a sponsor of a concert, sports contest, or other event. The goal is to create a positive image for the campaign by associating it with something perceived as popular or attractive by the target audience.	• Are typically turnkey promotional opportunities in which you can pay for services of staff to handle the event • Associate program's "brand" with well-liked celebrities, brands, or events	• Possibly expensive • Perception of negative association by some audiences • Creation of expectation of continued support that may not be possible • More limited reach than mass media
Collateral Materials		
Programs may create promotional materials (e.g., T-shirts, key chains, and refrigerator magnets).	• Can provide continued but limited exposure to target audience • Benefits people involved in activities	• Distribution required • High cost for limited exposure

what people wear can make a difference. In Florida's "truth" campaign, for example, the real Florida teens recruited for TV spots changed clothes before they went on the air. The program's ad agency worked with a wardrobe expert to select clothing that was more hip than the teens' own clothes.

Producing good creative is an art form. Beyond sending a clear message, advertising must be salient and interesting. The audience should feel understood and respected. Advertising can be tested to determine which concepts or finished ads have the highest likelihood of success, but just how it may work in the real world is always partly a mystery. The artistic expertise for which the creative firms are hired must be valued and appreciated, but it also must be balanced with the tobacco control experience and technical expertise that you bring to the process. You are ultimately responsible for ensuring that the ads that are approved have the highest likelihood of contributing to your tobacco control goal.

Managers evaluate potential advertising in different ways. The key is to think broadly and avoid nitpicking any product to meet your personal tastes. If you relate everything to what you know about your audience and your strategy, you can provide the creative firm with the needed perspective. Consider four key questions:

1. **Is the creative product something you can disseminate effectively to your audience?**
   For example, you may not want to produce

a TV spot if you don't have much money for a media buy; instead, radio might be a more cost-efficient option.

2. **Is the creative product on strategy?** For example, the product shouldn't dwell solely on health effects if your strategy is industry manipulation.

3. **Does the product reflect what you know about your audience?** Think about whether it communicates persuasively to your audience. Will they understand it? Will they feel understood? Is it persuasive? Will the audience respond to the actors in terms of age, diversity, and attitude?

4. **Might unintended negative consequences occur?** Advertising exposure can't be tightly controlled; other audiences will be exposed to these products. Consider the implications of that scenario. For example, teens who view a message aimed at adults about how many teens are smoking might begin to see smoking as the norm.

Types of Creative

Work with your creative firm to decide what kinds of products to use. Will billboards work? Should you buy radio time? What about a brochure? Does your budget allow for this advertising? The creative firm should present you with a plan to use several different types of advertising materials in a campaign. The materials should complement one another to completely reach members of your target audience, whether they watch TV, read newspapers, or only see billboards. (See Table 7.1 for a list of the most common types of advertising and the benefits and drawbacks associated with each product.)

Table 7.1 lists only some of the types of advertising available. Advertising messages are placed everywhere these days, from a banner flown above a beach to the well of a urinal. Your job is to determine the most appropriate and cost-efficient place for the audience to see your message, so it's clear, widely viewed, persuasive, and without unintended negative consequences.

You should also consider using creative materials that already exist. Even states with large campaigns that produce a large percentage of their own materials (e.g., California, Florida, and Massachusetts) have borrowed advertising executions from other states and countries. To help states share materials, the CDC Media Campaign Resource Center (MCRC) maintains an inventory of existing tobacco counter-advertising materials developed by a number of states, organizations, and federal agencies. By providing access to existing advertising materials, the resource center allows states, organizations, and government agencies to save the time and high cost of producing new ads. The MCRC collection includes ads for TV, radio, print, and outdoor use that address a variety of themes and target audiences. In addition, the MCRC negotiates rights and talent fees to simplify the process of using the ads in different states. (More information and a searchable database are available on the MCRC Web site, http://www.cdc.gov/tobacco/mcrc).

> **Media Campaign Resource Center**
>
> *E-mail:* **mcrc@cdc.gov**
>
> *Phone:* **(770) 488-5705, press 2**
>
> *Web site:* **www.cdc.gov/tobacco/mcrc**

In general, you'll want to select vehicles with the lowest cost per thousand audience members potentially reached (CPM). However, CPM should be balanced with the need for high-quality exposure. For example, showing ads to promote smoking cessation in a physician's waiting room may have a high cost and low overall reach, but the exposures are very high quality, because you have a captive audience consisting of people preparing to talk to their physician about their health.

Pretesting Creative

Advertising can be very expensive. Producing a high-quality, 30-second TV spot by using union talent can easily cost more than $250,000. Airing the spot can cost much, much more, so before major advertisers invest money in airing or placing an ad, they typically test it to determine whether it clearly conveys the intended message.

Pretesting can be performed at several stages in the creative process. You can pretest a concept, a script, a rough cut of a broadcast spot, or a storyboard (visuals and words that portray the actions in a proposed TV spot). (See Appendices 7.2 and 7.3 for sample storyboards.) Also, the finished ad itself can be used in a pretest. Pretesting won't tell you whether the ad will "work"; you'll find that out only after you place the ad and measure attitudinal changes or other results in the context of your entire campaign. However, pretesting can give you important information about whether your intended message is being communicated clearly to your target audience. The most common conclusions you can draw from pretesting are:

- **Overall reaction.** How is the ad likely to make the audience feel?

- **Communication of a message.** What message is your audience likely to take away from the ad?

- **Likes and dislikes.** What parts of the ad are likely to please or anger your audience?

- **Confusing aspects.** What parts of the ad are likely to confuse your audience?

- **Credibility.** Is your audience likely to find the ad believable?

- **Relevance.** Does the audience think this is a message for "people like them"? Does it apply to their lives?

- **Perceived motivational aspects.** Is your audience likely to think the ad will prompt them to change anything? Do they find the ad convincing? (Attempting to measure the ad's potential influence can be very misleading. People don't like to admit that advertising might affect their behavior. What's more, the ad may only need to affect an attitude as part of an overall program that will change behavior.)

Some pretesting efforts use larger sample sizes and try to measure people's intention to change behavior. On the opposite extreme, some pretesting can be abbreviated as a qualitative communication check. The testing measures whether the "take-away" (messages and impressions left with the audience after viewing of the ad) was what you intended.

Before you pretest, decide what you need to learn. You need to be realistic about what you can learn and whether you're learning something that can be the basis for some action. Don't ignore the results of your pretesting, but rather use them in your decision making.

As a program manager, you can require your creative firm to pretest (1) some or all of the ads you're considering for use in the counter-marketing campaign, (2) only the ads targeted at a specific group, or (3) only the ads that you believe could pose problems. You can also decide at what stage the testing would be most useful. The testing can be performed by the creative firm, a subcontractor to the creative firm, or another contractor you hire separately. Some people worry that creative firms won't test their own creative products fairly, but good firms know it's to their advantage to honestly pretest their products to find problems before they're widely distributed. You should understand and agree to the testing methods selected. You'll also want to observe the research, if possible, and fully understand the analysis. Firsthand observations will better prepare you to fight for the production of an ad or defend it once it's produced. (See Chapter 3: Gaining and Using Target Audience Insights for more information on pretesting.) You and the agency should be partners in the planning and execution of the research and in drawing conclusions from the results.

Creating a Standard Review Process

The final version of a creative product should not surprise you. A TV spot, magazine ad, or other creative product should be the result of a

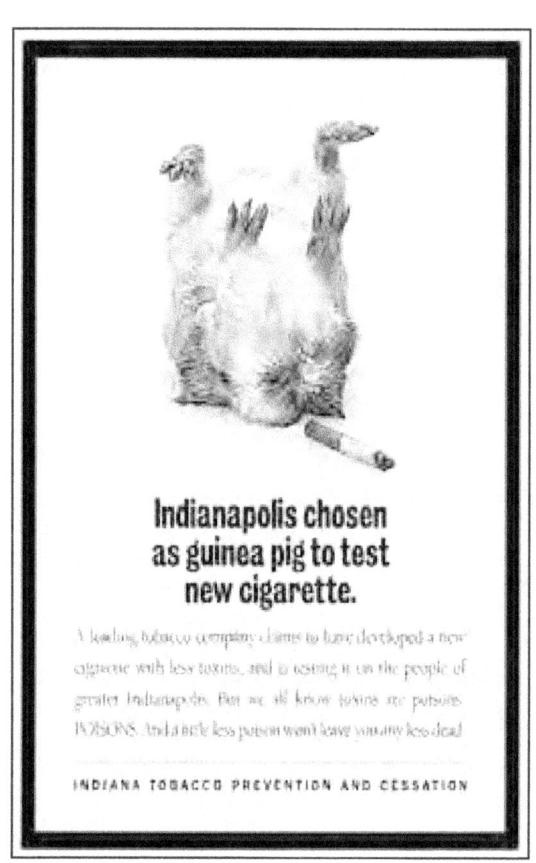

joint effort by the creative firm and you. Again, as a program manager, your role is to continually evaluate whether the product is persuasive and on strategy, can be disseminated to your audience, reflects what you know about your audience, and is not likely to cause unintended negative consequences.

You can make these judgments at several points in the creative process. You and your creative firm should agree on when your review is necessary. A list and discussion of the milestones for reviewing a TV spot are provided here. The TV spot is one of the more complicated and costly products a creative firm can produce and place. The process is similar for other creative products, such as print ads and radio spots. You may not have time to perform every step for every creative product, but you and your creative firm can decide jointly when your input would be most valuable.

The milestones are as follows:

- Read the creative brief.
- Review the scripts or storyboards.
- Attend pretesting focus groups or interviews.
- Attend or listen in on the preproduction meeting.
- Attend the shoot.
- View the first cut.
- View and approve the edited spot.

Read the creative brief. The first thing you should review when overseeing the production of a TV spot is the creative brief. You may even want to be involved in helping write the creative brief. Some ad agencies consider the creative brief to be an internal function of the ad agency, developed by agency planners and account staff, and shared exclusively with the creatives. However, you have the right and responsibility to ensure that it's strategically focused and communicates the key information and insights the creatives will need to do their work. This is the document that tells the agency's writers and artists—the people who create the ad—what you want. Because the function of the creative brief is to translate your strategy into specific guidelines for the creative team, you may want to help develop it or at least review it before it goes to the creative staff. (See Appendix 6.3: Elements of a Creative Brief and Appendices 6.4, 6.5, and 6.6 for samples of creative briefs.)

Review the scripts or storyboards. After the creative brief is shared with the creatives, they'll develop ideas for creative executions (e.g., the script or storyboards for a TV spot; see Appendices 7.2 and 7.3 for sample storyboards). The creative executions may be presented to you in a meeting. When you review the script or storyboard and see the intended visuals, think about how your audience might react and whether these creative concepts accomplish what you set out to do in the creative brief. This task won't always be easy. At first, you may not see how the proposed ad can accomplish your goal. Some advertising executions cannot be interpreted literally. In all cases, the firm should be able to explain how the ad can accomplish the goal(s) you set out in the creative brief. (See Appendix 7.1 for help in organizing your comments and questions about the creative concepts.) Raise any concerns you have about taste, language, or how you see the ad taking shape. Are the visuals reinforcing what's being said? Is the language appropriate and understandable for this audience? Is there anything that might unnecessarily offend the audience or mislead people? As the content expert, you must ensure that the "facts" in the ad are true and can be substantiated.

Attend pretesting focus groups or interviews. At this stage, the scripts and storyboards can be presented to members of your target audience to get their reactions. You should observe the pretesting to be sure that the audience understands the messages and finds the ad concepts relevant and clear. If you can't attend the testing, read the transcripts or the report of the findings, watch the video, or listen to the audiotape. The agency personnel (e.g., account service, research and planning, and creative staff) should also attend the sessions. You may also want other members of your staff to attend. Consider inviting key stakeholders to observe focus groups of specific populations that they represent. Even though these stakeholders share many characteristics with the specific population, they may differ in significant ways (such as education or income), and observing a focus group may help them to better understand the participants.

You may wish to pretest again after production of the TV spot, because storyboards don't always adequately convey the experience of seeing the finished ad. You can also pretest using animatics or a rough version of a spot or print ad. One caveat is that some creative concepts don't lend themselves well to focus group testing of a storyboard. For example, an ad that relies on clever special effects or a testimonial ad that relies on the candid emotions of a person negatively affected by tobacco use may not be convincing or engaging in focus groups where those special elements are missing. In these cases, you won't be able to judge the persuasiveness of the ad concepts, but you still should be able to determine whether the audience understood the messages and found them relevant.

Attend or listen in on the preproduction meeting. Shortly before the production of an ad (the shoot), a preproduction meeting is held for the agency's creative staff to meet with the people who will actually produce the spot. They discuss locations, wardrobe, talent, and other production issues. The meeting is often held where the shoot will take place. If you can't be there in person, it's a good idea to join the meeting by phone. Most production decisions are probably best left to the agency and the production crew, but occasionally you may want to address certain issues. For example, you would raise an objection if they were planning something you think might offend the audience or might not be appropriate for your campaign. If you have questions or concerns, don't be afraid to raise them. It's much harder to make changes once the shoot is complete.

Attend the shoot. Many marketing managers attend the filming of the ad (the shoot), though it's not a necessity. Your role usually will be limited, but your attendance will be more important in cases where you need to weigh in on unanticipated issues. For example, Florida and Minnesota developed ads using video of unscripted teens criticizing the industry's practices. It was important for the marketing manager to be present because the script was essentially being written and approved on the spot.

View the first cut. After the shoot and some editing, the agency can show you a rough cut of the production that may not yet include all the edits or production enhancements the creative firm is planning, such as color correction, sound adjustment, sound effects, and music. This step will give you a chance to review the spot before the creative firm invests a lot of time and money in postproduction processes. The agency can tell you what can be changed at this point. If you have concerns about some aspect(s) of the ad, you may also want to test the ad with the target audience to see if your concerns are valid. Sometimes ads are produced and never aired. This may seem wasteful, but it's smarter than spending a lot more money buying time to air an ineffective or offensive ad that will cause you problems. Many veteran marketers can tell you about an ad that never ran and how happy they are that it didn't run.

View and approve the edited spot. You should always review the version of the spot that you intend to air but try to avoid having to get clearance from a large number of people. Everyone is a critic, and sometimes it's difficult to remind your superiors that what really matters is how the audience sees the spot, not how it's viewed inside your department or agency.

In many states, a large number of reviews can't be avoided. Try to remind every reviewer what the ad is supposed to do and which audience it's intended to reach. Use the pretesting results to support the relevance of the message to your audience.

In the end, your role in the creative process is one of quality control. You're not a critic, an editor, or an artist, but you are the person ultimately responsible for ensuring that your advertising is on strategy and effective with the intended audience. You may not even like the ad. That's okay. You just need to believe it will work.

Exposure: Show the Message Enough for It to Sink In

Great advertising is worthless if nobody sees it. A program manager or marketing manager needs to ensure that the right people get the

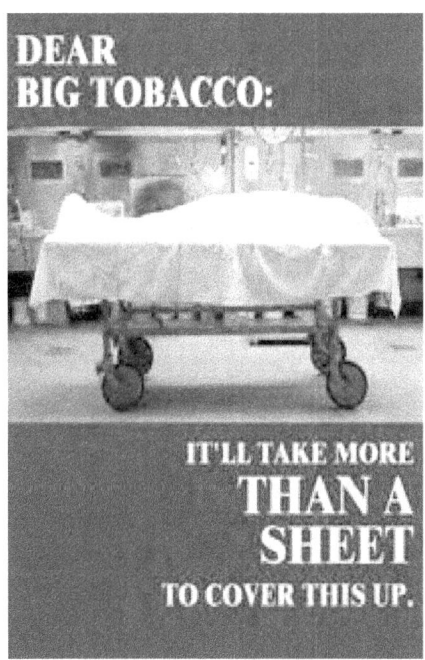

right message multiple times. You need your target audience to become familiar enough with your message that it raises awareness, changes an attitude, or prompts action. This means they have to see it more than once. Many advertising experts say that, in general, people won't even remember a commercial unless they've seen it at least three times. Others contend that TV spots must be seen three to seven times to be effective. In reality, the success of an ad largely depends on the quality of the creative execution and production. There are no set criteria, but one thing is for sure: Once is not enough.

Advertising is not a vaccine. In a global review of smoking cessation campaigns by CDC and the World Health Organization, successful cessation efforts required both a "strong" and "ongoing" media presence. When levels of advertising drop, so do the calls to cessation helplines. You can expect levels of ad awareness to mirror the schedule of your media buys. Awareness may be high while TV spots are on the air, but it will likely drop once the ads stop running.

You also need to think about when and how you reach your audience. The fact that you *can* reach the audience with your message at a certain time and through a certain channel does not mean you always should. For example, you might not want to run an ad on breast cancer during a Sunday football game. It's a bad "aperture" for a media message on breast cancer, because football fans aren't likely to change their thinking from rooting for a team to considering how the disease might affect them or their spouses. When Florida launched its rebellious youth antitobacco brand, the state could have disseminated its message in schools. After all, where better to reach teens? But the state shunned that dissemination approach. If teachers and principals promoted the "truth" brand, program managers reasoned, it would seem anything but young, cool, and rebellious. The approach would undermine the brand's value, and in the process, the strategy.

Exposure is usually measured by reach and frequency, which are typically translated into "rating points." A rating point is the percentage of the target audience potentially reached (reach) multiplied by the number of times the audience will potentially see the message (frequency). If, on the basis of your media buy, 50 percent of the targeted audience is expected to see your ad an average of three times, you've purchased 150 target rating points (TRPs). (The term target rating points is meant to convey that the rating points are specifically for your target audience.) Rating points are usually expressed in four-week figures, but you must always ask to be sure. An agency may add rating points together over a longer or shorter period. For example, an agency may talk about buying 1,200 rating points during the launch of your campaign. That statement may mean 300 points a week for four weeks or 150 points over eight weeks.

You may also hear media planners refer to "gross rating points" (GRPs). By definition, both GRPs and TRPs represent the total amount of rating points bought over a period of time in relation to an audience. Typically, a planner will use GRPs or TRPs to represent

Designing and Implementing an Effective Tobacco Counter-Marketing Campaign

rating points for your target audience, not rating points for a general audience, but you need to check to make sure.

Rating points vary depending on which audience is being targeted. For example, "Sabrina the Teenage Witch," a TV show produced by Warner Bros. Television Network, would have much higher rating points for adolescent girls than for 40-year-old men, and network news would have higher rating points for retirees than for teenagers.

Because buying media is so expensive, programs typically buy media in "flights" of three to six weeks, then go off the air for two to six weeks. If you're introducing a campaign, you should be on the air as continuously as possible during the first six to 12 months, and that strategy is even more important if you're trying to establish a brand. Awareness of the campaign will vary depending on how long a flight has been on the air, when it aired (e.g., time of day, season, programs), and how many flights were used over a period of time, but media are typically bought in a way that preserves some baseline level of awareness. Although ads are not on the air constantly, an effort is made to keep the program's message constantly in people's minds. The broadcast buy is supplemented by other vehicles, such as outdoor advertising, which is typically bought in month-long increments. These supplemental ads remain in place during the off weeks of a broadcast buy, and broadcast ads return to the airways before a dramatic dip in awareness occurs. You should be given a media flowchart (including dates, TRPs, and markets) that shows how each flight will take place for different audience segments. The media experts at your ad agency can advise you on how to maximize the impact of your budget.

Again, media messages aren't like inoculations: No audience becomes immune to an unhealthy behavior after a certain number of exposures to a message. Just as Coca-Cola must continue advertising even though the soft drink is very well known, tobacco control programs can't simply air a message, then disappear. A constant and evolving media program with new and engaging messages is needed to counter the competitive influences on the audience to smoke or chew tobacco.

How much exposure should you buy? That depends on your strategy, the stage of your campaign, the other counter-marketing activities, and your budget. Some strategies require more exposure than others. Some programs depend less on advertising and more on other interventions, such as smoking restrictions, education programs, or cigarette taxes. There's no one-size-fits-all formula.

Programs generally start with stronger media buys to win the audience's attention. When California launched the nation's first major tobacco counter-marketing campaign in 1990, the state was on the air almost continuously from April to November, buying 125 to 175 TRPs a week for adults and about 100 TRPs a week for teens. The program is now very well known inside the state, so media buys usually run three- or four-week flights of 100 to 150 TRPs per week, with breaks that last about a month.

"We have a maintenance level of 100 [TRPs] per week on the major networks," says Colleen Stevens, the program's marketing director. "If we have something new, we increase the buy to at least 150 [TRPs]. Admittedly, we'd like to air at higher TRP levels, but our budget doesn't allow for higher levels."

In some cases, the best guide to scaling your media buy is doing what commercial marketers with similar strategies do. When Florida decided to base its teen-targeted campaign on the creation of a hip, rebellious antitobacco brand, the state's ad agency looked at the media buys made during the launch of other youth brands. The state decided on a very aggressive buy, purchasing an average of 244 TRPs a week on TV alone for two months and supplementing this presence with radio ads.

Your creative firm's media-buying recommendation probably will be based largely on your budget. One reason Florida made such an aggressive buy was that the state could afford it. The state's tobacco settlement had specifically allocated tens of millions of dollars to the tobacco control program, about one-third of which was invested in marketing. Program staff also knew that many people were watching carefully to see whether the program would succeed.

It's probably a good idea to buy as much exposure as you can afford. If your strategy is sound, your message is effective, and your creative executions are clear and attention-getting, the only thing standing between your advertising and success is exposure.

Choosing a Media Approach: Paid Media, PSAs, and Earned Media

Typically, the most effective marketing campaigns use multiple communication approaches. This is true for selling soap, persuading drivers to buckle up, or encouraging people not to smoke around others. Paid advertising campaigns, public service announcement (PSA) campaigns, and "earned media" efforts all have advantages and drawbacks, but used in combination, they offer an opportunity to reach audiences with multiple yet complementary messages. In tobacco control, where significant media buys have been taking place for some time, this sort of combination approach is common.

Here's a look at these three approaches, along with discussions about using them in combination and using only PSAs and earned media when paid campaigns are too expensive.

Conducting a Paid Advertising Campaign

A paid advertising campaign is the most effective communication tool for reaching large audiences with a relatively simple message. It lets you target specific audiences with persuasive messages that can affect a person's awareness, attitudes, beliefs, and, potentially, behavior.

However, conducting a sustained paid advertising campaign is expensive. Successful paid media campaigns conducted by states have ranged in cost from approximately $.50 to $3.50 per capita a year, and a significant portion of those funds were for paid advertising.

A successful paid advertising campaign has a few key features:

- **Thorough campaign planning.** Before developing a paid media campaign, you must completely understand the members of your target audience, the messages that influence them, and how to reach them. You should outline the specific objectives you want to achieve and then determine which audiences, messages, and media vehicles are most appropriate for reaching those objectives.

- **Sufficient budget to achieve optimal levels of reach and frequency.** By working with a media planner, you can determine the levels of reach and frequency you can achieve with your budget. By analyzing what you can achieve with your resources, you can use them more effectively and efficiently. If you don't have the resources to conduct a paid advertising campaign properly, it may be better to use the resources on another form of communication or to limit the focus of the campaign to one target audience or one message strategy. When funding increases, you can focus more broadly. If you choose to focus very narrowly at first, you'll need to set expectations appropriately.

- **Advertising that is on strategy and breaks through ad clutter.** Spending millions of dollars on ad placement won't suffice if your advertising is off strategy or doesn't get noticed. Your ads must effectively communicate a message that will influence your target audience. Effectiveness can be determined by testing your commercials among the audience. With the amount of advertising in today's media vehicles, your ads must also stand out enough that the audience notices and remembers them, and they must be sufficiently persuasive to move the audience toward different beliefs, attitudes, and/or behaviors.

- **Initial, ongoing, and postcampaign evaluations.** To determine whether your campaign has achieved its objectives, you'll need to conduct multiple research studies. If possible, you should provide for:

    - A baseline measure of your audience's precampaign awareness, attitudes, beliefs, and behaviors

    - Midcampaign measures of your audience's response to the advertising and progress toward changing attitudes, beliefs, and other factors, so you can revise your ads or media strategy if necessary

    - A postcampaign evaluation to measure the results of your effort

Placing a Public Service Announcement

PSAs are typically useful only for reaching a general audience with a general message. Because stations are donating time, the sponsoring organization has no control over when, where, and how often the PSA airs. Tracking

Table 7.2: Media Characteristics

Paid Media	Public Service Announcement	Earned Media
Targeted	Not targeted	Somewhat targeted, but some audiences (e.g., low-literacy adults and teens) may be difficult to reach because they are not big consumers of news
Expensive to place	Inexpensive to place	Inexpensive to place
Total control of message	Nearly total control of message	Not much control of message but much more control when done well
Expensive to produce but existing ads can be reapplied inexpensively	Expensive to produce but existing ads can be reapplied inexpensively	Expense dependent on event or story Sometimes no financial cost other than time
Talent fees paid every 13 weeks	Talent fees paid yearly	No talent fees
Credibility depends on ad execution and audience's perspective	Credibility depends on ad execution and audience's perspective	Credibility typically greater for press stories than for ads Credibility somewhat dependent on media outlet

data from past PSA campaigns have shown that as many as one-half of PSAs are run late at night. This lack of control over the media placement makes PSAs ineffective for reaching specific or hard-to-reach audiences and makes their impact on audiences unreliable. PSAs are better used to raise the public's general awareness of an issue. For this reason, PSA placement is generally not recommended when states are trying to make a significant impact, unless they have no alternative because of funding limits.

You have a few options for trying to place your PSA. The Ad Council selects certain issues for which it will support the creative development and placement of PSAs. But the organizations selected must provide the funds to produce the ads, and often, only national organizations or national causes are chosen. You can also work directly with the public affairs directors at networks and local stations to persuade them to air your PSA.

PSAs are most successfully placed when they have the following characteristics:

- Strong public service appeal that will benefit most of the station's audience

- Local relevance to the station's viewing area (Relevance can be achieved by tagging the ad with a local organization's name, phone number, or both.)

- Coordinated as part of the bonus time of the paid portion of a campaign (See section on "Combining Approaches" later in this chapter.)

- High-quality production value

A little-known option for securing PSA placement is to work through state broadcasters' associations. These groups offer Non-Commercial Sustaining Announcement (NCSA) programs, in which you pay the association a fee to guarantee that your PSA will run. In one large state, for about $30,000 for a month-long program, the association will guarantee that 70 percent of its member TV and radio stations will each air the spot 15 times, with an equal split among prime time, daytime, and other times. This type of arrangement is officially considered PSA use, because the stations are donating the airtime. The program is available only to government agencies or nonprofit groups. At the end of the month, the association provides a performance report outlining when and where the ads ran. This option is often used when funding is insufficient to conduct a paid campaign.

Obtaining Earned Media

Having your campaign messages reported in the popular press can greatly enhance the effectiveness of your media campaign. This approach is called earned media, because your program staff must work diligently with reporters and editors to gain news media coverage of your issue. These efforts can give your campaign credibility and additional exposure. Because most audiences view news media content as more objective than advertising, they're often more receptive to the messages and perceive them as more credible. (See Chapter 8: Public Relations for in-depth discussion of earned media.)

How do you gain media coverage?

- **Identify the appropriate contacts within the media.** You can determine the appropriate contacts within the media by seeing who reports on your issue or by calling the news outlets. You may also want to note how the reporter frames the issue: Does he or she seem receptive to your message?

- **Establish yourself or your program as a resource for the media.** You can build a productive relationship with reporters and editors by providing data and background information. By positioning yourself as a resource for reporters and editors, you can help them in development of their stories. This relationship will increase the likelihood that they'll contact you when they're developing a future story on your issue.

- **Present newsworthy stories.** Mass media outlets are deluged with press releases and other suggestions for stories.

When you "pitch" a story to a media outlet, make sure the story has true value for its audience.

- **Provide supporting materials.** Doing the legwork for the writer or reporter will increase the chances of getting coverage of your story. Provide a press release, fact sheets, pictures, background information, video footage, short biographic sketches of key people, and other information, as appropriate.

- **Track your contacts with the media.** Keep notes each time you contact the media, listing the topics of your discussions, the information conveyed, the reporters and media contacted, and the angle used in covering your issue. This information will make your future efforts more effective.

Combining Approaches

As mentioned earlier, mass media campaigns work best when paid media campaigns, PSAs (primarily for cost-efficiency), and earned media are used together. In this scenario, the paid media campaign serves as the core tool for reaching your target audience(s) with a controlled, sustained message that is most likely to be influential. PSAs and earned media are then used to supplement the paid campaign by reaching secondary audiences and providing a broader context for your campaign.

With most paid media campaigns, you can negotiate bonus weight, which is extra media time or placements given free by the media outlets for your purchase of other media time or placements. This bonus time is usually given on shows for which the station hasn't sold all the advertising slots. Because you can't choose the time of your ad's placement, bonus time may not reach your exact target, so it's more suitable for a message to the general audience that supplements the messages of your paid campaign and increases overall public support for your issue.

Earned media allows you to target your primary and secondary audiences more precisely. Media outreach will give your paid campaign credibility by encouraging the media to reinforce your messages. It will also provide more detail and supporting information than can be communicated in a 30-second TV spot. You can use media outreach to target practically any segment that watches or reads news and informational media, such as opinion leaders through editorial pages and news talk shows or parents through specialty magazines.

Using these three approaches in combination will provide a greater opportunity for your audience to be exposed to and influenced by your message.

Working With Limited Resources

Not every organization has the resources to conduct a paid advertising campaign. When paid campaigns aren't possible, it's harder to target specific populations, but it's still possible to reach broad groups or the general public.

If you can't afford a paid campaign, you should consider reusing or producing one or more ads for PSA use for a general audience, to increase awareness of your issue; then use earned media to focus on specific aspects of your issue with different audiences. The process for PSA and media relations efforts will be generally the same even if you don't have a paid campaign, though you may have to work harder to persuade the media to cover your story. You can do this by conducting newsworthy events (e.g., press conferences), releasing new data, and taking advantage of any chance for media attention when your issue is raised by some outside influence (e.g., a well-known figure dies relatively young of lung cancer). Without a paid campaign, you'll have to adjust your objectives to account for your lack of control over placement of your message.

Evaluating Advertising Efforts

Advertising is often the most expensive and time-consuming component of a tobacco counter-marketing campaign. With so much invested, several stakeholders will want to know whether you're making a difference and whether funds are being used wisely. To demonstrate the success of your efforts, you should consider using three types of assessment: formative, process, and outcome evaluation. It's also very important to involve an evaluation expert to help you develop and implement a rigorous evaluation appropriate for your campaign.

Rigorous evaluation can help you to justify your spending to stakeholders by showing that the ad campaign, not other factors, accounted for changes in the target audience. Formative evaluation can help you to determine whether you have the right strategy, message, and creative products, before you invest in media buys. Process evaluation allows you to keep track of what your ad agency and other contractors are implementing and to ensure that those activities meet your guidelines and objectives. Once your ads have been run, the outcome evaluation can help you to monitor the exposure of the target audience to your message(s), their awareness of the ads, and their ability to recall the message(s). Most important, you can use outcome evaluation to help you determine whether changes have occurred in the tobacco-related knowledge, attitudes, beliefs, intentions, or behaviors of your target audience.

How To Evaluate the Advertising Campaign

Depending on the scope and costs of your advertising effort, you should consider using formative evaluation during planning of your advertising campaign, process evaluation during implementation, and outcome evaluation during follow-up. Conducting formative evaluation during the *planning* phase will help you to learn which communication strategies and ad concepts have the highest likelihood of being effective and whether the communication pieces you're developing leave the audience with the messages and impressions you intended. This evaluation can include research such as exploratory focus groups for audience insights, expert reviews, pretesting messages and materials, and pilot testing of an ad campaign that uses several communication channels (e.g., TV, radio, print, and billboards).

Process evaluation should be conducted as you *implement* your advertising activities, to make sure your efforts are on track and in line with your guidelines and objectives. You'll need to conduct rigorous monitoring by regularly completing or reviewing logs and other documentation tools. For example, if your contractor agrees to pretest an ad by a certain date, a log can show whether all the steps to conduct the pretest were completed and whether they were done on time.

Process evaluation should also include monitoring your target audience's exposure to your advertising. You can obtain data on exposure, usually measured in reach and frequency, from your ad agency's reports on your media buy. These reports show information such as when and where your ads were aired, how many members of your target audience were exposed, and costs. Reports from companies such as Nielsen, Arbitron, and the Audit Bureau of Circulations are other sources of data on exposure. The reports can also tell you the demographics of the audience reached, when the ad ran or was aired, and the format of the stations that ran the ad.

Outcome evaluation will help you to learn what effect your advertising is having. As noted earlier, you'll at least need to conduct initial, ongoing, and postcampaign evaluations to determine whether your efforts are meeting your objectives. You and your evaluation expert will need to make certain decisions about methods to be used in conducting an outcome evaluation that's right for you. First, to design the evaluation, you'll have to decide which groups will be studied (e.g., smokers and nonsmokers) and when. Then you'll need to determine who will be in your sample and how it will be selected. Next you should decide what questions to ask your sample and what methods to use to get the data you need. Finally, you must determine how the data will be analyzed to obtain the answers you need for your evaluation.

Using Evaluation Results for Decision Making

If the evaluations are conducted well, your efforts can yield results that provide a sound basis for making project decisions. For example, the findings from your ad agency's reports on the media buy can help you to make decisions about ad placement over time. You can use the findings to compare results across markets in your state to see what worked and where. Also, reports that show ad placement by week can help you to decide how to time your outcome evaluation so you can gauge your audience's awareness of your advertising.

Tracking a target audience's awareness and message recall of an ad, as well as their overall reactions, can allow you to analyze the data by subgroups (e.g., age and race/ethnicity), to determine whether the ad has different effects on different groups. You can then make decisions about ad design and future placement of ads directed to these subgroups. If you're doing several types of advertising (e.g., TV, radio, and billboards), efforts to track awareness, recall, and reaction for each type can help you to determine which is the most effective and where to spend your advertising dollars. If you track your target audience's tobacco-related knowledge, attitudes, beliefs, and behaviors at several points during the flights of an ad, you also can gauge the ad's effectiveness over time.

Resources for Evaluation

This chapter covers some of the basics of evaluating an ad campaign. You also should review Chapter 5: Evaluating the Success of Your Counter-Marketing Program for more information about how to assess the impact of your whole counter-marketing program. CDC's Office on Smoking and Health (OSH) is also preparing a manual that focuses on outcome evaluation for paid counter-advertising campaigns, which is scheduled for publication in late 2003. (Check http://www.cdc.gov/tobacco for updates on the availability of this manual.) Another publication offering evaluation information is CDC's *Introduction to Program Evaluation for Comprehensive Tobacco Control Programs*, published in 2001.

Points To Remember

Although creative firms produce advertising, a manager within the tobacco control program must be the ultimate authority on what kind of advertising to produce. To effectively manage a creative firm, while still encouraging innovative ideas, the manager should focus on a handful of critical questions in four areas—logistics, strategy, creative, and exposure.

Logistics
- What contractual arrangements (e.g., incentives, results-based payments, and penalties) might encourage the creative firm to focus on your goals of behavior change?
- What guidelines are needed to set common expectations and ensure quality control of creative materials, media buys, billing, scope-of-work restrictions, and other important issues?

Strategy
- Have you and your agency developed a clear, written set of message strategies for each audience?
- Do the advertising strategies coordinate with other parts of the program at both the local and state levels?
- Considering that the tobacco industry, voluntary health organizations, the American Legacy Foundation, and other groups may already be reaching your audience, how does your campaign fit into the overall context of what your audience is hearing? How might you need to alter the campaign to be most cost efficient and effective?

Creative
- Is each creative product, from a TV spot to a T-shirt, on strategy?
- Can each product be disseminated effectively to your audience?
- Does each product reflect what you know about your audience?
- Once people are exposed to this creative product, could unintended negative consequences occur?

Exposure
- Are you reaching your audience effectively (i.e., gaining their attention and clearly communicating a message) and efficiently (i.e., for a reasonable price)?
- Are you reaching your audience through the right channel, at the right time, and in the right place?

Bibliography

American Legacy Foundation. *Getting to the Truth: Assessing Youths' Reactions to the "truth" and "Think. Don't Smoke" Tobacco Countermarketing Campaigns. Legacy First Look Report 9.* Washington, DC: American Legacy Foundation, June 2002.

Flay BR, Cook TD. Three models of summative evaluation of prevention campaigns with a mass media component. In: Rice RE, Atkins CK, editors. *Public Communication Campaigns.* Newbury Park, CA: Sage Publications, 1989, pp. 175–95.

Fletcher AD, Bowers TA. *Fundamentals of Advertising Research,* 3rd ed. Belmont, CA: Wadsworth Publishing Company, 1988.

Freimuth V, Cole G, Kirby S. Issues in evaluating mass-media health communication campaigns. In: Rootman I, editor. *Evaluation in Health Promotion: Principles and Perspectives.* WHO Regional Publications. European Series No. 92. Copenhagen, Denmark: WHO Regional Office for Europe, 2001, pp. 475–92.

Kotler P, Armstrong G. *Principles of Marketing,* 9th ed. Upper Saddle River, NJ: Prentice-Hall, 2001.

MacDonald G, Starr G, Schooley M, et al. *Introduction to Program Evaluation for Comprehensive Tobacco Control Programs.* Atlanta, GA: Centers for Disease Control and Prevention, 2001.

Miller A. Designing an effective counteradvertising campaign—Massachusetts. *Cancer* 1998;83:2742–5.

Mitchell PK, Smith WA, editors. *Social Marketing Lite and Energy Efficiency: A Practical Resource Book for Social Marketing.* Washington, DC: Academy for Educational Development, 2000.

Popham WJ, Potter LD, Hetrick MA, et al. Effectiveness of the California 1990–1991 tobacco education media campaign. *American Journal of Preventive Medicine* 1994;10:319–26.

Siegel M. Mass media anti-smoking campaigns: a powerful tool for health promotion. *Annals of Internal Medicine* 1998;129:128–32.

Sly DF, Heald GR, Ray S. The Florida "truth" anti-tobacco media evaluation: design, first year results, and implications for planning future state media evaluations. *Tobacco Control* 2001a;10:9–15.

Sly DF, Hopkins RS, Trapido E, et al. Influence of a counteradvertising media campaign on initiation of smoking: the Florida "truth" campaign. *American Journal of Public Health* 2001b;91:233–8.

U.S. Department of Health and Human Services. *Reducing the Health Consequences of Smoking: 25 Years of Progress. A Report of the Surgeon General.* Atlanta, GA: U.S. Department of Health and Human Services, Public Health Service, Centers for Disease Control, Center for Chronic Disease Prevention and Health Promotion, Office on Smoking and Health, 1989.USDHHS Publication No. (CDC) 89-8411.

U.S. Department of Health and Human Services. *Smoking and Health: Report of the Advisory Committee to the Surgeon General of the Public Health Service. A Report of the Surgeon General.* Atlanta, GA: U.S. Department of Health and Human Services, Public Health Service, Centers for Disease Control, Center for Chronic Disease Prevention and Health Promotion, Office on Smoking and Health, 1964.

Chapter 8

Public Relations

While the advertising in California's tobacco education media campaign has received a lot of positive recognition, the public relations component has been the unsung hero of the campaign. The public relations work is equal in importance to the advertising.

— Colleen Stevens, Tobacco Control Section, California Department of Health Services

Like advertising, public relations (PR) is a way of reaching people with a message. But while advertising space or time must be bought or donated, PR exposure is "earned" by working with the news media, opinion leaders, or others. That's why the media coverage generated from PR is dubbed "earned media": You must *earn* the coverage by developing materials, by working with reporters, and by expending resources through a continuing, systematic process.

Enhancing the credibility of your message is a key feature of PR. Because audiences know that an ad is designed to influence them, they may evaluate its message more critically than the information that's received through the news media, which is often seen as less biased. Although audiences may question some of what they read in newspapers or see on the news, most still consider these sources to be more objective and accurate than advertising, and they generally accept the information more readily. For example, many would believe the information released in an article in the *Wall Street Journal*, yet may not be convinced by an ad on the same topic with the same message. The same is true of other credible sources. The job of PR is to encourage the dissemination of your messages through others, most notably the news media.

In This Chapter

- Setting Goals and Selecting Tactics
- Preparing for Implementation of Your Public Relations Program
- Working With the News Media
- Developing Press Materials
- Responding To Negative News Stories
- Evaluating Your Public Relations Efforts

To help you create an effective PR campaign, this chapter covers four main topics:

1. Setting goals and selecting tactics for your PR activities, including efforts to reach your target audiences and important stakeholders.

2. Preparing for the implementation of your PR program, including developing a PR plan and managing a PR firm.

3. Working with the news media, including creating press materials and responding to negative news stories.

4. Evaluating your PR efforts.

Setting Goals and Selecting Tactics

PR is an essential component of a tobacco counter-marketing program because it offers credibility, objectivity, and a de facto endorsement of your campaign (as long as the media coverage is positive). When you have a small paid media budget, PR becomes your primary method of communicating with various audiences. Even if you have a large paid media budget, PR will complement and support your paid media efforts. Without an effective PR effort, even the most expensive and creative paid media campaign can founder.

What PR Can and Can't Do

PR can

- Provide quick responses to hot issues and sudden events
- Establish relationships with media, stakeholders, opinion leaders, and others
- Reach audiences on an ongoing basis with information that may be seen as more credible than advertising messages
- Enhance the credibility of your advertising/paid media messages
- Gain public support and create an environment conducive to your other tobacco control initiatives
- Expose the practices of your competitors (i.e., the tobacco industry, smokers' rights groups, and others) and provide a contrasting perspective
- Provide a framework for effective crisis communication

PR can't

- Guarantee your message placement, focus or slant, specific content, or accuracy in the media or other venues
- Substitute for other components of an integrated and comprehensive program

In general, PR complements your counter-advertising program and other efforts by:

- Reaching your target audience with in-depth messages that elaborate on your key points in ways that ads can't

- Helping to create positive views of your campaign and your organization among the news media, stakeholders, policy makers, and opinion leaders

- Helping to influence policy change through long-term relationships, partnership and coalition building, and consistent efforts to expand the support base

An integrated counter-marketing program will use PR to serve all three of these functions. This section discusses the first two functions: (1) using PR to reach your target audience and (2) using PR to promote your program with opinion leaders and stakeholders. The third function, discussed in another chapter, is changing policy. (See Chapter 9: Media Advocacy for more information.)

Target Audience Public Relations

PR can be a strategic communication tool for sending key messages to targeted audiences and for complementing advertising messages. This use of PR will be referred to in this manual as "Target Audience PR."

Developing Target Audience PR activities is similar to developing an advertising campaign: You need to clarify your overall goal, determine target audience(s), set specific objectives, select key message strategies, and select the best channels. Much of your advertising research will also apply to your Target Audience PR activities. However, rather than buying ad space, you'll be working with reporters and editors to encourage them to run stories, op-eds, and editorials that convey the key messages of your campaign. These stories can provide additional context—and additional credibility—that will make the advertising component of your campaign more powerful.

For example, if your goal is to increase cessation and your key audience is adult smokers with children, your message strategy might be to highlight the pain that smokers may cause their families if they die or get sick. Your advertising efforts might include running TV spots of testimonials from a smoker's relatives about how they have suffered from the smoker's tobacco-related death or illness. Your Target Audience PR might include directing reporters to "real-life" human interest stories about local families who have suffered with this situation, possibly even the individuals who are featured in your ads.

In addition to working with reporters to get the message out through the news media, you might also coordinate a lunch meeting with chamber of commerce members to discuss various ways to help working parents gain access to cessation support in the workplace. You might also make a presentation at a Parent Teacher Association (PTA) meeting about smoking cessation support groups or quitlines, and bring fliers with recommended steps for quitting and the local quitline phone number.

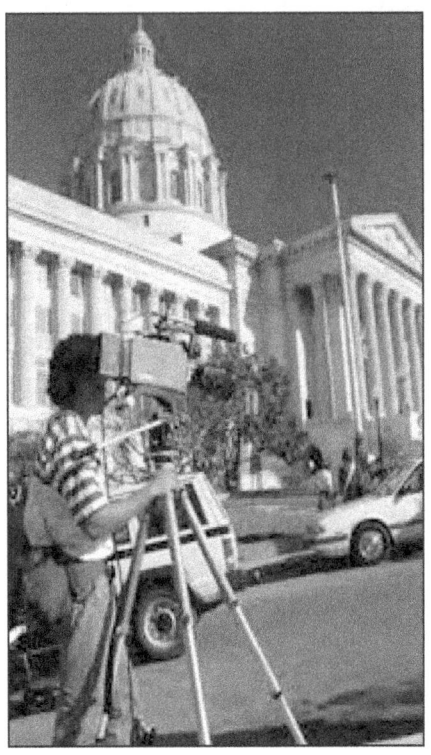

How do you make Target Audience PR a reality in your program? Once you know your goals, audiences, and messages, you or your PR firm should first identify the organizations or news media outlets that reach your target audience. Second, you should determine how you can encourage those organizations or media outlets to disseminate your messages.

Finding Media Outlets That Reach the Audience

One easy way to find media outlets that reach your target audience is to examine your advertising media buy. The newspapers, magazines, and other outlets included in the media buy will have been analyzed by the media planners and buyers to ensure that they reach your core audience. They also may be ideal for your Target Audience PR activities. You should also consider the media that weren't part of the media buy. For example, even if your ad campaign doesn't include Web advertising or newspapers, you may want to use these outlets in your PR effort. Depending on your target audience, you may also want to consider community-based media, such as church bulletins, newsletters, and fliers from local organizations. If you're working with a PR firm or consultant, they'll be able to identify the optimal media outlets for your target audiences based not only on efficiency (how many target audience members they reach for the resources expended), but also on the quality of communication (e.g., how credible the sources are and how appropriate they are for the message).

Gaining Exposure Through Media Outlets

Once you identify the outlets that reach your target audience(s), you must generate those intermediaries' interest in disseminating your message. In Target Audience PR, the most common intermediary is the news media. The best way to get your message in the media is to help reporters make that message appear new and interesting to their audience (readers, listeners, or viewers). Here are some of the most common tactics:

- **Create an event.** Reporters will often cover your newsworthy campaign events, including summits, community activities, rallies, and so forth.

- **Set up interviews with program participants.** Everyone loves a good personal story (witness Art and Entertainment's "Biography," VH1's "Behind the Music," and Lifetime's "Intimate Portrait"). Some participants in your campaign may have interesting personal stories related to tobacco. These personal profiles work well for magazines and newspapers' lifestyle sections, and they humanize your efforts.

- **Set up interviews with local residents affected by the issue.** In addition to campaign participants' stories, you might want to identify local residents affected by your issue who can talk to the media. The resident is more likely to generate news coverage if he or she is a prominent member of the community, such as a sports celebrity or an elected official. But remember that these community members must appeal to your target audience—if you're targeting teens, don't use the authoritarian, middle-aged mayor.

- **Offer reporters "behind-the-scenes" access.** You can give reporters a look behind the scenes of making an ad, or let them follow one of the actors during the shoot (similar to MTV's "Making the Video").

- **Try a stunt.** You can conduct unique events for the sole purpose of getting news media coverage. Mississippi set up its own version of MTV's "The Real World" and placed a group of smokers who wanted to quit in a house with Web cameras so that people could see who gave up smoking first. This tactic received national exposure and educated the audience about cessation.

- **Create a speakers bureau.** A speakers bureau will help make your subject matter experts more easily available for speaking engagements with associations, groups, and businesses at conferences and other events, and prepare these speakers for media interviews.

- **Announce the results of a study or survey.** Sometimes when you do this, you'll get featured twice: once when you announce the launch of the study or survey and again when you announce the results.

- **Develop a publication or Web page.** You can develop publications or add information to your Web site that will encourage readers to pass on your message to other interested parties or to those who could benefit from the information. Your tobacco control campaign's Web site can include copies of and links to the media coverage that you've received, which will increase the reach of this coverage. These efforts will need to be coordinated with your advertising activities.

You can also leverage your advertising spending to create Target Audience PR opportunities. Many media outlets offer "bonus weight time," which is extra space or time given to you as an incentive for purchasing advertising with them. This bonus weight time can be used for communications other than additional ads. For example, you can work with the outlet on promotional or sponsorship opportunities. For the national "truth" campaign, the American Legacy Foundation worked with teen magazines to include "truth" gear in their

"What's Cool" fashion sections, rather than run additional ads. You can also work with media outlets to get interviews for campaign leaders and others involved in the campaign.

These are just a handful of the ways that programs win attention for their messages. Pick the ideas that may work for your program. There are plenty of other possibilities—try inventing your own.

Capitalizing on Outside Events To Increase Exposure to the Message

Events independent of your tobacco control campaign may generate news stories that offer opportunities for media coverage. These stories can either undermine or support your campaign. In either case, you should respond to related stories to ensure that your campaign messages are heard. It's especially critical that you respond to any challenges to your campaign messages. Even if you don't get equal coverage for your response, you will have educated the reporters about the issue, which will be to your benefit for future stories. How to respond to negative news stories is covered later in this chapter.

For example, if you're targeting teens and a positive story about the Philip Morris "Think. Don't Smoke" campaign runs in a publication that reaches this audience, you can submit data to the reporters on how "Don't Smoke" efforts are ineffective and how other approaches (such as those used in your campaign) are more effective. In these cases, it may be helpful to contact local nongovernment organizations, such as the American Cancer Society, the American Lung Association, the American Heart Association, the Campaign for Tobacco-Free Kids, and others, to see if you can coordinate your responses.

Your counter-marketing program will be conducted in the context of national tobacco control efforts. You'll need to anticipate events, such as the release of a Surgeon General's report, newly published scientific findings, the American Legacy Foundation's campaigns, state or federal tobacco legislation, and the advocacy efforts of volunteer and nonprofit organizations (such as the Campaign for Tobacco-Free Kids). Staying abreast of these activities may involve subscribing to national tobacco news services, signing up for various tobacco-related e-mail distribution lists, and participating in national forums (such as the Centers for Disease Control and Prevention's Media Network).

You can also piggyback on national PR events, such as the Great American Smokeout, Kick Butts Day, and World No-Tobacco Day. When you're planning your PR campaign, do some research on these national events and include tie-ins to the events that are appropriate for your audience. Using these events to gain exposure for your messages can be a more efficient tactic than creating your own events. A Tobacco Control Media Events Calendar, along with accompanying media materials, is available on the CDC's Office on Smoking and Health Web site at http://www.cdc.gov/tobacco/calendar/calendar.htm.

You'll also need to monitor the competition's PR activities. You can track news releases issued by the tobacco industry by searching the PR

Target Audience PR in Florida's "truth" Campaign

With $70 million from its landmark settlement with the tobacco industry, Florida launched the Florida Tobacco Pilot Program in 1998. It was the nation's first antitobacco education program funded with tobacco industry money. The program's "truth" campaign is designed to create an antitobacco brand that appeals to teens the way that the major tobacco brands do.

Target Audience PR played a key role in the "truth" campaign. Much of the media coverage resulted from the efforts of Students Working Against Tobacco (SWAT), the program's youth advocacy group. The group's activities were designed to engage teens and to garner media coverage that complemented the ad campaign's messages and tone. Examples of their PR activities include:

- In the summer of 1998, the campaign offered the "truth" tour, a 10-day, 13-city whistlestop train tour and concert series across Florida. Then-Governor Lawton Chiles rode the train, joining the teen spokespeople who conducted their own press conferences at every stop. SWAT members trained their peers in advocacy and media relations along the way, empowering teens throughout the state to join in the movement's rebellion against the tobacco industry.

- During the fall of 1999, SWAT took on tobacco magazine advertising with "Big Tobacco on the Run." SWAT members tore cigarette ads from the magazines they read, plastered them with a neon-orange "Rejected. Rebuffed. Returned." sticker and mailed them to tobacco company executives along with a request to meet with SWAT to discuss youth marketing guidelines. The Brown & Williamson Tobacco Corporation accepted the invitation and sent a representative to meet with the SWAT board of directors.

The media coverage of these and other events, handled by the PR firm supporting the Florida Tobacco Pilot Program, resulted in more than 845 million media impressions (the combined audiences reached by all of the media vehicles covering the events). Coverage included stories on "Good Morning America" on the American Broadcasting Company (ABC); on the "Evening News' Eye on America," "60 Minutes," and "CBS News Sunday Morning" on the Columbia Broadcasting System (CBS); on the Cable News Network (CNN) and network affiliates throughout Florida, as well as outlets in New York, Chicago, Los Angeles, Dallas, Cincinnati, Indianapolis, and elsewhere. Print coverage included *The New York Times, The Wall Street Journal, The Washington Post, USA Today, Seventeen,* and *Teen People,* as well as every major-market Florida newspaper and numerous minority outlets.

newswire (http://biz.yahoo.com/prnews). Another comprehensive source of tobacco-related news is at http://www.tobacco.org, which e-mails daily news briefings to subscribers. These briefings will help you to stay informed about the latest national and state tobacco-related news.

Stakeholder Public Relations

A comprehensive PR program will reach not only your target audience(s), but also your stakeholders, which may include opinion leaders, business leaders, policy makers, local advocates, and the public. While the primary goal of your Target Audience PR is to reinforce your campaign messages, the primary goal of your Stakeholder PR efforts is to garner support for your program and its funding. By demonstrating your program's effectiveness and value, Stakeholder PR may help to increase your program's longevity.

To conduct effective Stakeholder PR, you must:

- Identify your stakeholders
- Identify ways to reach those stakeholders
- Identify and capitalize on media opportunities to reach stakeholders
- Involve stakeholders in the campaign—and keep them involved

Identifying the Stakeholders

The first step in Stakeholder PR is identifying your stakeholders. You must determine whose support is critical to your campaign and who can add to the credibility of your campaign. These are your core stakeholders. You'll probably want the public's support as well because policy makers may follow public opinion if the support—or lack of support—is great enough. Think beyond the state level and identify stakeholders at the community level, especially if your program provides grants or funding for activities at that level.

You should identify your stakeholders before you begin planning your program because one of the best ways to win support is to involve key stakeholders early in your planning. Think of ways to encourage them to have a stake in the program or to view it as partly *their* program. You may also want to include your potential detractors in certain meetings so that you can understand the opposition and develop a response or modify your plans. These accommodations, if they don't detract from your goals and objectives, may be the key to turning a detractor into a supporter. For example, if you're going to focus on smokefree workplaces (including bars and restaurants), you'll want to include some restaurant and bar owners and workers in your effort. By seeking their input and making adjustments to address their concerns, you could earn their support up front and help your initiative.

There are many individuals and organizations that you should consider as potential stakeholders, including local businesses and employers, business associations, chambers of commerce, volunteer and community-based organizations, places of worship and faith-based groups, hospitals and health care facilities, neighborhood associations, social clubs, health and other professional groups or associations, state and local government officials, school boards and PTAs, public and private universities and community colleges, vocational and continuing-education schools, and daycare and childcare centers.

Identifying Outlets That Reach the Stakeholders

Once you have identified your stakeholders, you will need to find ways to connect with them through various communication channels. These channels will include not only media outlets, but also conferences, personal meetings, and other communication opportunities. The media outlets are likely to include traditional news outlets (daily newspapers, TV and radio news programs, and TV and radio talk shows), along with health- and tobacco-related publications, Web sites, and policy-related publications. You may also consider community-based media, such as bulletins published by local, faith-based, and other organizations.

Mass media may not be the most appropriate way to reach your core stakeholders. Some people and groups will require more personal forms of outreach, including phone calls, meetings, and individualized letters. Other ways to communicate with your stakeholders are through customized outlets, such as the following:

- **Newsletters.** You can create a campaign newsletter to inform and entertain supporters and to recognize their efforts. You can also send print or electronic bulletins on the campaign to partner organizations so that they can include them in their newsletters. (See Appendix 8.1 for a sample printed campaign newsletter and Appendix 8.2 for a sample online newsletter.)

- **Speaking engagements.** In-person communication is valuable because stakeholders can ask you questions directly. Not only can you provide them with the information that they want, but you can also learn the issues that are most important to them, which will help you tailor future outreach. Set up a yearly schedule of opportunities to deliver messages to your stakeholders at their meetings; you should also hold meetings of your own and invite them.

- **Web sites.** You can create a Web site solely for stakeholders. For example, Legacy created two Web sites for its "truth" campaign. One site is for teens (http://www.thetruth.com) and focuses on campaign messages. The second site is a password-protected site (http://www.truthpartners.com), specifically for stakeholders; it disseminates research, strategies, and other information to the campaign's partners. It has a mass e-mail function that can be used to notify partners of important announcements or updates.

Identifying Media Opportunities To Reach Stakeholders

Certain kinds of campaign activities are more likely to attract the attention of large groups of stakeholders:

- **Campaign launch.** This is your prime opportunity to get significant news media coverage about your campaign. All of your main stakeholders and policy makers will be interested because the campaign is new. You'll want to focus on the campaign's goals and create a sense of excitement.

- **Specific advertising flights.** Although less of an opportunity than the campaign launch, releasing a collection of ads can garner news media coverage, especially if the ads are unique or controversial. A flight or set of ads also demonstrates progress toward the campaign goals. However, it is important to notify particular stakeholders (such as the local programs and volunteers) of new ads *before* they are run, so that the stakeholders can be prepared for inquiries from reporters or the public.

- **Events.** Related summits, speaking engagements, health fairs, and other events are opportunities to reach out to stakeholders and gain coverage.

Stakeholder Involvement in California's PR Campaign

California has been at the forefront of integrating many components of a comprehensive tobacco countermarketing program. One California PR effort illustrates how to successfully meld local programs, grassroots efforts, and advertising with stakeholder involvement to disseminate campaign messages in the news.

In the spring of 1995, California's tobacco education program worked with local programs throughout the state on Operation Storefront. More than 700 trained youth and adult volunteers surveyed more than 5,700 tobacco retailers throughout California, including grocery stores, supermarkets, drugstores, convenience stores, small pharmacies, gas stations, and liquor stores. These volunteers documented the number of indoor and outdoor storefront tobacco ads in the retailers' establishments, including window signs, posters, banners, display racks, decals, clocks, neon signs, doormats, ashtrays, counter mats, and other items that included tobacco brands or slogans.

The survey found a significantly higher average number of tobacco ads and promotions in stores near schools (within 1,000 feet) than in stores not near schools. Tobacco retailers near schools were more likely to place tobacco advertisements close to candy racks or less than 3 feet from the floor, where children were most likely to see them.

The survey's results were released at 19 local press conferences throughout the state. With the coordination by the PR staff at the state health department and at the PR firm, each local program was able to attract local press coverage and to contribute to the powerful statewide and national impact of the results. The survey results were subsequently incorporated into ads that exposed tobacco industry advertising tactics directed toward children.

- **Evaluation reports.** Stakeholders as well as detractors will be interested in whether your campaign is working. If your results are positive, you'll definitely want to spread the word. If your goals aren't met, you will still want to share with your core partners the results as well as the reasons why you believe that the results were not as strong as hoped, so that your stakeholders can help you develop new directions and defend your efforts from attacks.

Capitalizing on Media Opportunities

Responding to attacks on your campaign is essential to maintaining its credibility and support from stakeholders. Be prepared to work quickly with reporters and to draft news releases, editorials, and op-eds in response to attacks. When you respond to the attacks, it is important to use the right tone. Sometimes a forceful approach is appropriate, while, at other times, you should present a calm, non-confrontational response. In either case, don't sound defensive and be sure that your responses are supported with appropriate data. If you've built good relationships with your partners, ask them to support your program by issuing their own responses to the attacks. Quick decision making and action are essential in these situations.

As with Target Audience PR, you'll also want to monitor the activities of the tobacco industry. Keep an eye out for fake grassroots efforts organized by the tobacco industry or other opponents. You should counter these efforts by exposing them as coordinated by the tobacco industry. For example, a smokers' rights campaign may successfully cloud the issue of secondhand smoke by claiming that free choice is being threatened. If you have concrete evidence that these efforts are funded or coordinated either directly or indirectly by the tobacco industry, then you may provide that information to the news media to ensure that they have all of the facts. If you're not completely sure of the information, don't risk your credibility by speculating.

Don't forget to look for good news about counter-marketing efforts (even in other states) that support your campaign. Highlighting the successes of similar efforts will show stakeholders that you're following a proven path.

Involving Stakeholders in Your Campaign

Once you have identified potential partners or stakeholders, directly involving them (especially local coalitions and advocates) in your counter-marketing effort can be an excellent method of retaining their interest and support. You'll also gain the benefit of their insight and expertise. Stakeholder involvement may be valuable in:

- Campaign planning (especially when working with specific populations)

- Research and evaluation planning

- Key phases of implementation (for example, invite stakeholders to be part of your proposal review committee after you issue a Request for Proposals for work to be done by contractors)

- Advertising development
- Visibly supporting your campaign when it's facing a threat from detractors
- Planning and implementing media advocacy and grassroots events

The more that you genuinely involve key stakeholders in your efforts, the more time, resources, and effort they'll invest in protecting your program and ensuring its success.

Defining the stakeholders' role in your efforts helps them understand the rationale for their involvement and will motivate them to become involved and stay involved. These reasons will differ, depending on the interests and focus of each stakeholder. For example, the business and labor sectors have a significant interest in the health of local families and communities. In addition, private sector industries are interested in being "good neighbors" in the communities in which they operate, since the community supplies their workforce, and often, their markets. However, because each entity has a different agenda, you'll need to tell them individually why they need to get involved with your cause and how they can help. Consider the ways in which the participation of partners will help them. What incentives and benefits exist or can be created to help win their support? Consider what these people and their institutions are already doing to help the community. Building community goodwill, for example, can be a motivating factor for some partners.

Preparing for Implementation of Your Public Relations Program

The first section of this chapter provided a conceptual framework for organizing your PR activities into Target Audience PR and Stakeholder PR. This section provides information on preparing for the implementation of your PR activities, including developing a PR plan and managing a PR firm.

Developing a PR Plan

Because your PR efforts should be conducted in the context of a strategic communication effort, you should develop a PR plan for each of your major tobacco control program initiatives. As you develop the plan, you'll need to be mindful of what role your organization plays in tobacco control (e.g., public education, advocacy, lobbying, and health care). Outlining the goals, objectives and associated tactics, and timing for each effort will ensure that no steps are overlooked. Tracking the activities as they are implemented will provide you with a record of what was done, which will help you to evaluate your efforts and to improve future PR outreach.

The PR plan should answer four basic questions for each outreach effort:

1. **What do you want to accomplish?** Describe your goal in as much detail as possible so you'll be able to determine whether you are moving toward this goal.

2. **How will you accomplish it?** Detail your objectives and associated tactics, including activities that you plan to

undertake, materials that need to be developed in support of those activities, a materials dissemination plan, a list of intended media contacts, follow-up contact plans, planned press events, and spokespeople. You may want to outline partners who will assist and what their roles will be.

3. **When will you accomplish it?** Create a timetable that shows when each of your activities will be completed.

4. **How will you determine if your goals were met?** Describe how you're going to measure your effort. You should decide up front what indicators you'll use to measure the results and how you'll collect the information. Indicators may include the number of media "hits" that you received or the number of people exposed to your messages through the news media. Other key indicators include the focus, slant, and placement of news stories in which you've tried to communicate your key messages. For example, if the stories written have a pro-industry slant, then you may not have met your goal, even though you have received substantial media coverage.

As part of your overall PR plan, you should develop a crisis communications plan that outlines the process for dealing with attacks on your campaign. Because you'll have to respond quickly to such attacks, you may need to develop a shortened review process to replace the usual lengthy review process. Your shortened process may include having your head PR person craft a response and having it quickly approved by the program manager or the marketing director. Receiving a call from a reporter for your response to an attack is a valuable opportunity to convey your campaign messages that you will not want to miss. Planning ahead will allow you to include recommendations of experts and partners who can support your efforts. If you don't develop such a plan proactively, you may find yourself being attacked without time to do the necessary planning to provide a strategic response. (Responding to negative news stories is covered later in this chapter.)

Your program is likely to be scrutinized by the media, the public, and the tobacco industry. To help prevent criticism, you should proactively consider how your messages and activities may be perceived by these audiences. Hold yourself and your program to high standards of ethics, accuracy, and accountability about how you position your messages and what activities you choose to conduct.

Managing a PR Firm

PR firms provide a range of services and can be valuable for conducting target audience and stakeholder outreach in support of large campaigns. Although your PR firm will have staff who can handle most, if not all, of the communication functions, you should stay well informed about all PR activities so that you maintain the lead role in decision making.

Many firms like to set a monthly retainer for their services that is based on the expected level of services to be provided, while others will establish a yearly budget for your program, then bill only the incurred labor and other costs each month under some maximum annual ceiling. With large counter-marketing programs, the latter arrangement may be preferred because each monthly invoice reflects the level of the work actually performed and allows for easier tracking of the specific costs.

If you want to reach specific populations in your state (e.g., African Americans; Hispanics/ Latinos; Native Americans; the gay, lesbian, bisexual, and transgender community; and people with disabilities or other special needs), then you may want to look for one or more firms that specialize in reaching these populations. The firms may recognize specific communication challenges with these groups and may have stronger and broader relationships with the media and stakeholders that are important to them. Often, these specialty PR firms can subcontract with your primary PR firm, removing the need for separate competitive bids.

If you do arrange for subcontractor PR firms, make sure that you can establish direct contact with each firm when needed and that you stay fully informed about their activities. Although most of the work may flow through the prime contractor to the subcontractors and back, there may be times when it's critical to have direct access to a subcontractor. Keep in mind, though, that the prime contractor is legally responsible for all work done on the contract, even by subcontractors, so make sure that they're aware of any contact that you have with subcontractors.

To locate specialized firms in your area, you can review directories such as the *Directory of Multicultural Relations Professionals and Firms*, which is offered by the Public Relations Society of America.

Key PR Firm Functions

A PR firm can perform several functions for you:

- **Strategy**—helping you to develop your overall image and supporting communication strategies to reach your goals

- **Counsel**—giving you advice on how to handle issues and situations to maintain image and reputation and to support your messages

- **Research**—conducting research on the target audience, messages, and public opinion

- **Message and materials development**—developing messages to fit your strategies, developing materials for the news media and others

- **Media relations**—working directly with the media to get coverage

- **Spokesperson training**—identifying and training spokespeople who support your campaign

- **Stakeholder relations**—facilitating meetings with partners and other key stakeholders

- **Issues monitoring**—reviewing the news to see how your issue and campaign are covered

- **Event planning**—creating events and holding press conferences to attract media coverage

- **Creative**—creating "collateral materials" (items such as posters, brochures, and fliers that are given to your target audience), Web sites, and other communication tools to convey your key messages

You may not need all of these services from your PR firm. For example, you may rely on your ad agency for strategy development and on a contract with a state university for research. However, you should be aware that PR firms offer a perspective that differs from most ad agencies or other vendors, so you'll probably want to tap PR expertise when making crucial strategic decisions. If you are relying on multiple sources for support, make sure that all of the sources are coordinating their efforts while you maintain the lead for overseeing the work. Coordination among all of the individuals and entities involved is essential to avoid a PR crisis that could occur if everyone is not on the same page.

Coordinating Your PR Firm With Your Ad Agency

Many of the services offered by PR firms overlap with those offered by ad agencies, event management firms, and others. Be sure to designate a lead agency for certain functions, like establishing your overall strategy. Many people on the counter-marketing team, including those at the advertising agency, will have opinions on what will generate news coverage. Listening to these opinions is important because you may get some great ideas, but give special consideration to the advice of the PR firm staff on news media issues. They have worked with reporters and know what is more likely to attract coverage and how that coverage can be managed. Because you are ultimately responsible for the activities of your organization, it's important that you consider all of the input and advice and make the final decisions on major issues yourself.

Bring in your PR staff early in the development of the whole counter-marketing program. Involvement from the start will help PR agencies develop ideas and give them time to plan effective outreach and events to achieve your goals. Calling a PR firm a few days before you release a new ad campaign will not give you or the PR firm time to maximize media opportunities or to plan for other components of a comprehensive approach. Therefore, you may not have the necessary partner support and media relationships in place to complement an ad campaign. With these components in place, your campaign will be more likely to gain valuable media coverage and collaboration among partners. Involvement during the campaign's development will also allow the PR experts to identify potentially negative or controversial issues and to develop contingency plans for them.

Handling PR In-House

Although PR firms are uniquely qualified to conduct outreach to media, stakeholders, and others, you can also handle the public relations functions in-house if you have the right staff and resources. You'll need to designate someone to manage the PR tasks. Major tobacco control programs often employ full-time staff solely to manage news media relations, especially in the program's initial stages. In Florida, for example, the counter-marketing program employed a press secretary, a deputy press secretary, and two interns to manage the news media when the campaign was most visible. If you choose to handle all of your PR in-house, you will need at least a press secretary and probably others to work with reporters, develop materials, train spokespeople, and develop strategies that include partnership building and special events planning.

Working With the News Media

The news media can be difficult to work with if you don't understand their needs and if you don't develop good working relationships with them. However, successfully working with the news media can greatly support your programs and enhance the image of your campaign and organization. To work effectively with the news media, you will need to consider:

- What the media want
- What they consider newsworthy
- Who they are specifically and how you can reach them
- How you might gain their attention and pitch a story
- How to keep them interested in the program though press conferences, editorial board meetings, and Web-based "press rooms"
- How to place your messages in the media through letters to the editor, op-ed pieces, and calendar items
- How to respond to their unsolicited inquiries
- How to develop spokespeople
- How to develop the optimal materials for the news media
- How to meet media deadlines, which often are short

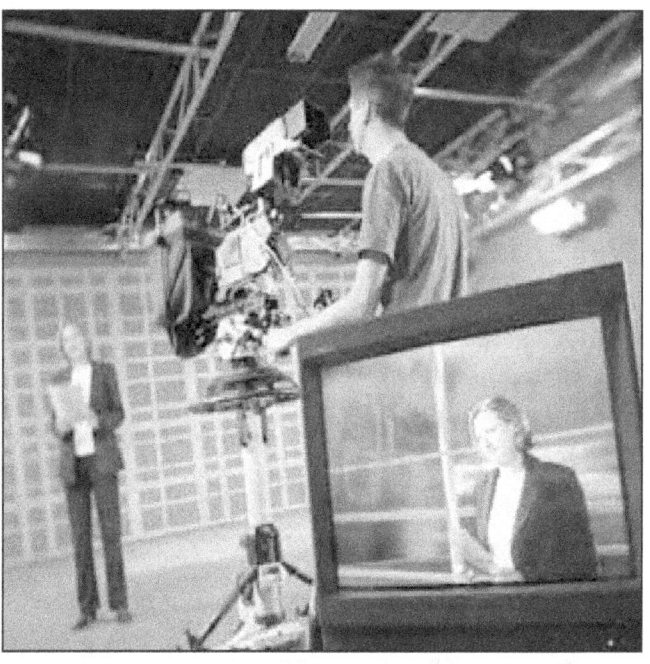

Checklist To Determine Newsworthiness

❏ Is the story timely? Is new information being offered, perhaps newly collected data?

❏ Is the story distinct, unusual, or unexpected? Is the issue or some aspect of it new to the public?

❏ Does the story indicate a trend or relate to other breaking news?

❏ Is the information essential? Does it convey something people want or need to know?

❏ Will it affect many people in the community? Does it hit close to home? Localizing a national story by adding local statistics, spokespeople, and experts significantly increases a story's chances of being picked up.

❏ Is the information useful to readers?

❏ Does the story have emotional appeal? A human-interest element?

❏ Do you have compelling visuals to accompany the story? Offering a reporter visuals may increase the appeal of a story and may increase its chances of being run.

❏ Does the story involve a national or local celebrity?

Knowing What the Media Want

Most media companies are in business to make a profit. They make money by developing and disseminating accurate, informative, and sometimes entertaining media content (for newspapers, magazines, TV programs, and radio stations) with two goals in mind: (1) attracting or retaining readers, viewers, or listeners; and (2) selling advertising. The more readers, viewers, or listeners that they have, the more they can charge advertisers for advertising space or broadcast time, and the more money they can make. Competition among media outlets for consumers is intense, as is the continuing search for compelling information and high-quality entertainment. Keep the media's goals in mind when you're developing stories that you want placed.

Determining What Is Newsworthy

To attract coverage of your issue, you must have something newsworthy to say. You're competing with countless other issues and organizations for scarce space or airtime. Before you pick up the phone or write one word, put yourself in the place of a reporter, editor, or producer and ask yourself why people should be interested in your story at this time. The same facts can produce entirely different stories. You'll need to have a new "hook" or "angle"—some piece of information that's new or could be examined in a new and interesting way. To gauge the potential of the story idea that you want to pitch, check the proposed news hook against the criteria in the checklist provided. If your story is timely and if you answer "yes" to at least two other criteria,

> ### *Typical Entries for a Media Contact List*
>
> - Date when the information was most recently updated
>
> - First and last name and title of the reporter or the editor
>
> - Name of the media outlet
>
> - Complete mailing address: street, city, state, and ZIP code
>
> - Telephone, fax, and e-mail
>
> - Field of interest or beat
>
> - Deadline and schedule
>
> - Other relevant information, such as ABC network affiliate, radio, monthly magazine, or daily newspaper
>
> - Reach and circulation

the odds are that the media professionals will consider it newsworthy.

Developing and Maintaining a Media List

Maintaining up-to-date media outlet lists for your area is key to a functioning PR program. Media lists contain key information about all of the journalists that you work with or would like to reach.

If you are putting together a media list yourself, one easy way to get started is to look on the Internet for listings of media outlets in your area. For example, you can find listings of established media outlets at http://www.emonline.com/links/index.html and http://newsdirectory.tucows.com/news/press/na/us. Other sources for information about media outlets in your area include chambers of commerce and the yellow pages. You can also purchase publications that provide listings of media outlets. Don't forget to perform searches for the media outlets that reach the various ethnic communities and diverse populations within your area. Your partner organizations may be able to provide you with the media lists that they've used.

The PR firm or consultant with whom you are working should be able to identify the optimal media outlets for your target audience(s), based not only on audience reach, but also on the credibility of each outlet with your audience(s). Most PR firms have access to databases of reporters and editors and can generate media lists quickly. You will probably want your PR firm to develop a custom database and to track your contacts with key reporters and what they like to cover.

Your media list will likely include:

- Newspapers (dailies, weeklies, and monthlies)

- Local trade and business publications

- Other local publications, such as university papers, bulletins from places of worship, and community newsletters

- Local TV and radio stations (including college and university networks)

Working with Minority Media

Many state programs include a focus on specific populations disproportionately affected by tobacco use. (See Chapter 4: Reaching Specific Populations for more information.) To reach these populations, you often have to augment your general media selection with minority news media. Specialized PR firms can provide media lists and contacts for media that reach specific audiences. However, some minority media outlets may be less likely to publish tobacco control articles if they accept and depend on money from the tobacco industry for advertising, events, or promotions. When working with minority media, you must be aware of their position on the issue.

When pitching a news story to minority media outlets, be sure to:

- Highlight the toll that tobacco use has on their audience
- Explain the positive role that they can play in solving the problem
- Provide them with information on your efforts
- Include members of the relevant stakeholder organization(s) on your team when holding in-person meetings

As mentioned, the minority media outlets that you're approaching may be accepting advertising, event, or promotional dollars from the tobacco industry. Many minority media outlets are on tight budgets and rely on tobacco advertising as part of the revenue mix that supports their publications. You should sympathize with their situation so that they don't feel chastised by you or your program, but you should not condone or support their receipt of this money. If your campaign includes paid placements in their media outlets, mentioning this when you meet with them may show that you value their outlets as paid media channels.

- Local cable stations
- Public broadcasting stations (which may have community-affairs programming)
- Public information officers at military bases (many bases have broadcast stations and newsletters that reach service members and their families)
- Freelance writers who may be looking for stories to feed to media outlets

If you are conducting a paid advertising media buy, be sure to include all of the newspapers, magazines, TV and radio stations, and other media outlets in your advertising buy.

Once you have collected the media listings, you must determine who your contacts are with these outlets. You will not have much success if you simply collect media outlet fax numbers and send unannounced news releases and advisories. You must call the media outlets and ask who in their organization covers topics related to tobacco. Don't limit yourself to health reporters, although they will be key. You may be interested in the reporters who cover stories related to restaurants and other businesses so that you can prepare them for your smokefree restaurants campaign. You may also want to know who covers education, family, recreation, and other relevant areas. Staff turnover is frequent at many media outlets, so update your contact list or database often.

The next step is to contact the identified reporters to introduce yourself. Become a "source" for them—someone who can tip them off to news about tobacco, explain the context, provide background information and additional data, and connect them with relevant people for interviews or quotes.

If you want your story to run nationally, you should know that many newspapers are members of one or more wire services (e.g., Associated Press [AP], United Press International [UPI], and Reuters), and rely on these services to provide their readers with national news and features. A story that goes over the AP wire is commonly picked up by 200 or more newspapers. That's a quick way to get national coverage of your story. Often, larger circulation papers feed stories to wire services. You can contact the services directly or develop media contacts with the larger papers in your area to gain access to these services.

Another idea often used in larger media markets is to join a press association and network to find reporters who will competently cover your issue.

Developing and Cultivating Good Media Relationships

Reporters are inundated with information every day. You'll need to take steps to attract the reporter to the information that you have to offer. Make it as easy as possible for the reporter to write the story that you want without having to contact you. Make your information concise and to the point. Be available to give the reporter direct quotes and additional information; the reporter is likely to need these for most major news or feature stories. When you talk with reporters, be sure to:

- **Treat reporters as respected individuals.** Learn their beats and interests. Journalists are almost always pressed for time. To cultivate positive coverage, be courteous, concise, timely, relevant, and objective. Ask how they prefer to get information (e.g., by fax or e-mail) and abide by their request. Don't send large e-mail attachments with big graphics.

- **Be prepared and credible.** Have backgrounders, fact sheets, and lists of experts ready to discuss the issue, and fax the information to the media outlets before contacting the journalists.

- **Respect deadlines.** All media outlets operate on deadlines. When you call the assignment editor to learn who covers what, find out when the deadlines are and respect them. Information sent too early may be forgotten. A hot, last-minute story can be pitched on the phone. In general, mail news releases so that they arrive three to five days before an event. This extra time will allow the editors to assign someone to your story. If you are phoning in a story, do so at least one day ahead of time.

- **Be polite.** If the journalist just isn't interested, accept it. The reporter may suggest that someone else at the media outlet cover the story, be interested in the next story idea that you offer, or learn that you are a source and come to you for information or ideas in the future. Don't burn any bridges.

Pitching Your Story to Reporters

Pitching a story means contacting reporters to persuade them to cover a story or event. Journalists want to hear about good story ideas because your ideas can help them put together more compelling stories. When pitching a story to a reporter, you must:

- **Be succinct.** Jot down a few sentences that clearly and briefly state what you want to tell the reporter. You can use these notes as a script to prompt you. The purpose of a story pitch is to pique the interest of a journalist, not to communicate everything there is to know about a subject. In most cases, less is more.

- **State clearly who you are and why you're calling.** Then convey the essence of your issue or event in the first 15 seconds. Think about what you're pitching as though it were a headline that will grab the journalist's attention immediately. The first sentence of the conversation should emphasize why people will care about this story.

- **Ask whether the reporter has time to talk.** If the answer is "no," inquire about a better time. If the reporter agrees to chat for a moment but is rushed, be brief and get to the point quickly. Journalists will elect to keep you on the phone longer if they're interested in your story. They'll also make themselves more available to you in the future if they feel assured that you will be respectful of their time.

- **Be sensitive to the time of day.** Different media outlets work on different schedules and deadlines. Find out the best time to contact each outlet on your media list. A general rule of thumb is that newsroom editors are the most open to discussing story ideas after the morning meetings have concluded—usually after 10:30 a.m. Avoid calling newsrooms after 3 p.m. because journalists are often focused on meeting tight deadlines at the end of the day.

- **Position your story as one that is receiving attention right now.** Then ensure that your pitch includes an angle that's timely, topical, and pertinent to a current news peg.

- **Whenever possible, humanize a story.** Providing compelling visuals, personal storylines, and interesting anecdotes with the initial pitch will afford journalists the luxury of acting on a story idea quickly without having to do a lot of homework.

- **Preserve your credibility.** Avoid making claims about a story that won't hold under further scrutiny. Making claims that can't be substantiated will compromise your credibility and limit your success with future pitches.

- **Avoid repackaging the same old information.** If a story does not reveal new information, do the necessary research to find a fresh hook, a recent statistic, or a different angle to justify running the story again. For example, if you're pitching a story on smoking cessation programs that have been covered in the past, narrow your pitch to include a timely news peg, such as recent statistics on smoking among teenagers and adapt your message points to support that angle of your story.

- **Become an ally to the news media.** News outlets want stories that will appeal to their audiences. Understanding the audience base of a news organization will help you to pitch stories that will interest them.

Conducting a Press Conference

Holding a press conference is a great way to get information to the media. Before planning a press conference, determine if there's a compelling reason to have one, such as a release of new information or another significant event. If you can create a local angle for a story or create a local link to a nationally breaking story, you are more likely to get local media outlets to attend your press conference and to cover the story. To make sure that your press conference goes smoothly, take these steps:

- **Choose a location.** If you choose a public location, make sure that you apply for any necessary permits or get permission from the appropriate person.

- **Set the date and time.** Midmorning on a Tuesday or Wednesday is generally the best time to attract reporters.

- **Select speakers.** Determine who will speak at the press conference, what each person's topics will be, and how long the press conference will last (usually 30 to 45 minutes). Generally, you'll want someone to make an opening statement (five to 10 minutes), followed by other speakers who can share different perspectives or secondary information (10 to 15 minutes). The remaining time should be used for a question-and-answer period. You should have a moderator who can direct the questions to the appropriate participants and can maintain order—especially if you are dealing with a controversial topic.

- **Invite public figures**. Invite "VIP" guests, such as the governor, the mayor, or other public figures, well in advance to increase the likelihood that they can attend. Having such public figures in attendance can provide an implicit endorsement of your message. Follow up as the date gets closer in case there are cancellations. You don't want to promote their attendance if they can't make it. Make sure that you coordinate with their PR staff.

- **Decide which pictures or visuals will best convey your message.** You can create enlarged photos or giant posters that show your findings. Use your logo and make your organization's name visible on a big sign.

- **Prepare a news advisory.** Include a point of contact and phone number on it, and mail or fax it to reporters on your media list early enough to arrive one week before the event.

- **Encourage reporters to attend.** A few days before the event, phone the reporters to remind them of the press conference and encourage them to attend.

- **Assemble media kits or handouts.** Include summaries of the topic that you're presenting, prepared statements to be read, and photos and graphics illustrating the topic of the press conferences.

- **Set up the room.** On the day of the event, leave enough space for TV cameras on the sides or in the back of the room. Be sure that there are functioning electrical outlets available where the reporters will set up.

- **Have all members of the media sign in.** Give them a copy of your media kit or handouts.

- **Prepare an agenda.** Give all attendees an agenda for the press conference that includes key speakers and timing for the event.

- **Be punctual.** Start and end the press conference on time.

- **Say thanks.** Thank the media and your guests for attending.

- **Follow up.** Contact reporters who request additional information.

Meeting With Editorial Boards

One way to add to your program's credibility is to encourage favorable editorials. Editorials are articles that express opinions and are usually not signed by an individual because they are seen as representing the official position of the newspaper. To educate a newspaper about tobacco control and to properly introduce major elements of your campaign, consider meeting with newspaper editorial boards. The editorial board sets the paper's general editorial policy and includes the people who write the editorials that appear in the paper. The editorial board of a major metropolitan newspaper usually consists of the publisher, the editor, the editorial page editor, and some columnists and editorial writers. However, most editorial board meetings include only the editorial page editor, the editorial writers, and/or the columnists. At a smaller paper, a single person may handle the entire editorial page.

Editorial boards each have their own schedules and procedures, so call the one that you're

Checklist for Press Conference Planning

Facility Accommodations and Appearances

Be sure to select a location with

- ❏ Adequate space for attendees and equipment, including tables and chairs
- ❏ Enough electrical outlets for equipment
- ❏ Adequate parking available
- ❏ Accessibility for senior citizens and people with disabilities
- ❏ Adequate lighting
- ❏ Properly functioning air conditioning or heating
- ❏ Good acoustics for speaking and recording

Be sure to have alternative plans in case of bad weather.

Other accommodations and equipment that you may want to consider include:

- ❏ Lectern and/or platform and stage
- ❏ Reception area
- ❏ Videotape equipment
- ❏ Microphones and amplifier
- ❏ Recording equipment
- ❏ Audiovisual aids (e.g., screens, charts, easels, chalkboards, slide projectors, computers, and projectors)
- ❏ Photographer and video crew

Test all of the equipment in advance and allow time to get any needed replacements.

Before the Event

- ❏ Conduct a "walk-through" to determine the appearance of the facility
- ❏ Check the condition and location of the signs
- ❏ Before the press conference, test the equipment again with the actual material that you plan to use

Materials

Make sure that your spokespeople and staff are equipped with the materials that they need to effectively deliver your messages and to meet event objectives. Examples of materials include the following:

- ❏ Agenda, schedule, and program
- ❏ Gifts or awards
- ❏ Brochures
- ❏ Media kits
- ❏ Direction signs
- ❏ Name tags
- ❏ Host badges or ribbons
- ❏ Guest book or sign-in sheet
- ❏ Posters or banners
- ❏ Placards for speakers or guests of honor

Staffing

Make sure that staff are available to oversee these functions:

- ❏ Rehearsal
- ❏ Parking and traffic control
- ❏ Registration and guest sign-in
- ❏ Master of ceremonies
- ❏ Photography and/or videotaping
- ❏ Audiovisual arrangements
- ❏ Decorations and catering
- ❏ Setup/cleanup

NOTE: If your event involves a presentation or demonstration, you may wish to have prepared questions for designated questioners in the audience to facilitate a question-and-answer discussion.

targeting to find out how it functions. Many editorial boards hold regular meetings with outside groups. If you can get on the agenda for one of these meetings, make sure that you're thoroughly familiar with the media outlet and its position on tobacco. Also, you should:

- Attend the meeting with no more than three people

- Prepare a 5- to 10-minute presentation (no longer) that states your main message and the importance of your issue to the community

- Take materials to hand out, including a succinct explanation of the issue, a fact sheet on your issue, and the names and contact information of people who can be reached for more information

- Be prepared for a pointed group discussion in which everyone asks questions and voices opinions

If you can't meet with the editorial board, you can write an editorial board memo. This memo will contain the same basic information that you would have presented in person. If a hot issue is in the news, you can use editorial board memos to target columnists by providing an interesting point of view on the issue.

Letters to the Editor

Letters to the editor are an effective way for you to voice an opinion to policy makers and to educate the community about your tobacco-related issues. Use these letters to correct facts in an inaccurate or biased news article, to explain the connection between a news item and your activities, or to praise or criticize a recent article. Your program may send the editor as many different letters on the same subject as you have allies to write and sign them. To increase your odds that your letter will appear with little or no editing by the paper, consider these guidelines:

- **Avoid general salutations.** Whenever possible, use the actual name of the editor. If you don't know the name, address your letter to Dear Editor. Do not use general salutations like "Dear Sir" or "To Whom It May Concern."

- **Keep the letter short.** A maximum of three to five short paragraphs or 200 to 300 words should be sufficient. Some newspapers have length restrictions. Some newspapers also reserve the right to edit for length and may not edit a letter the way that you would want. Find out about these policies before submitting a letter.

- **Keep it simple and succinct.** Make sure that your first sentence is short yet compelling. Don't be afraid to be direct, engaging, and even controversial.

- **Get personal.** Demonstrate local relevance with your letter. Use local statistics, personal stories, and names to make your point. If you are going to tell someone else's personal story, be sure to get his or her permission in advance.

- **Be timely.** Capitalize on recent news, events, editorials, and public-awareness campaigns. If you are responding to a recently published article, refer to the headline of the article and the date that it was published at the beginning of your letter.

- **Correct but don't emphasize inaccuracies.** If the letter is to correct an inaccuracy, very briefly mention the misconception or inaccuracy, but do not give it much space (you don't want to introduce the negative point to an even wider audience). Then set the record straight in no uncertain terms and back up your statements. In the last paragraph, draw a conclusion or ask for an action, such as "call a toll-free number for more information or visit a Web site."

- **Don't forget to give your full name, address, and telephone number**. The editor may want to confirm your identity and organization/affiliation, or to clarify some point in the letter. Include a phone number where you can be reached in the evening, especially if your issue is urgent.

- **Follow up.** Don't be discouraged if your letter isn't printed. Keep trying. You may want to submit a revised letter with a different angle on the issue at a later date.

Op-Eds

The op-ed ("opinion/editorial" or "opposite the editorial page") expresses a forceful opinion on an issue, backed by well-researched and documented facts. While a letter to the editor often provides a concise and direct response to a specific article or broadcast, the op-ed may be more detailed. Here are some suggestions for content and format:

- **Be timely.** Connect the op-ed to the release of a new survey, a recent article, or a community event. Timing is key for an op-ed.

- **Follow the standard format.** Provide the author's name, title, and occupation. Mention the author's connection to your organization. Double-space the text and keep the article between 500 and 800 words. Localize the article with statistics and stories that provoke discussion and provide practical solutions to the issue. End with an overview of your group's mission.

- **Select a messenger.** Identify the best author or signer for the op-ed. Selection of the most appropriate author is critical in getting the article published and maximizing its impact. Even if you collaborate on the research and writing, ask a board member or a local influential politician to sign the op-ed. The more prominent the signer, the more likely the piece is to be published.

- **Follow up.** Call the paper three to 10 days after sending your op-ed to ask if it is being considered for publication. The follow-up call is also an opportunity to educate your contact about your tobacco-related issue, even if the op-ed isn't published.

(See Appendix 8.3 for a sample editorial, Appendix 8.4 for a sample letter to the editor, and Appendix 8.5 for a sample op-ed.)

Calendar Items

Newspapers, radio and TV stations, and local access/community cable TV channels often mention special events and meetings. This publicity is free and easy to obtain. When your event or meeting is open to the public, send the calendar editor a one-paragraph description of the program, plus information about the event's time, date, place, and cost, along with a contact name and phone number. This information is best sent two to three weeks in advance of the event. Respect the media outlets' deadlines.

Developing a Web-Based Pressroom

Making information about your program easily accessible to reporters will help you get more accurate coverage. Members of the media are increasingly turning to the Web for information about the topics that they cover, and creating a Web-based pressroom will make it fast and easy for reporters to get information about your effort.

Although your general Web site may contain a wealth of useful information, it may not include your latest news or clearly address what a reporter will want to know. Creating a special section tailored to reporters' needs can make it easier for them to get the story right.

Some tips for creating your online pressroom:

- **Post the same elements online that are in your media kits.** These include news releases, media advisories, fact sheets, backgrounders, speeches or articles by organization leaders, biographies of key people, an annual report, a calendar of events, photos with identifying captions, and contact information. (See the Media Kit section later in this chapter for more information on the contents of media kits.)

- **Put your ads online.** Digitize your ads and put them on the Web site so that reporters can see them. Be sure to secure all of the necessary permissions and pay all of the required talent fees before you place any ad online. The Web version of the ad should be low resolution so that it can't be downloaded to ensure that reporters or others don't use the ad in a news program or for any other purpose without your knowledge and express permission. Provide information on the Web site about how a reporter can quickly receive a videotape with your latest ad(s) for use in a news story.

- **Include screen captures of your TV ads.** Place screen captures (stills from a video) of the ads on the site so reporters for print publications can download them to use with their story. Screen captures should be of a high enough quality to be used in a publication. Contact your ad agency or the CDC's Media Campaign Resource Center in advance to make sure that all of the permissions are secured and that the talent fees are paid.

- **Make the links easy to navigate.** Make sure that the link to the pressroom is on the main page of your Web site. Don't create several layers of links in the press area; every key piece of information should have a link from the first pressroom page.

- **Make it easy for a reporter to contact your organization.** Each page should have a link where the reporter can send an e-mail to your organization's media contact for more information.

- **Track usage.** Use a log-in function to track who is using the pressroom and when.

- **Send automatic e-mail updates.** Consider programming an automatic e-mail notification function that sends a message to reporters when new information is posted.

- **Keep the Web site current.** All news releases and other information should be posted to the pressroom at the same time that they are distributed by fax, e-mail, or another method.

- **Continue your other media activities.** Realize that the online pressroom only supplements—but doesn't replace—regular phone calls, faxes, and other contact with reporters.

Responding to Unsolicited Media Inquiries

When you get a call from a reporter for information about your campaign, you should

- **Ask for particulars.** Find out what news outlet the reporter represents, what the full story is about, when the story will run, what questions the reporter has, and who else he or she plans to interview.

- **Ask about deadlines.** You are under no obligation to respond on the spot. However, it is important to respond to the reporter in a timely fashion. You may want to find out more or discuss the question with others before responding—before the reporter's deadline.

- **Determine who is the best source and respondent.** If it isn't you, brief the person who is the best source and have that person return the call.

- **Note the reporter's name, affiliation, phone number, and deadline.** If you're unfamiliar with the media outlet, do a little research, perhaps on the Internet.

- **Check the information.** Check all the facts carefully and collect your thoughts before you return a call.

- **Always call back.** Respect deadlines. Set a time to return the call, and make sure that you don't keep a reporter waiting.

Selecting and Training Spokespeople

Selecting and training spokespeople who will carry your message to your audiences are essential for disseminating your messages and for creating and maintaining a positive image for your campaign and organization. Your spokespeople should be ready to speak on the record and on the air with reporters. Make sure that they understand that discussions with reporters should always be considered "on the record." Many organizations have full-time spokespeople, although the role often falls to

> ### Bridging Statements
>
> "Bridging" is responding to a question by answering the question that you want to answer, not the one that was asked. You should never have to say "No comment." Bridging is a way to keep the interview on track, to control it, and to get your message out. Here are just a few examples of bridging statements:
>
> - "I think it's important to know…"
> - "We see it from a different perspective…"
> - "What I'd like people to remember is…"
> - "Let's talk about what's happening…"
> - "Our perspective is…"

the director of a program. When selecting spokespeople, you should choose spokespeople who have the following characteristics:

- **Represent the image that you want to project for your message, campaign, or organization.** They may be friendly and energetic, scientific, or very polished or casual in their appearance. Your selection depends on the message and image that you are trying to convey. It helps if your spokespeople are viewed as likable as well as credible.

- **Represent your target audience.** You want the spokesperson to be seen as credible. If your target is kids, you may want a youth spokesperson; if it's policy makers, you may want a respected leader of a community organization.

- **Are well spoken, articulate, and fast thinkers.** However, do not assume that people who are articulate in conversation will be "naturals" at being spokespeople. Make sure that you provide training and that they are prepared to deliver your messages.

It is helpful to have a list of spokespeople that you've trained so that you can quickly refer reporters to them for quotes and interviews. You can record key information about your trained spokespeople by using a spokesperson profile sheet. (See Appendix 8.6 for an example.) When you want to refer reporters to your spokespeople, you can use these profiles to help select the most appropriate person to contact.

All of your spokespeople should go through media training to perfect their on-air presence. Most PR agencies offer media training as a core service. Many independent media trainers are also available and can be hired as freelancers. Most media training sessions include videotaping mock interviews and then critiquing the performance. Most people improve significantly with just a few practice sessions. When reviewing a taped mock interview, look for:

- Clear and believable answers
- Main points repeated in quick, appealing sound bites
- A relaxed and comfortable interviewee

General Interview Tips

- When working with reporters, try your best to correct factual inaccuracies; otherwise, they will be accepted as fact.

- Pair the use of statistics with personal stories or case studies that bring them to life.

- Repeat important information to reinforce key message points.

- Know your campaign goals and objectives, and be prepared to provide information and answer questions in depth.

- Don't speak to issues that are not your area of expertise. If a reporter asks you about another unrelated health issue, refer the reporter to an appropriate subject matter expert if you are not knowledgeable on the subject.

- Don't speculate or lie to reporters. Always be honest and stick to the facts. If you don't know an answer to a question, say so, and offer to find the answer or refer the reporter to someone who can.

- Always make your own statement. If a reporter asks, "Would you say . . . " and then adds a quote for you to agree to, don't take the bait. Instead, succinctly state the main message you are trying to convey.

- Assume that everything is on the record and that everything is for attribution. Don't confide in a journalist. Say only what you would want to appear in a headline or lead of a story.

- Don't offer personal opinions when speaking on behalf of your organization.

Tips for Print Interviews

- Take notes during the interview, mainly about points that you want to address. Interviews are high-pressure situations; don't count on keeping it all straight in your head.

- Smile, stand up, and move around. You'll be more animated, and it will come through over the telephone.

Tips for Radio/TV Interviews and Talk Shows

- Before the appearance you should:

    - Become familiar with the show.

    - Role-play with a stand-in for the host.

- Jot down likely questions and answers.

- List three or fewer key points that you want people to remember. Keep them simple and be prepared to repeat them using varied wording throughout the interview.

- Prepare anecdotes, examples, or research to support your messages.

- During the appearance, you should:

  - Be confident, personable, and honest. If you don't know an answer, say so.

  - Talk more slowly than usual and speak in short sound bites.

  - Dress for success. For TV, wear medium tones; don't wear stripes, bold plaids, or wild prints. Stay away from bright white, too. Keep jewelry and ties simple.

  - Always assume that a microphone is live. Never say anything within earshot of a microphone or a reporter that you wouldn't want to be broadcast or recorded.

Developing Press Materials

If you want to get your message in the news media, you'll need to make your message—and your supporting points behind it—very easy for the media to find and use. Over the years, PR professionals have developed a standard way of organizing information into materials to suit this purpose. These materials are often packaged together in a media kit (also called a press kit, a press packet, or an information kit).

Media Kit

A media kit generally contains a lead or main news release and related elements (brochure, fact sheet, and photos) that tell a complete story. Effective media kits offer an appropriate amount of unduplicated information, arranged in the order of importance to the recipient. The most recent news release should be the first thing visible when the kit is opened. The contents should be compiled with the needs of the intended audience(s) in mind.

Media kits usually take the form of a two-pocket folder with a cover label featuring the name of the organization providing the information. (Use a computer-generated label to identify your organization and the kit's contents if customized printed folders are unavailable.)

Media kit components include:

- Table of contents

- Pitch letter (described below)

- Media advisory (described below)

- News release(s) (described below)

- Fact sheet or backgrounder on the issue and your organization (described below)

- Photo(s) with identifying captions

- Business card or label with contact information for your organization's main media contact

- Additional information, such as the following:
  - Printed brochure
  - Reprints of speeches or articles by organization leaders
  - Biographies of key people
  - Press clippings from previous coverage of the organization
  - Annual report
  - Calendar of events
  - Video news release

Pitch Letter

The pitch letter is designed to persuade reporters to cover a specific story. More than a phone call, a pitch letter or e-mail lets you outline what you're doing and why it is newsworthy. A good pitch letter has staying power. (See Appendix 8.7 for a sample pitch letter.) If it doesn't generate a story today, it may tomorrow. Here are some format and style suggestions:

- **Target pitch letters and news releases.** Send correspondence to one journalist at each publication or media outlet. Avoid having two journalists at the same outlet compete for the same story.

- **Be timely.** Play off recent or anticipated events.

- **Be concise.** The pitch letter should be one typewritten page or less. Aim for no more than four or five paragraphs.

- **"Sell" the story idea's newsworthiness.** Propose a news hook, state why it's a hot story, and suggest photos or other possibilities for visuals. Providing good visuals is especially critical to a TV pitch.

- **Skip the hype.** Forget cute leads, flowery text, and self-congratulatory language.

- **Organize the letter like a news story.** Don't beat around the bush. Make the opening tell the story, then provide background information.

- **ALWAYS include a contact name and a phone number.**

- **Advance the story.** Offer the names of interview subjects and experts who complement the contents of the accompanying news releases or materials.

- **Localize.** Generate local statistics and provide local anecdotes to tie your story to a national story on the same subject.

- **Conclude with your intention to follow up by phone.** Include your phone number.

- **Follow up.** Phone in a few days to explore different angles, but don't be pushy. Your job is to let reporters know what's going on, and their job is to decide whether it's newsworthy. Always thank reporters for their time. If the idea is rejected today, it may be more relevant tomorrow.

- **Use organizational letterhead and hand address the envelope.**

Common Traps

There are some common "traps" that people fall into when giving interviews. Sometimes, reporters will intentionally set up the interviewee to get a better quote; sometimes, these happen spontaneously. In either event, keep them in mind when being interviewed. Always keep your cool and never argue with or be condescending to a reporter.

- **Off the record.** You are never off the record. Consider anything that you say to a reporter as a potential quote.

- **The long pause.** Sometimes, a reporter will pause after you've answered in an effort to keep you talking. When you've finished answering a question, don't feel compelled to fill a silence by continuing to talk.

- **The derogatory remark.** If a reporter makes a derogatory remark, don't take the bait. Ignore the comment and bridge to your key message.

- **The phantom authority.** The reporter makes a vague reference to a study or a quote by an unnamed authority. Don't respond unless the reporter can provide exact information about the study and author.

- **Badgering.** The reporter asks the same question over and over or asks the same question in several different ways in an effort to get the response for which he or she is looking. Don't concede the point. Bridge to your message.

- **Irrelevant questions.** If a reporter asks a question that's not relevant to the topic or your area of expertise, bridge to your message.

- **"A" or "B" dilemma.** The reporter gives a dilemma, "Do you prefer X or Y?" Don't let the reporter limit your choices. State what you think is best and don't hesitate to state several options if that's preferable.

- **Multiple or rapid questions.** A reporter asks several questions in rapid order or asks questions with multiple parts. Respond by taking the issues one at a time. If the reporter has asked several questions, answer the one that you want to answer and ignore the other ones.

Media Advisory

A media advisory telegraphs basic information about an upcoming event and may catch a busy editor's attention when a longer news release may not. It should be very simple and can even be written in bullet format, like an invitation showing who, what, when, where, why, point of contact, phone number, and date. Send media advisories to all local media outlets, as well as to the AP wire service, which maintains a daily log of events that is sent to all subscribing news outlets in a particular city or state.

Be sure to indicate a time and a place for the interview or photo opportunities, especially if the event is an all-day affair. Make sure that you also provide a contact name and phone number on the advisory for reporters who want to get more information or schedule interviews.

News Release

The news release (also called a press release) is the workhorse of media relations. It communicates an issue's newsworthiness in a matter of seconds. If it doesn't, it will be tossed. Although news releases are sometimes used as submitted, they most often provide the foundation for a story or interview.

Just as important as the content of the news release is the format or look. Neatness counts. Make sure that the release date, your organization's logo, and the necessary contact information are shown clearly and prominently. Here are some guidelines for the format:

- **Style.** Indent paragraphs five spaces. Double-space and leave wide margins.
- **Fonts.** Choose one font. Don't mix fonts or type sizes.
- **Length.** Try to keep your news release to no more than two double-spaced pages, about 400 to 500 words.
- **Pagination.** For releases that run more than one page, type "more" at the bottom of the first page. Avoid carrying forward single words or lines of text. Make sure that the name of your organization, an identifying phrase (or "slug"), and the page number appear at the top of subsequent pages.
- **End.** You can denote the end of a release in two ways: Type "—30— "or "###" after the final paragraph.

(See Appendix 8.8 for a sample news release.)

Also note that you can prepare print news stories with images and pay to have them distributed to the media. Agencies that provide this kind of service include PR Newswire, North American Precis Syndicate, and News USA.

Video News Release

The video news release (VNR) is essentially a prepackaged 90-second TV news story sent to TV stations. You should ask your regular media contacts whether VNRs are useful before investing money in creating them. VNRs are useful when you're conducting an event that TV stations can't attend but would be interested in covering. TV stations often take sections of a VNR and use them with footage of their anchors. VNRs are often transmitted to TV stations via satellite. You can also digitize them and place them on your Web site so others can see the story.

Some major media outlets have a policy of not using VNRs because VNRs do not meet their broadcast standards. An alternative to a VNR is to send a satellite video feed featuring sound bites and background footage (B-roll) that the TV station can use to create its own story. This approach is more cost-effective and easier to put together because you supply just the raw materials instead of a fully packaged news story with a voiceover. To let the stations know about the feed, you can send a media advisory with the time and satellite information, then follow up with calls to the news editors.

Criteria for an Effective News Release

- Does it grab the reader's attention from the start?
- Does the headline inform the reader? Does it presell the story?
- Does the lead paragraph single out at least two of the five "Ws" (who, what, when, where, and why) that explain why the story is important?
- Does the second paragraph address all of the other "Ws"?
- Have you put the most important information up front?
- Have you put the most important quotes up front?
- Have you clearly and accurately provided the title and affiliation of the people being quoted?
- Does it use the inverted pyramid style? Start by giving the reader the conclusion, follow with the most important supporting information, and end with background information. This allows editors to cut from the bottom and still retain the newsworthy kernel of the release.
- Does the closing paragraph succinctly restate the purpose of your campaign or organization?
- Is the text concise, readable, and easily understood?
- Is the information accurate? Have you double-checked all of the facts and figures? Are all of the attributions and sources complete? Are the names, titles, and all of the text spelled correctly?
- Does the release avoid jargon and spell out acronyms in the first mention?
- Are quotations used properly to express opinions, offer ideas, and explain actions, and not merely to puff up the story?
- Is a pertinent Web site or other reference information provided?
- Have you provided a date and a point of contact with a phone number at the top of the release?
- Does the release clearly indicate when the information can be published (e.g., "For release at 10:00 a.m. Thursday, Nov. 17" or "Embargoed until noon, Feb. 1")?

Fact Sheet

The fact sheet or backgrounder provides basic, objective, and detailed information on an issue or subject. Fact sheets are usually a single page. A fact sheet supplements the information in a pitch letter or a news release. It adds credibility to any accompanying advertisements, media kits, op-ed pieces, or other timely materials. Follow the news release format guidelines to create your fact sheet. You may also want to use bullets or boldface for key points. If appropriate, use a question-and-answer format. (See Appendix 8.9 for a sample fact sheet.)

Responding to Negative News Stories

Sometimes, despite your best efforts to communicate accurate information and messages that support your program, a news outlet will run a negative or inaccurate story. It is important to respond calmly and strategically.

Tip 1: Remain calm.

- **Stay calm and don't take the negative story personally.** When you talk to the media, you are speaking for your agency or organization. No matter how angry you are, reacting thoughtlessly or attacking the reporter will not only reflect negatively on both you and your organization, but it will also hinder your efforts to communicate your messages.

- **Try to understand the reporter's point of view.** Reporters do not always have the time to get all of the facts before their deadline, or they might fear that if they continue to spend time on research, a competing reporter might release the story ahead of them.

- **Look at the situation as an opportunity.** Always try to think in terms of educating the media, thereby building bridges to promote accurate stories in the future.

Tip 2: Analyze the situation.

- **Look at your relationship with this reporter and media outlet.** Following up on a negative news report is usually not the best time to work with a reporter or media outlet for the first time. Expressing your complaint to someone who knows you and knows that you're credible is easier and more productive.

- **Keep in mind that reporters don't work for you.** Reporters have no obligation to report only positive stories for you—although they do have a responsibility to inform their audience with accurate information. You can and should appeal to their sense of community service if the stories that they're running are inaccurate or not in the best interest of the public.

- **Remember whom you're trying to reach.** You're not trying to win a contest with media representatives. You're trying to reach your target audience(s). If the reporter or media outlet is unwilling to hear your position, consider trying to get your point across to your audience(s) through alternate news sources.

- **Determine whether the story you saw or heard attempted to express both sides of the issue.** To many reporters, a balanced piece is one that examines the opposing sides of a story, even if you perceive one point of view as an extreme position and the other as the generally accepted point of view. As long as reporters attempt to present both sides, they will likely consider this to be fair reporting.

- **Determine whether there truly was an inaccuracy or if the reporter simply presented the facts with a negative slant.** Correcting a factual error is relatively simple and straightforward. However, a difference of opinion about a subject isn't as easy to counter. Statements that you may perceive as biased, uninformed, or sensational reporting may not be viewed by reporters as an error on their part. You can still respond to the piece, but your strategy will be different than if you're simply correcting a factual error.

- **If the story is basically true with only minor factual errors, you may choose not to comment.** Quibbling with a reporter over a minor point when a news item is otherwise accurate will not help you build bridges for future positive stories. However, you may still want to contact the reporter to establish a dialogue and offer yourself as a source, which may result in more positive stories in the future.

Tip 3: Know what to request.

Once you have analyzed the situation and have decided that action is necessary, know your options. Reporters only have a few possibilities for how to respond to your complaint. Decide ahead of time your ideal solution as well as your minimal solution. Think of this as a negotiation. Here are some actions that you may request:

- **Ask for a retraction or correction.** This is reasonable when a grievous error has been made and you have supporting material to refute the facts or statements reported. Ask for a correction immediately, and request that it be run as prominently as the original piece. Al-though this is not likely to happen, you may be able discourage the editor from burying the retraction in a section that's not widely read.

- **Ask for another piece to air that presents your perspective on the issue.** A follow-up response is a reasonable request if your point of view was completely ignored or misrepresented in the original report. Reporters are not likely to present a follow-up piece that simply contradicts a story that they have recently run because they will not want to lose credibility. They will be more likely to work with you if you give them a fresh perspective or a new angle, or supply some "new information" (thereby giving them a way to maintain credibility).

- **Ask for an apology.** Sometimes reporters make mistakes unintentionally. If the errors are not egregious enough that they will significantly hinder your communication efforts, perhaps an acknowledgment of the mistake over the phone by the reporter is enough. If this is the case, you may use this as an opportunity to develop rapport with this reporter and to establish yourself as a source that the reporter can contact to confirm the accuracy of information in the future.

- **Ask that a correction note be placed in the permanent record.** Ask the reporter or editor to place a written correction on file with the original piece in the permanent record and to tie the correction to the original report. If the mistake is a factual one, you do not want to see it repeated. Reporters often go back to do research, and may report the mistaken information again if they don't realize a correction was made.

- **Ask that a letter to the editor or guest editorial be printed.** A letter to the editor may be an effective response because these letters are widely read and publications are often very willing to print opposing views. Before releasing your letter, be sure to coordinate with your PR staff and seek concurrence from subject matter experts within your agency. See tips on writing letters to the editor earlier in this chapter.

Tip 4: Know whom to contact.

- **Talk to the reporter first.** Always give the reporter the first opportunity to respond to your concerns before moving up the chain of command. Give the reporter the benefit of the doubt. An editor may have changed a piece without the reporter's knowledge. A producer putting together the nightly news teaser may have misunderstood the message that the reporter was communicating in the piece, or "sensationalized" an originally balanced report. Let the reporter have an opportunity to respond and explain. Know the reporter's position before taking any further action.

- **If talking with the reporter doesn't result in the desired action, then speak to the news editor or the producer.** Keep going up the chain until you are satisfied with the response or until you are convinced that you will not get the desired action.

- **Consider going to an alternate media outlet.** If you have doubts about the integrity of the media outlet that presented the negative or inaccurate report concerning your issue or organization, you can go to an alternate media outlet to present your information and point of view. Of course, go to the alternate source with a great story idea, not just a complaint about the other media outlet.

- **Consider reaching your public through many alternate outlets.** If all else fails in your efforts to set the record straight with the original media outlet, redouble your efforts to get your message to the public through alternative means. For example, set up a public forum, make your presence known on the Internet, and invite partners to write letters or make phone calls. Offer articles for community newsletters. Work to establish contacts in competing media outlets.

Tip 5: Know what you want to communicate.

- **Remember who your ultimate audience is.** You are ultimately trying to reach specific target audiences and stakeholders. Keep them in mind as you craft your messages and responses.

- **Develop your message.** Have your messages reviewed by advisors and subject matter experts in your organization and partner organizations.

- **Frame messages in a positive way.** Don't focus on criticisms or negativity. Don't get distracted by the arguments or concerns of your critics unless they're substantial enough to truly be creating obstacles to communicating your messages.

- **Include a call to action.** If appropriate, include specific information about what audiences can do to respond or become involved in the issue.

Tip 6: Prevent and plan for future attacks.

- **Be ready to voice objections quickly.** When a surprise negative news story hits that relates to your effort or attacks your program or tobacco control efforts in general, you need to respond very quickly (often the same day of the story) to take advantage of it. Thus, you may need to develop a shortened review process to replace the usual lengthy review process. Your shortened process may include asking your head PR person to craft a response, then having it quickly approved by the program manager or marketing director. Having a crisis communications plan on hand will facilitate your response.

- **Prepare responses in advance.** Because you know the important issues as well as the basic arguments of your critics, you and your PR staff can prepare messages and responses ahead of time, especially for potentially controversial issues. Draft letters to the editor that could be altered slightly and sent within hours of the airing or printing of an inaccurate or negative story.

- **Attempt to prevent negative stories.** Staying in contact with your media list and providing them with the most recent and accurate information will help keep reporters informed about your issue and will likely prevent inaccurate or negative stories.

- **Let the media outlets know that you're paying attention.** Because you are part of media outlets' audience, they have a stake in responding to your needs. Let them know that you watch or read their stories. Maintain regular contact. For example, you may call a reporter to praise a good story. Build bridges with the media at every opportunity.

- **Let the media know that you're a potential source for information.** Invite reporters to call on you for interviews or information verification in the future. Make sure that you're available to give credible and constructive interviews and information. Identify and train spokespeople that you can offer as contacts for reporters to interview.

- **Coordinate with your PR team.** Make sure the team is aware of any ongoing issues with the media and are involved in planning responses.

Evaluating Your Public Relations Efforts

As discussed in Chapter 5: Evaluating the Success of Your Counter-Marketing Program, evaluation is an essential component of a successful counter-marketing program. Evaluation will help you report to stakeholders about what you're doing and will give you valuable insight into how to adjust and improve your efforts. More specifically, evaluation can help you answer questions such as the following:

- How is the funding for PR being used?
- What activities have you conducted?
- What are the results of your efforts?
- Did you identify, reach, and involve key stakeholders in the PR activities?
- Did they view your campaign as effective?
- Did you identify and reach your target audience(s)?
- How can you use the evaluation results to adjust your PR plan, reach more of the target audience, and contribute to the success of the counter-marketing program?

How To Evaluate Your PR Efforts

First, in a process evaluation, you'll need to monitor your efforts by tracking exactly what you have done. As indicated in Chapter 5: Evaluating the Success of Your Counter-Marketing Program, you or your PR firm will need to regularly complete logs, call sheets, and other tools to track the activities that are linked to the goals and objectives of your PR plan. If, for example, one of your process objectives is to reach a specified list of journalists by a certain date, a call sheet should be created to allow you to document what journalists were reached and when. (See Appendix 8.10 for an example of a media contact record.) If process objectives specify that certain events (e.g., press conferences, radio and TV appearances, and meetings with editorial boards) will be held or materials (e.g., news releases, pitch letters, and a Web-based pressroom) will be developed and/or distributed within a certain time frame, event and materials logs should be designed and used regularly to document your efforts. This tracking system may be time consuming, but it's important to have these data on hand. You can use the records to respond to inquiries from stakeholders and for planning purposes.

Your process objectives may also specify your intention to achieve a certain amount and quality of media coverage and target audience exposure. To measure media coverage, you'll probably need to use a clipping service, such as Burrelle's, Bacon's, or Luce. These firms search a list of publications that you identify for key words related to your efforts. They clip the stories that contain these words, compile them, and send them to you on a regular schedule. Each clip will contain a slip that indicates the source publication, the publication's audience, and other information. You usually pay a set-up fee for these services, then pay for each clip. You can then analyze the clippings to determine whether the slant of each story supports your efforts. For an additional fee, some clipping services will provide reports analyzing the coverage for you. Larger newspapers are often available online and can be searched electronically, either by visiting their individual Web sites or by using a search service like Lexis-Nexis.

You can also track video coverage through firms such as VMS and Bacon's. If you know that your topic was covered by the broadcast media, you can tell them the name of the program and station, and they can get a tape for you. They can also search the transcripts and provide you with a report of all broadcast coverage, including the text transcripts of each "hit." These broadcast-tracking services usually charge by each search, with tapes costing extra. You should consider using one of these services because it's generally the only way to track your earned media efforts.

Conducting an outcome evaluation to determine how your PR efforts have affected the target audience (i.e., change in awareness, attitudes, beliefs, and behaviors) requires considerable time and resources and may include surveying the audience exposed to the counter-marketing messages. One cost-effective way to do that is to collaborate with those who are conducting a target audience survey to evaluate counter-advertising and include PR evaluation questions in that survey.

Using Process Evaluation Results for Decision Making

After you have compiled the news coverage that your PR efforts have generated, analyze it to see what adjustments and improvements you should make. Are certain reporters not covering your issue? Perhaps you should pitch a different reporter or a different media outlet, or perhaps you should consider using a different angle. Are your key messages not getting into the coverage? Maybe you need to retrain your spokespeople or try new PR tactics. After each PR opportunity, determine and then document what did and didn't work so that your next opportunity will be more fruitful. By regularly evaluating your efforts, you'll learn which stories will likely get good play and which approaches will most likely succeed in getting the maximum coverage in support of your messages and campaign.

Points To Remember

- Create an annual PR plan. For both your Target Audience PR and your Stakeholder PR, create a yearly calendar of all the PR opportunities that you plan to pursue. Include national events that you'll tie in to (e.g., Great American Smokeout, World No-Tobacco Day, and Kick Butts Day), holidays and times of the year that lend themselves to certain stories (e.g., New Year's for cessation and back to school and spring break for youth prevention), and your own campaign events. See what gaps are in your calendar, and decide how to fill them so that you maintain a high level of coverage year-round. Create a PR plan for each activity that indicates the target audience(s), specific objectives, key messages, media channels, tactics, and timeline.

- Stay on message. Getting news coverage helps only if the coverage promotes your message. To make sure that you stay on message, create a limited set of standard talking points and key messages that will be used in all PR activities, whether planned in advance or done in response to an unplanned PR opportunity.

- Respond quickly to unplanned PR opportunities. When a surprise news story hits that relates to your effort, you will need to respond very quickly (often the same day of the story) to take advantage of it. This means that you may have to skip the campaign's usual lengthy review processes and let your head PR person craft the response and have it quickly approved by the program manager or marketing director. In many cases, you may receive a call from a reporter for your reaction. These opportunities require quick thinking, quick decision making, and quick action.

- Integrate PR with other counter-marketing activities. PR is most effective when it works in synergy with other components of your program. For this to happen, the PR staff must know everything about the campaign well in advance so that they can plan the appropriate outreach. Involving PR staff in the planning of advertising, grassroots activities, and other efforts will allow them to identify potential PR issues, both positive and negative, and to plan appropriately.

- Evaluate your PR efforts. For each event or activity, track the coverage you get. You'll learn quickly what works and what doesn't in getting the coverage that you want. Modify your annual PR plan accordingly. If you have the resources, perform a formal content analysis of the coverage to document the campaign messages to which your audiences are being exposed. At a minimum, review all of the key news stories to make sure that they reflect your campaign messages.

Bibliography

ASSIST, Site Trainers Network. *Advanced Media Advocacy Module Trainer's Manual.* Rockville, MD: National Cancer Institute, 1998.

Campaign for Tobacco-Free Kids. *Kick Butts Day 2000 Activity Guide.* Washington, DC: Porter Novelli, 2000.

Catacalos R. Online media room is new part of public relations mix. *Houston Business Journal,* Sept. 17, 1999, Available at: http://houston.bizjournals.com/houston/stories/1999/09/20/focus4.html. Accessed October 30, 2002.

Office of National Drug Control Policy. *Media Tool Kit for Anti-Drug Action.* Washington, DC: Office of National Drug Control Policy, 2000.

Public Relations Society of America. *Directory of Multicultural Relations Professionals and Firms.* New York, NY: PRSA, 2000.

Saffir L. *Power Public Relations: How to Master the New PR,* 2nd ed. Lincolnwood, IL: NTC Business Books, 2000.

Schultz D, Barnes B. *Strategic Brand Communication Campaigns,* 5th ed. Lincolnwood, IL: NTC Business Books, 1999.

Stevens C. Designing an effective counter-advertising campaign—California. *Cancer* 1998;83 (Suppl. 12):2736–41.

Chapter 9

Media Advocacy

*Once you "get" media advocacy, you have to do it.
Or live with the fact that you're not doing everything
you can to make a difference.*

— Makani Themba-Nixon in *News for a Change:
An Advocate's Guide to Working With the Media* (1999)

In This Chapter

- Coordinating Media Advocacy Efforts
- Elements of Media Advocacy: Focus on Strategy
- Media Advocacy in Action: the Art of Framing
- Evaluating Your Media Advocacy Efforts

Media advocacy is defined as the strategic use of mass media and community advocacy to advance environmental change or a public policy initiative. The concept has been used broadly on tobacco control and other issues, and it has many applications. One key application is as a response to issues involving well-financed opponents who use money to shape the political and social environment. Compared with public relations, media advocacy is more focused on a particular policy goal, resulting in social change. It's also more decentralized, community based, and community owned.

The information in this chapter focuses on the strategy behind media advocacy and why it's important. Practical "how-to" steps for developing materials and working with the media are outlined in Chapter 8: Public Relations. These steps should be reviewed before you read this chapter.

Traditionally, health communications used the media to re-create, on a large scale, the instructive relationship of a physician to patient or a teacher to student. In contrast, media advocacy doesn't try to persuade individuals to make specific behavior changes, but instead seeks to use the media to change the *social environment* in which individuals make personal behavior decisions. Media advocacy focuses on the social forces that shape behavior—that is, on public and private policy—rather than on personal behavior. The goal is to attain a more sweeping and permanent change in society at large.

What Media Advocacy Does and Doesn't Do

Does	Doesn't
• Rely on collaborative message development	• Rely solely on professional message development
• Reinforce social responsibility for the problem of tobacco	• Emphasize individual responsibility for the problem of tobacco
• Focus on advancing policy change	• Tell individuals what they should think
• Give people a voice	• Give people a message
• Train the community in media skills	• Take care of the media for the community
• Help communities create long-lasting environmental change	• Guarantee individual behavior change based on new information

Media advocacy is based on an understanding that the media are a tool, not a goal, and that media coverage is a means to an end, not an end in itself. Through the media, advocates gain access and a voice in the social decision-making process. But the use of media alone won't accomplish the goal of change. Media advocacy efforts should be used in combination with other communications and policy initiatives.

Media advocacy is a crucial component of a comprehensive media campaign because it empowers the community and targets policy makers. It's a way of getting your message heard and inspiring others to join in your cause. It can change attitudes and create a flood of support. Media advocacy begins with the premise that those closest to a problem are the best positioned to fix it and takes advantage of the fact that most media are local. It can extend the reach and penetration of any statewide media campaign by piggybacking national stories and extending the reach of a scientific report or finding.

There are no specific "recipes" for media advocacy. The successful use of media advocacy requires flexibility and being in tune with community issues, needs, and resources so that opportunities are embraced when they arise. Media advocacy is a learning process, and skills are developed through practice. Media advocacy requires long-term thinking and not being discouraged by short-term setbacks. When media advocacy efforts begin to succeed, you may face greater challenges as the opposition responds.

Coordinating Media Advocacy Efforts

Unlike other counter-marketing components, the role of the state health department in media advocacy is to support the policy efforts of local coalitions, which are often led by advocacy groups. A major challenge for the counter-marketing team is coordinating efforts so that everyone is working toward common or complementary goals and that each partner is working in the appropriate role. For example, public officials may need to avoid lobbying, but other partners may focus their attention in this area. Some partners may be better at collecting data and analyzing results of initiatives to inform changes in strategies.

To ensure that media advocacy efforts and your broader counter-marketing program are consistent with, and supportive of, each other, your counter-marketing team should coordinate its efforts with those of local coalitions as it conducts activities that are best delivered from a central source. Your team should:

- Identify potential statewide and local advocacy groups and individuals that can support your efforts

- Invite representatives from advocacy groups to be part of your campaign advisory board; their involvement in planning and implementation of key strategies ensures that everyone's efforts support a common goal

- Share campaign materials with advocates so that they can comment on these materials, help improve them, help promote the campaign, and deflect criticism and attacks from the tobacco industry and others

You also should consider operating an intra-state media network that includes programs aligned with state goals. Through your network, you can offer:

- Technical assistance, including access to national experts

- Information sharing, particularly on your program's effectiveness and industry opposition

- Networking, which offers the opportunity for brainstorming

- Training in areas, such as message development and spokesperson training

- Evaluation and feedback, which are part of the on-the-job learning that makes advocates better at what they do

- Tools, such as press releases and talking points, that advocates can customize for their communities

- Tie-ins to paid media campaigns, which can help support a program's paid campaign and generate earned coverage

- "Action Alerts," e-mails that describe key opportunities and how local advocates can take advantage of them

Sharing activities and events through a media network will allow local media advocacy efforts and your program to complement and support each other. Information on how to develop and use media materials and tactics can be found in Chapter 8: Public Relations. The primary pitfall to avoid is providing grants or other funding for local advocacy groups or coalitions without central support, training, technical assistance, and coordination. Without this support, you may find that funds aren't spent efficiently and you may not see the results that indicate progress toward your state's goals.

Interviewing With the Media: When Less Is More

Anyone who has been interviewed for a local television news program knows the drill. First, you get the call from a producer asking if you're available. Then, you set up an appointment for the video crew to come and tape the interview. In the intervening time, you might pore over fact sheets and background materials to ensure that you're familiar with the latest information. You might talk to your colleagues and co-workers about what you should say, straighten up your office (and yourself), and maybe call friends and relatives to let them know that you're going to be on TV. When the crew arrives, you drop everything to help them set up. While they're framing the shot and adjusting the lights and the camera, you talk with the producer and/or the interviewer.

Finally, the interview begins. Under the hot lights, you're asked a few questions and give the best answers you can. You may be asked to repeat a few statements. The interview may be over in five minutes, or it may last as long as 20 minutes, but half of your day has been devoted to it.

After all of this investment in time and energy, if you did a really good job, you may be given 10 seconds of news time. If the interview was with a newspaper reporter, the process has been similar (except for the lights and camera) and you might be given a one- or two-sentence quote in the finished story.

Is this tiny payoff worth your time and effort? Don't you have more important things to do? You have so much to say on this important topic! How can they reduce it to 10 seconds or a few sentences?

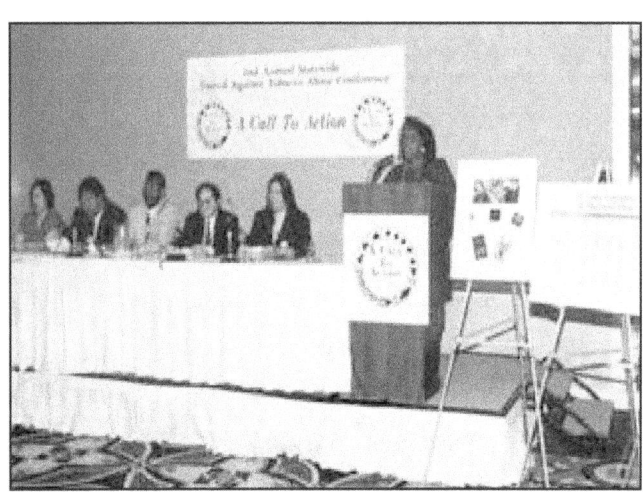

It may seem like you've invested too much effort for so little in return, but a few well-chosen, well-placed words can have a greater impact than a long treatise. The key is knowing how to use those 10 seconds or those two sentences strategically by framing your message well and aiming it at the right audience.

Considering the Industry's Response

Media advocacy has been used on a variety of social issues, such as housing, alcohol control, childhood lead poisoning prevention, and violence prevention. Tobacco control advocates were generating headlines that reframed society's view of tobacco use from a personal decision to a public health problem decades before dedicated cigarette tax increases, successful lawsuits, and the Master Settlement Agreement provided significant funds for sophisticated advertising campaigns. They did this for a very practical reason—it worked!

When people think of using the media to help solve public health issues, too often their imaginations are limited by what they've seen or done before. Posters, bumper stickers,

The Roper Report

The following are excerpts from the 1978 "Study of Public Attitudes Toward Cigarette Smoking and the Tobacco Industry," *conducted for the Tobacco Institute by the Roper Organization. This study was one of the first internal industry documents to be revealed to the public after it was subpoenaed by the Federal Trade Commission in the 1980s.*

Implications of the Findings

The original Surgeon General's report, followed by the first "hazard" warning on cigarette packages, the subsequent "danger" warning on packages, the removal of cigarette advertising from television, and the inclusion of the danger warning in cigarette advertising were all "blows" of sorts for the tobacco industry. They were, however, blows that the cigarette industry could successfully weather because they were all directed against the smoker himself. While the overwhelming majority of the public has been convinced by the antismoking forces that smoking is dangerous to the smokers' health, this has not persuaded very many smokers to give up smoking.

The antismoking forces' latest tack, however—on the passive smoking issue—is another matter. What the smoker does to himself may be his business, but what the smoker does to the nonsmoker is quite a different matter. . . .

This we see as the most dangerous development to the viability of the tobacco industry that has yet occurred. . . . The issue, as we see it, is no longer what the smoker does to himself, but what he does to others.

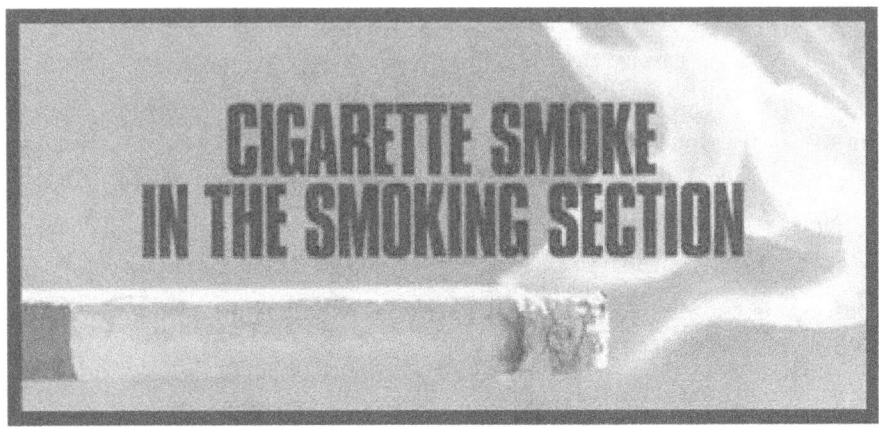

pamphlets, and public service announcements often have been the media tools of choice, not because evidence suggested that these were effective options, but because these products were most familiar to advocates. By looking carefully at how the industry responds to media advocacy initiatives, media advocacy practitioners are now better able to identify the efforts that are the most threatening to the tobacco industry. Until recently, tobacco control advocates seldom had sufficient funds for solid evaluation research. However, tobacco companies have been able to reach into their own deep pockets to research their opposition carefully. If tobacco companies fight against a tobacco control initiative, it's probably effective; conversely, if tobacco companies support or don't fight against an initiative, then you should probably analyze it well to ensure that it's truly effective before using that tactic in your program.

One example of evolving to tactics that presented a greater threat to the industry relates to the positioning of media messages. Through most of the 1970s, antitobacco media messages tended to be antismoking messages, focusing almost exclusively on persuading people to either quit or not start smoking. Beginning in the early 1980s, advocates reframed the issue to focus on the rights of nonsmokers and the need to regulate and counteract the tobacco industry's behavior. In other words, individual-focused antismoking messages became industry-focused antitobacco messages. As revealed by the 1978 Roper Report (see sidebar on previous page) and by many other internal industry documents that were subsequently uncovered, this strategy was exactly what the industry feared the most because it posed the greatest threat to its economic future.

The Eclecticism of Media Advocacy

Because many successful media advocacy interventions have produced confrontational, hard-hitting news stories, many people assume that any controversial news story is media advocacy, and that media advocacy is always combative.

Media advocacy does focus on policy change or environmental change. However, it doesn't have to be confrontational, and it isn't limited

CAUSES CANCER IN THE NON-SMOKING SECTION.

It's time we made smoking history

to earned media. Media advocacy can refer to a wide range of activities, including:

- Initiating calls, faxes, and e-mails to reporters ("pitching" stories or angles)

- Responding to calls and e-mails from reporters

- Designing good visual images for TV cameras

- Helping to develop messages for targeted paid media campaigns

- Helping to identify or develop good storylines that will appeal to media representatives

- Staging strategic media events

- Developing long-term relationships with editors, producers, and reporters (known as "media gatekeepers")

- Alerting the media about important political or other policy-related developments and framing these developments for the media

- Meeting with newspaper editorial boards

- Writing opinion/editorial (op-ed) columns and letters to the editor

- Conducting creative research to educate the media and to generate media attention

This list could go on. Anything that is done strategically to use the media to advance policy change or policy enforcement could be called media advocacy. Like other communication strategies, media advocacy works best when it's designed to advance a specific goal and when it's part of a comprehensive media plan that employs a variety of tactics, including paid media. (See Chapter 7: Advertising and Chapter 8: Public Relations for more information about earned and paid media strategies and tactics.)

Elements of Media Advocacy: Focus on Strategy

As noted earlier, media advocacy is the *strategic* use of media and community advocacy to create policy or environmental change. Those who work with the media face a range of options requiring strategic decisions whenever they have (or create) a piece of news:

- Should I share this information with the press?

- Should I call all of the reporters that I know or offer the story as an exclusive to one reporter?

- Is this development worthy of a press conference?

- Should we stage a press event and hope that the media will cover it?

The answers to these questions vary according to the history, the surrounding circumstances, and the goal of each media advocacy intervention. In every case, the answers should be based on what makes the most strategic sense at the time. For example, holding a press conference may be a wise choice, but only if doing so will be an efficient and effective way to advance toward the overall goal.

The basis for success in every media advocacy intervention is disciplining yourself to answer five important questions:

1. **What do you want?** This first question forces you to begin at the end and work backward by defining your policy goal or purpose in terms that are as realistic and specific as possible. Define the problem that you want to solve in terms that can be addressed by policy change (or policy enforcement), and state the solution that you seek in terms of specific policy action. You don't need to articulate a comprehensive solution to the problem, just the next concrete step along the path to your goal.

2. **Who can give you what you want?** Define your target audience. Do you need cooperation from local merchants? Action by the city council? Help from the governor? Who has the power to provide what you need to accomplish your goal? What is their self-interest? Who or what influences them? Are there secondary audiences that you can reach more easily who can influence the primary target? These policy decision makers, not the general public, are typically your primary target audience for media advocacy.

3. **What do they need to hear?** Once you've determined who has the power to provide what you want (i.e., your target audience), you need to determine what types of messages will most likely resonate with them. Begin developing your message by learning what your audience is thinking; don't assume that they'll accept your premises. Will they be influenced by new health information? By popular opinion in the community? By examples of success stories in other states?

4. **From whom should they hear it?** Identify your messenger by determining who'll have the greatest chance of influencing your target audience. State legislators may be more responsive to a

concerned parent who is also a constituent than to a trained epidemiologist who comes in from out of town. Conversely, a local board of health may be more responsive to a scientific expert. Learn about the decision-making process that you seek to influence so that you can choose your spokespeople strategically.

5. **How can you reach your target audience?** What kind of media coverage will attract your target audience's attention? Will a letter to the editor be noticed? Will TV news coverage of the results of a new scientific study reach them? Will a staged media event be effective?

Case Study: X Marks the Target

This case study is excerpted from News for a Change: An Advocate's Guide to Working With the Media *(Wallack et al. 1999).*

"X" was a proposed cigarette brand that many activists believed appropriated the strong, positive sentiment that young African Americans have for Malcolm X for use in selling cigarettes. The brand was manufactured by a small Massachusetts company, Star Tobacco Corporation, and marketed and distributed by Duffy Distributors. The packaging, marketing, and low price seemed lethal weapons in the tobacco industry's efforts to hook more young African Americans.

The effort to stop X brand cigarettes evolved out of a network of activists who had been mobilizing communities of color around the targeted marketing of tobacco and alcohol products. Brenda Bell-Caffee, director of the California African American Tobacco Education Network, saw a message about X on a computer mailing list for tobacco control advocates and immediately alerted her colleagues. In the group's assessment, the two small companies that manufactured and marketed the product were more reachable, winnable targets than any relevant public agencies. The strategy was, therefore, crafted to mobilize pressure and shame these companies into revoking the brand.

The group worked to shame the targeted companies by emphasizing two messages: X brand, whether purposely or not, defamed an important leader and cultural icon—Malcolm X; and it was packaged in a way that was sure to attract African American youth. The group gave the companies 10 days to withdraw the brand.

Media played a critical role in pressuring the companies to respond. Activists got the word out to both African American and corporate-owned media outlets, and articles on X appeared in more than 100 newspapers nationwide. Succumbing to national pressure, Duffy Distributors issued a statement one day after the deadline, which—without any admission of wrongdoing—announced that it had decided to withdraw the X brand cigarettes from distribution.

Answer these questions *before* you begin planning each media advocacy event. Review your answers often during the planning and evaluation process.

Sometimes the best media advocacy option is counterintuitive. For example, if someone asked, "What do you do when a reporter asks you a question?" most people would probably say, "Answer it." But the most obvious response may not be the best. Consider the following options:

- The reporter's question may not lead to the best information or to information in the best "frame" (more on framing later). You probably know more about the issue than the reporter does. If you're asked a badly framed question (e.g., one that presumes tobacco control is a battle between smokers and nonsmokers), it may be strategic for you to suggest a different question and then answer that one instead (e.g., one that reframes the issue as a battle of smokers *and* nonsmokers against corporations that sell a lethal and addictive product).

- You may not be the most strategic person to answer the question. There may be someone else whose knowledge, skill, reputation, or personal experience makes that person a better choice to answer the question and a better messenger for the information. The strategic choice may be to refer the reporter to this other source and explain why.

- Perhaps you don't know the answer or don't know as much as you would like to answer the question. The most strategic response may be that you'll investigate and get back to the reporter with the best information available.

If you decide to simply answer the question, you still have a range of choices. Consider the different responses to the question, "What does your organization do?"

- "We fight cancer and heart disease caused by tobacco use."

- "Right now, we're trying to help encourage local restaurants to go smokefree."

- "We support the community's efforts to reduce tobacco use by young people."

- "We fight to counteract the damage done by tobacco companies as they try to addict a new generation of customers."

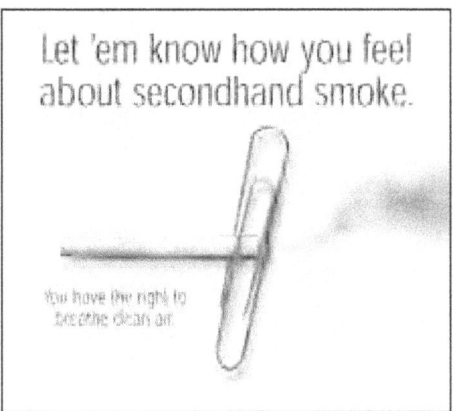

Even when you're having a casual conversation with a reporter, you might be faced with a dozen or more questions, each of which produces its own range of strategic options. Whether deciding if you should stage a major media event or answer a simple question from a reporter, good media advocacy is always driven by strategic thinking. Always keep your eyes on your policy goal.

Community Empowerment

The second important part of the definition of media advocacy is "community advocacy." True media advocacy does not exist without community advocacy. Many traditional media strategies are aimed at trying to change individual behaviors or beliefs. Media advocacy works with the community to change the environment within which individual decisions are made. For example, instead of using the media to try to convince people that smoking is expensive and dangerous, one media advocacy approach would be to try to persuade building owners to ban tobacco use on their premises.

Working with the community is an important part of a media advocacy approach. In many other parts of your counter-marketing program, specialists or experts can be hired or appointed to plan and execute the strategy for you. However, community-based social change can't be contracted out or delegated; if the community doesn't want to change, change won't happen. When the community does want to change, media advocacy is a way that community members can make the change happen themselves.

Media Advocacy in Action: the Art of Framing

Ask a group of tobacco control advocates whether tobacco receives enough coverage in the news media, and most will tell you that it doesn't. Ask that same group whether they've ever seen any news stories about tobacco that distorted the issue or otherwise didn't help advance tobacco control, and they will tell you that they've seen many such unproductive stories. One of the most common complaints

---

When issue advocates sit around a table to talk 'message,' they invariably rush to hatching catchy slogans and clever sound bites. Or they concoct elaborate arguments put forward by their adversaries. Good sound bites and slogans—and speeches, policy solutions, meaningful statistics, arguments—all support and reinforce your message, but they aren't what communications experts mean by 'message.' To communications professionals, your message is your organizing theme. And no media advocacy campaign can succeed without a powerful, coherent organizing theme, a theme that is at the same time logically persuasive, morally authoritative, and capable of evoking passion. A campaign message must speak at one and the same time to the brain and the heart.

— Ethel Klein,
political scientist

Framing Example: Same Question, Different Answers

Before you talk to a reporter, you should define your goal and how you hope to accomplish it. Do you want to generate publicity for your organization? Are you trying to advance a specific policy? Are you trying to focus media attention on the role of tobacco companies?

Consider this common question: Why do teens smoke?

Tobacco companies suggest that smoking is normative with this typical answer: "Peer pressure. Teens smoke because they want to fit in with their friends." Through this response, the tobacco companies are trying to divert attention from their well-financed marketing programs and draw resources away from prevention programs that really do work. This question has many better answers. Each answer brings a slightly different focus to the problem or the solution.

- **Answer:** Teens smoke because we make it easy for them to get cigarettes. Therefore, we need to keep cigarettes out of the hands of our children.

- **Focus:** Youth access laws

- **Answer:** Teens smoke because the tobacco industry needs them to replace dying older smokers. No one knows how to market to a target audience more effectively than this industry.

- **Focus:** Industry behavior

- **Answer:** Actually, teens aren't smoking as much as they were several years ago. We're doing a much better job of keeping teens away from tobacco.

- **Focus:** The effectiveness of your tobacco control program

- **Answer:** Not all teens are smoking more. African American teens, for example, smoke at a much lower rate than whites or Asians. We need to put our resources into the areas that need the most help.

- **Focus:** Disparities

- **Answer:** Teens experiment with a lot of things. They continue to smoke for the same reason that adults do—nicotine is highly addictive. We need to give teens the same kinds of cessation services that we give to adults.

- **Focus:** Youth cessation

Even though the reporter is asking the questions, your answers have the power to influence the story and how it's framed. By answering strategically, you can help increase the chances that they get the story right.

about the news media is that "they don't get the story right."

Getting the media interested in a story and helping to ensure that they get the story right are what *framing* is all about. These two facets of framing are called "framing for access" and "framing for content."

Framing for access is what you do when you're trying to get the media interested in your story. By gaining the attention of journalists, you gain access to the media. When you're framing for access, you "pitch" a newsworthy aspect of your story that will make the reporters want to attend your event, interview your spokesperson, and so on. Use the "Checklist to Determine Newsworthiness" found in Chapter 8: Public Relations when selecting the best news angle for each story idea. Consider what each reporter will be the most interested in covering. If you're trying to educate the community about secondhand smoke to lay the groundwork for clean indoor air policies, and you're approaching a reporter for the newspaper's business section, perhaps you can emphasize the economic costs that the restaurant and bar owners incur when their employees become ill from breathing secondhand smoke. If you're approaching a TV reporter who covers family-related issues, emphasize the risks of secondhand smoke to family members, especially children, who live with smokers. Once you have access to the media, you shift to framing for content. When framing for content, you focus on the perspective of the story and the information that you want to be conveyed. The reporters, editors, and producers who create news stories have to be selective about what they include and what they leave out of a news story.

The advocate doesn't make the decisions about what's included within the frame of a story and what's left out, but the advocate can influence those decisions. In every interview, meeting, and conversation with a journalist, the goal of the advocate is to frame the story so that it includes the needed information to promote the policy or environmental change goal.

When helping to frame or reframe a story for content, always keep your overall strategy in mind. (Review the answers to the five questions listed earlier in the chapter.) Work constantly to frame stories in ways that help advance your policy goal by delivering the right message to the right target audience. For example, if your goal is to strengthen the enforcement of youth access laws, you might generate some interest by telling a reporter that you have a story about youth smoking rates in your community. You'll have a better story if you say that you know several teenagers who can tell their personal stories about how easy it is to buy tobacco in the community. You'll have a great story if you say that you know teens who are organizing to pressure merchants and law enforcement agencies to do a better job of enforcing youth access to tobacco laws.

Developing the Message

All of the elements of your message—the content, the tone, the messenger, and the medium that delivers it—should be determined by your answers to the five strategic planning questions.

Effective Media Bites

What makes a good media bite? By definition, media bites are short—10 to 15 seconds, or one or two sentences, or sometimes just a phrase. Good media bites can capture complex concepts in simple ways. They paint mental pictures. They evoke strong feelings. They are memorable or witty. But most important, good media bites help advance your strategy. Being quoted isn't worth much if the quotes don't help you accomplish your goals.

Here's one example of an effective media bite:

> "Smoking a 'safer' cigarette is like jumping out of the 10th story of a building instead of the 12th story."

This quote addresses the tobacco industry's efforts to create products that seem relatively safe to consumers, such as low-tar cigarettes. This issue can be tricky for advocates because, at first glance, removing some of the harmful ingredients in cigarettes seems like a good idea. The following media bite is a clever way of conveying the idea that no matter what you do to a cigarette, it remains a lethal product:

> "Tobacco is the only consumer product that, when used as directed, kills the user."

One of the tobacco industry's stock arguments is that tobacco is only one of many products (e.g., alcohol and fatty foods) that can be unhealthy. According to this argument, if public health advocates succeed in regulating tobacco use, it will only be a matter of time until they also regulate the use of these other products. The quote points to a crucial distinction: alcohol, fatty foods, and similar products kill when abused or consumed in excess, whereas tobacco products kill when used in their customary, intended way.

You can brainstorm good media bites ahead of time to have them ready when you need them in an interview. Start by anticipating the questions that you might be asked. Then do some research. What have advocates said on this issue before? Modernize bites that have been used in the past by tying them to current developments. Try out different approaches and new ideas. Practice saying your answers out loud. Ask yourself two questions:

(1) Would this response be likely to make the news?
(2) Does this answer help advance my goal?

When developing your message, keep it short, simple, and direct. Plan as if your audience will only remember one thing from your media advocacy intervention (think of it as the headline). Decide in advance what that one thing should be, and base your entire communication around it.

Whenever possible, use research techniques, like opinion surveys and focus groups, to develop and test your message. (See Chapter 3: Gaining and Using Target Audience Insights for more information.) If you don't have access to these methods, talk to friends and relatives who don't work in the health field. Discuss the message with members of your target audience (e.g., friendly legislators) who can tell you what the message means to them and how it might influence their actions.

Monitor the media to see how they treat the issue that your message addresses. (See the evaluation section of Chapter 8: Public Relations for details on tracking media coverage.) Monitoring the media will allow you to understand how your issue is being covered and which tobacco control and tobacco industry spokespeople reporters are contacting. Understanding how the media covers your issue is necessary to inform your message strategy. Different audiences may respond to different messages. Your message may (and probably will) have to change over time in response to a changing environment. If you keep your strategic plan in mind, you can adapt effectively to these changes. Once your messages have been developed, it's important to share them with your fellow advocates so that your message will penetrate the market. It takes many different people saying the same thing to have an impact on policy makers.

Link your message to widely held cultural values. Most Americans have a common core set of values, including concern for health, equality, fairness, protection of children, respect for science, intolerance of deception, and belief in the right to a safe and clean environment. You don't have to convince your audience that these are good things. You only need to show them how these values relate to your message.

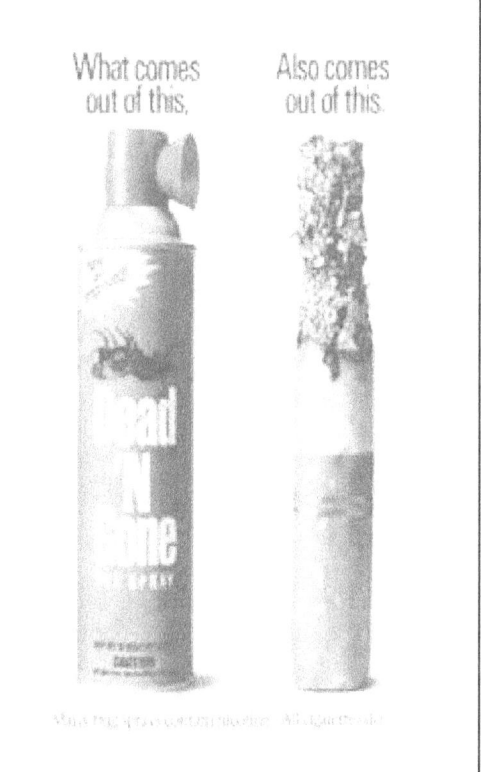

Case Study: Giving the Target a Choice

Tony Schwartz provided the paradigm of effective targeting. He made cassette tapes of the following message and sent them to the members of the New York City Council's Health Committee:

> To the members of the Health Committee of the New York City Council. We'd like to have you listen to the following two commercials, and tell us which one you will give us the opportunity to run. We are People for a Smoke-Free Indoors. Here's the first commercial.
>
>> You know the people in the New York City Council have the power to do a lot of good or a lot of bad. Just a few Committee Members can see to it that a bill gets immediate attention by the whole City Council. Or they can bottle up a bill forever, keeping the City Council from acting on it. Well, the City Council Committee on Health just took an action that all New Yorkers can be proud of. They just voted the smoking pollution control law out of committee, giving the whole City Council a chance to act on it. Despite intense lobbying from very powerful cigarette companies, they took this action for the health of New Yorkers. And so, with real pride and admiration for what they've done for New Yorkers, we say thank you Chairman ___, thank you ___, thank you ___. Thank you all for caring enough about the health of New Yorkers to not give in to the special interests. People for a Smoke-Free Indoors, Inc., paid for this ad to show our appreciation.
>
> Here is the second ad.
>
>> You know the people in the New York City Council have the power to do a lot of good or a lot of bad. Just a few Committee Members can see to it that a bill gets immediate attention by the whole City Council. Or they can bottle up a bill forever, keeping the City Council from acting on it. Well, the City Council Committee on Health just took an action that shows they care more about special interests than about the people of New York. They just voted down the smoking pollution control act, giving in to the powerful cigarette companies and preventing the City Council from acting for the health of all New Yorkers. If this makes you mad, write or call the Health Committee members and tell them how you feel. Tell ___, ___, ___. Tell them all that you don't appreciate it when they show they care more about special interests than they do about the health of New Yorkers. And if you don't tell them now, tell them next election day. Paid for by People for a Smoke-Free Indoors, Inc.
>
> So call me at ___, and tell me which one you'd like us to run.

People for a Smoke-Free Indoors had already purchased the radio time to run one of these ads. The bill passed out of committee and was eventually approved by the full council. The first ad was aired.

A good message does three things:

1. **States the concern** (e.g., secondhand smoke is dangerous to nonsmokers)

2. **Evokes a widely held value** (e.g., it's unfair to impose health risks on nonsmokers while they're trying to earn a living or to enjoy public accommodations)

3. **Presents a solution** (e.g., because nonsmokers have a right to breathe clean air in public places and at work, clean indoor air policies should be supported)

Targeting the Audience

When you aim at the whole world, you often hit no one. Strategic use of the media includes knowing exactly whom you want to reach and how to reach them.

All stations and publications that sell advertising know the demographics of their audiences. They base their programming on that information and use it to sell advertising. You can use that information to communicate your message to target audiences. Tobacco companies use it with precision to sell their deadly products. For the purposes of media advocacy, don't think of the media as a way to broadcast to the whole world. Rather, think of the media as a way to "narrowcast" your message—to have a personal conversation with your specific target. When narrowcasting is done well, it can function as "guerrilla media." Tony Schwartz is one of the great masters of guerrilla media, producer of some of the first and most powerful tobacco counter-marketing efforts, and the author of *The Responsive Chord*, which is a seminal contribution to media advocacy. He prefers radio for precision targeting because it's ubiquitous and inexpensive, and it accompanies many commuters to work. When the message is crafted well enough to reflect what's already in the audience's mind, radio is especially effective in piercing the consciousness. As Schwartz points out, "People don't have earlids."

Evaluating Your Media Advocacy Efforts

Changing tobacco policy through media advocacy can take a long time. It's a complex process that requires balancing focus and flexibility. By evaluating your efforts, you can continue to improve how you work with reporters and become more effective in working with them, thus helping to advance social change.

Evaluation can help you respond to the inquiries of various stakeholders. Your funders may want to know whether media advocacy is a worthwhile investment. Media advocates will want to know whether what they did was consistent with their plan and whether their actions produced the results that they wanted. Other media advocates may want to draw from the lessons that you've learned to become more effective themselves. Evaluation of your media advocacy efforts can help answer questions such as the following:

- What happened?

- Did you do what you intended?

- Was your issue covered by a media channel that your target audience sees, reads, or listens to?

- Was your story told in the way that you wanted; that is, did your frame the coverage?

- Were you able to build relationships with media gatekeepers so that you're now a trusted source for them?

- How did those who can effect change (e.g., policy makers) and their constituencies react to the media advocacy effort?

- Did your media work help you build community support for the overall policy or program goal?

- What didn't go well? What will you change in the future?

How To Evaluate Your Media Advocacy Efforts

You may want to review Chapter 5: Evaluating the Success of Your Counter-Marketing Program, which addresses the evaluation process in depth. Be pragmatic in developing your evaluation, and use an approach that's geared to the intended use of the results. To do this, you'll want to involve the intended users in shaping the evaluation from the start.

Evaluating media advocacy will be somewhat different from evaluating other components of a counter-marketing program. Measuring media coverage by counting column inches or by calculating air time won't tell you whether your efforts have helped to advance your policy goals. Moreover, each media advocacy effort is unique, influenced by circumstances and shifting to respond to unplanned events and breaking news. Many media advocates have used case studies to evaluate their efforts. Case studies can provide in-depth examinations of how media coverage on a particular topic was framed and how community advocates were involved in the media advocacy initiatives.

To conduct a process evaluation, you should focus mainly on documenting what you did, what the media did in response, and whether the message was framed in the way that you intended. You can use logs and other documentation to track your activities and to mea-sure whether you've achieved your process objectives and followed your program plan. To document what the media have done, clip relevant articles from print sources (or electronically search print sources that are also published on the Web) and record the TV and radio news coverage. Assess whether the stories have framed your issue in a way that advanced your policy goals. Try to understand why certain news releases or media calls generated better coverage than others. Review the coverage with colleagues, friends, and critics, and reflect on how the issue was framed. You can also hire media tracking services to compile the news stories and editorials that appeared during a certain period of time and to categorize them by slant, placement, and other factors. In addition, interview key parties, such as reporters and policy makers. If you find that a story didn't capture the interest of reporters, ask them why. These discussions and interviews can help you improve what you do.

To conduct an outcome evaluation, the most important measures relate to changes in social norms and policies, and the specific measures will depend on your media advocacy goal. For a social norm change, you'll want to survey the knowledge, attitudes, and behaviors of those among whom you hope to effect change. For a policy change, you'll want to track any actions taken by the key parties to adopt relevant policies. Because these changes often take a long time, you can also measure short-term outcomes, such as whether public officials recite your key messages, facts, or survey results in public forums.

Using Evaluation Results for Decision Making

Once you've analyzed the news coverage with your colleagues and collected feedback from reporters and your target audience, you'll want to use the information to adjust your strategy. Results may tell you, for example, that you need to use different communication channels because your information isn't reaching your target audience. Or your review may show that you succeeded in accessing the media, but the information wasn't framed in a way that would advance your intended policy objectives. This finding may indicate that you need more practice in defining and articulating your frame. Using evaluation in this way can help you stay focused, keep the message consistent, reach your target audience, and impact policy to produce the environmental change that you seek.

Points To Remember

The following is adapted from *News for a Change: An Advocate's Guide to Working With the Media* (Wallack et al. 1999):

- **You can't have a media advocacy strategy without an overall strategy.** Think of media advocacy in support of and in addition to other approaches, rather than instead of or in isolation from them.

- **If you want to be taken seriously as a credible source for reporters, you need to take the media seriously.** If you want to work effectively through the media, you'll need to know the media. You must pay attention to whether and how your issue is covered so that you can be more effective in your own media efforts.

- **Understand the conventions and values that drive journalists.** Journalists are professionals. Learn how they go about their business and use the common ground that you share to give them good, newsworthy stories while advancing your issues.

Continues

Points To Remember (cont.)

- **Pitch stories, not issues.** Tobacco control has been around for a long time. You need to look for new ways to make your issues compelling to journalists and news consumers. Journalists think in terms of stories. Issues can be vague and bloodless; advocates need to make issues come alive by crafting stories.

- Supply journalists with creative story elements that illustrate the policy solution that you support. These include good visuals, media bites, and "authentic voices" who can tell compelling personal stories. These elements will help you focus on your solution. The problem may be easier to talk about than the solution, but the solution is more important.

- Make your news events count. Plan carefully. Make sure that the speakers, materials, and the setting all reinforce your key message. Know what you want to say, say it, repeat it in different ways, and have others say it.

- An interview is not a conversation. Think of interviews as potential vehicles to get your message out. Stick to your agenda, not the reporter's. Don't get lulled into casual thinking. Be purposeful and make your point.

- Use the opinion pages to reach policy makers and opinion leaders. An editorial page strategy, including op-ed columns, should be part of your media advocacy efforts. It can be more effective than some news events in reaching the people who can make a difference to your issue.

- Consider all kinds of media in your strategy. Paid TV and radio advertising, as well as alternative media outlets, all have unique uses and can be effective in advancing your goals. Be sure that you know why a particular media outlet or approach is right for you now. Whatever media you choose, reuse the news: Send copies of articles, op-ed pieces, and letters to the editor to supporters and policy makers (know that all of the policy makers keep clipping files of your issue).

- Use evaluation to refine your media advocacy strategy and to improve your effectiveness. Despite your best planning and most rigorous efforts, your approaches will not always work. Take setbacks as a challenge: rethink your strategies, try different messages or messengers, but don't give up.

The following Web site provides a comprehensive set of tobacco activism resources that you may find helpful when developing your program: http://www.tobacco.org/Resources/lbguide.html.

Bibliography

ASSIST, Site Trainers Network. *Advanced Media Advocacy Module Trainer's Manual.* Rockville, MD: National Cancer Institute, 1998.

Chapman S, Lupton D. *The Fight for Public Health: Principles and Practice of Media Advocacy.* London: BMJ Publishing Group, 1994.

Health Promotion Resource Center, Stanford Center for Research in Disease Prevention. *Shaping Policy through Appropriate Communication Channels.* Palo Alto, CA: Stanford University School of Medicine, 1973.

Jernigan DH, Wright PA. Media advocacy: lessons from community experiences. *Journal of Public Health Policy* 1996;17(3):306–330.

Minnesota Department of Health,, Tobacco Prevention and Control Section. *Minnesota Youth Tobacco Prevention Initiative: , Communication Planning Resource Kit.* St. Paul, MN: Minnesota Department of Health, Tobacco Prevention and Control Section, 2000.

Patton MQ. *Utilization-Focused Evaluation.* The New Century Text. 3rd ed., Edition 3. Thousand Oaks, CA: Sage Publications, 1997.

Pertschuk M, Wilbur P. *Media Advocacy: Reframing Public Debate.* Washington, DC: The Benton Foundation, 1991.

Schwartz T. *The Responsive Chord.* Garden City, NY: Anchor Books, 1973.

Wallack L, Dorman L, Jernigan D, Themba M. *Media Advocacy and Public Health: Power for Prevention.* Thousand Oaks, CA: Sage Publications, 1993.

Wallack L, Woodruff K, Dorman L, Diaz I. News for a Change: *An Advocate's Guide to Working With the Media.* Thousand Oaks, CA: Sage Publications, 1999.

Wilbur P, Stewart K. *Strategic Media Advocacy for Enforcement of Underage Drinking Laws.* Bethesda, MD: U.S. Department of Justice, 1999.

Chapter 10

Grassroots Marketing

We never said 'don't smoke.' Teens aren't looking for more preaching; they're looking for the opposite, actually— a chance to be independent and rebellious. So that's what Students Working Against Tobacco was all about. We didn't preach to our friends. We got a bunch of kids together to make a statement to the tobacco industry—to rebel against them.

— Jared Perez, founding marketing director
Florida's Students Working Against Tobacco

In This Chapter

- Getting People Involved
- Helping Those Involved To Become More Engaged
- Using Community Partners To Reach Your Audience
- Evaluating Your Grassroots Marketing Efforts

Grassroots marketing encourages people to participate in your counter-marketing program. It gets new people involved, increases the involvement of those already reached by your campaign, and employs those already engaged to increase your target audience's exposure to key messages or services. A collection of tactics falls under the heading of grassroots marketing: events, community organizing, partnerships, and some forms of "permission marketing" (offering benefits to audience members in exchange for permission to continue marketing to them). What brings them together is their purpose: they're all about establishing and using participation. (For information on grassroots efforts for policy change, see Chapter 9: Media Advocacy.)

Involving people isn't easy, but it can help you significantly in achieving your goal of decreasing tobacco use or exposure to secondhand smoke. People involved in antitobacco activities are less likely to smoke or chew tobacco themselves and are more likely to urge their friends or family members to quit. Through grassroots marketing, you can build community support for your cause—which is critical to every part of your effort—and you can use community partners to carry messages to your target audience, enhancing exposure (how many people get the message), relevance (whether they care about it), and, in certain cases, credibility (whether they believe it). For example, a father might care more about what his wife says ("The smoke in restaurants bothers our son. I'm going to a rally for smoke-free restaurants. Want to come?") than what he hears on television ("Secondhand smoke is harmful to children"). The key is to remember that different people offer credibility on different topics for different audiences. For example, you may trust your doctor for health information, but you'd turn to a mechanic for information on car repair.

Keep in mind that community partners aren't commercial spokespeople. They're not under your control, and they don't always follow the script. However, grassroots activities work best when community participants are treated as partners, at least to some extent. The freedom to make choices is part of what makes an activity powerful for the participant. A clear example is when grassroots marketing is tied to media advocacy. When community members are treated as partners in creating an advocacy activity, the activity may not be as polished as one that's organized entirely by professionals. However, being part of the decision making draws the people involved deeper into the issue. They emerge more committed and more credible on the issue to other community members, not because they know every message verbatim, but because they believe in what they're saying. This doesn't mean that you want them to be off strategy, saying or doing things that aren't in line with your central messages or goals. The constant challenge for the manager of a grassroots marketing program is to find the right balance between choices and control.

This chapter describes some of the tactics that successful counter-marketing campaigns have used to address the following three goals of grassroots marketing:

1. Getting people involved

2. Helping those involved to become more engaged

3. Using partners to extend the reach and frequency of your messages

What Grassroots Marketing Can and Can't Do

Can	*Can't*
▪ Involve people	▪ Substitute for strategy
▪ Create interpersonal exposure to a message	▪ Be tightly controlled
▪ Channel some feedback	▪ Expose a broad audience to a very specific message
▪ Build community support	

Keys to Involvement
- Decide whom you want to involve.
- Offer them something that they want.
- Make it easy for them to participate.

Getting People Involved

What's true about marketing in general is also true about grassroots marketing: If you want people to get involved, you need to offer them something that they want. You will also need to make it easy for them to participate. To use commercial marketing terms, you will need to offer potential participants high value at low cost.

Tobacco counter-marketing programs have gotten people involved by offering benefits like glamour, recognition, and—quite simply—fun. Programs hold activities when and where people can easily attend. This may mean scheduling an activity after work or school and in the target audience's neighborhood or, better yet, holding an activity at another event that is already drawing the kind of people that you want.

Start with identifying the audience that you want to reach: Is it young children? Policy makers? Hispanic parents? Women? The answer will depend on your overall program goal and specific grassroots goal. If your program goal is to reduce exposure to secondhand smoke and your specific grassroots goal is to change the social norms around tobacco use, you may want to include policy makers with influence over smokefree restaurant ordinances as one of your target audiences.

The audience(s) you select will help determine the character of the tactic that you use. Offering recognition may draw involvement from policy makers; a contest may interest young children. Be creative: You may want to invent something new, but you don't have to start from scratch. Here are tactics that some counter-marketing campaigns have used and that others have replicated.

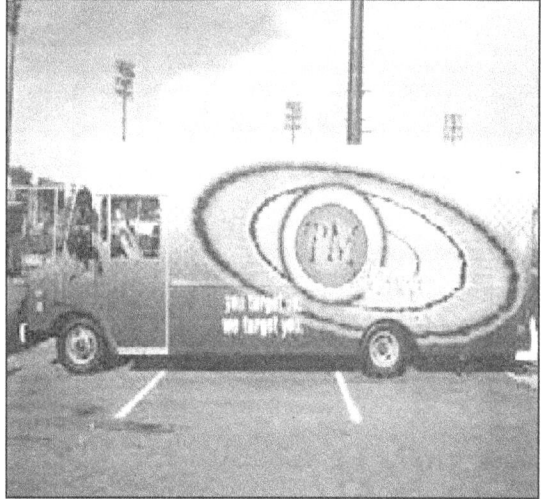

Recognition events. Some of the most important people to recruit in a counter-marketing campaign are those with a lot of influence over potential and current smokers. These "influentials" may be role models or people in a position to control widely distributed tobacco-related images, such as entertainers, reporters, and publishers. Recognition events are one way to earn the attention of such influentials in the news media and the entertainment industry. By honoring people who do the right thing (portray tobacco honestly) or by exposing people who do the wrong thing (glamorize tobacco), you can offer a benefit that many in-fluentials seek—positive publicity. For example, California presents its "Thumbs Up! Thumbs Down!" awards for tobacco use in movies, and the National Institute on Drug Abuse presents its PRISM awards for the accurate portrayal of drug, alcohol, and tobacco use in entertainment. These types of events might help you recruit influentials to be part of a campaign.

Glamour events. Building excitement is one way to attract people. You can piggyback on news events to make your campaign seem current and important or invite celebrities to participate. The key is to make sure that you stay focused on one of your messages. The American Lung Association in Sacramento, California, does just that to teach media literacy, piggybacking on the Emmy Awards to illustrate how tobacco is glamorized and normalized on TV. The American Lung Association's Flemmy Awards are presented each year to TV shows that inaccurately depict tobacco. This event draws considerable media attention and highlights a message about how smoking isn't as glamorous or as common in real life as it is depicted on TV.

Advocacy events. Activities that advocate for better tobacco policies, such as restrictions on smoking, are not only valuable tools for changing policies, but also a way to get more people involved in tobacco control. Among other advocacy activities, tobacco control advocates have urged restaurants and bars to go smoke-free, pleaded with magazines to refuse tobacco advertising, and campaigned to limit tobacco advertising in stores. States can also piggyback on national advocacy events, such as the Campaign for Tobacco-Free Kids' "Kick Butts Day."

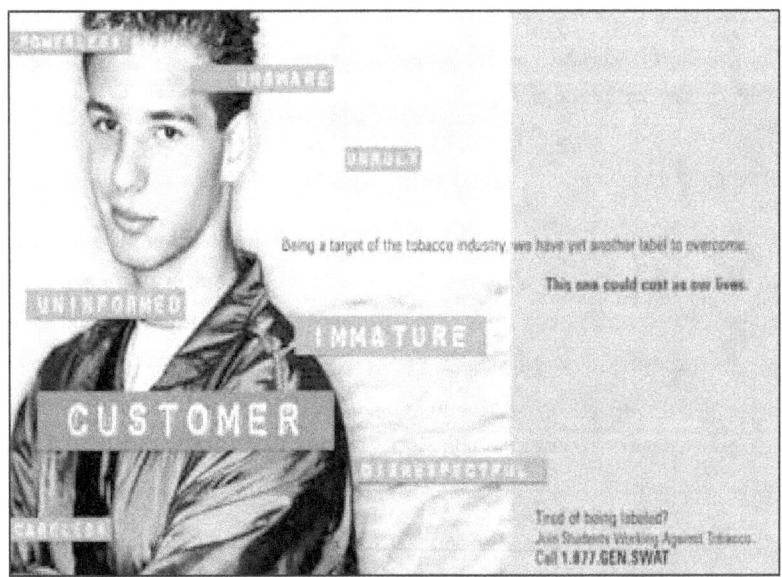

Activities within events. Drawing a crowd—or the media—is no easy task. Sometimes, instead of trying to create an event, programs piggyback on existing events. Activities can range from setting up a booth at an ethnic festival to distributing materials at a rock concert. Florida's "truth" campaign sent its "truth truck" to rock concerts sponsored by tobacco brands to offer a needed counterpoint and to recruit youth volunteers. The "truth" campaign also set up booths at concerts to collect signatures petitioning Hollywood stars for more accurate portrayals of tobacco. California distributed its "Gold Card," which was designed to look like a gold credit card and contained the state's quitline number on it, at numerous events. People placed the cards in their wallets and, therefore, had the quitline number available when they needed it. The Gold Card is now the fourth-ranked source of calls to the quitline.

Research activities. Hearing about something is one thing; learning about it is another. Some tobacco control programs create community activities in which people collect data about their own environment—and become more aware of what's around them as a result. California's Operation Storefront, for example, recruited local youth to collect information about the amount and type of point-of-purchase advertising done in grocery and convenience stores. Then the youth publicized the results. Although youth might not gather information that is as reliable as what can be gathered by evaluation professionals, the community involvement and subsequent publicity can help engage more people in tobacco-related issues. The Montana "Most of Us" project relied on grassroots marketing activities to enhance and broaden the reach of its media campaign. Students in a high school math class conducted a school survey on tobacco use, demonstrating for themselves the campaign's message that the majority of teens don't use tobacco. Another example from Contra Costa County, California, involved coalition members who conducted informal opinion polls, surveying community members about their dining preferences (i.e., smoking or non-smoking section), as a way to personalize attitudes and convey them to local officials during hearings on smokefree restaurant ordinances.

Contests. A prize is one of the most common benefits offered in exchange for involvement. Poster contests often are used to encourage young people, typically those in middle school and younger, to think about the downside to tobacco use. Unfortunately, young people often are asked to create these messages in a vacuum: they have no information about what kinds of messages might work. Messages developed without the benefit of research are less likely to be effective. Using these messages in a campaign (e.g., by buying space on local billboards) is risky. The most effective contests are those that stick to your strategy. In Florida's teen-oriented "truth" campaign, the program emphasized its messages about industry manipulation by creating a contest that asked teens what they might say to a tobacco executive. The teen who submitted the winning answer received an award from Music Television (MTV).

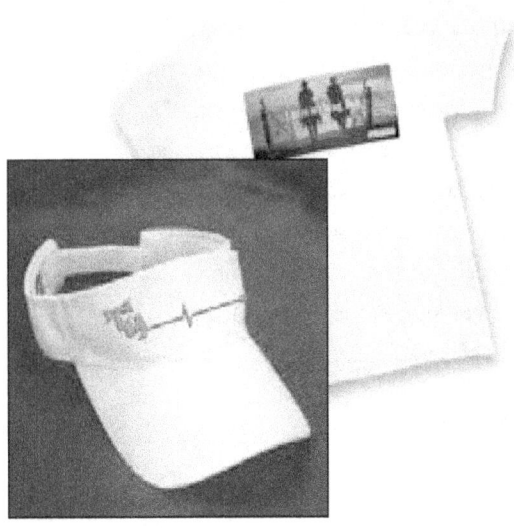

Using specialties and giveaways. Grassroots activities often lend themselves to advertising specialties and giveaways, such as pens, T-shirts, and stickers. If you plan to use these types of materials, first make sure that they fit with your strategy (e.g., California distributed Gold Cards to promote its quitline). Second, don't let each community or group create their own materials. To maintain a consistent message and to create efficiencies of scale, you'll want to produce the materials centrally and then distribute them to your partners for dissemination.

Helping Those Involved To Become More Engaged

Successful events are good ways to involve people initially, but you'll make a bigger impact if you become a more regular part of their lives. You'll want some people to become truly *engaged* in your campaign—to feel a part of it. This is critical if one of your goals is policy change. A tobacco control program can go only so far, especially if it's managed by a government health department that can't lobby for policy changes. At some point, people in a community need to press for change or it won't happen, which is why community programs are included as a critical component in the Centers for Disease Control and Prevention's *Best Practices for Comprehensive Tobacco Control Programs* (CDC 1999).

Different people will be interested in different levels of involvement. You should try to accommodate as many levels of involvement as possible, then "sell up"—encourage them to become more involved over time. In marketing, this relationship is sometimes called "permission marketing": You offer benefits to audience members in exchange for permission to continue marketing to them. The goal is not to make a single "sale," but to develop a longer-term relationship that will involve many "sales" or interactions over a lifetime. For example, sometimes marketers send useful information by e-mail in exchange for information about your purchase preferences, then follow up with an offer to sell you something customized to your needs. The difference with tobacco control advocacy is that you're not selling a product; rather, you're "selling" the idea of actively supporting the program. Grassroots counter-marketing campaigns have several general levels of engagement:

- **Sampler.** The lowest level of engagement is when people agree to participate in one activity based on the benefits of that activity. One example is a child who will participate in a poster contest because he likes to draw. He may not have bought into the larger antitobacco effort.

- **Ally.** An Ally is someone who agrees with your overall goals and will be part of an activity if it seems interesting, fun, or important.

- **Believer.** A Believer wants to help your cause and is probably thinking of ways to involve others. Believers will participate in almost any activity that they think will further the goals of the effort.

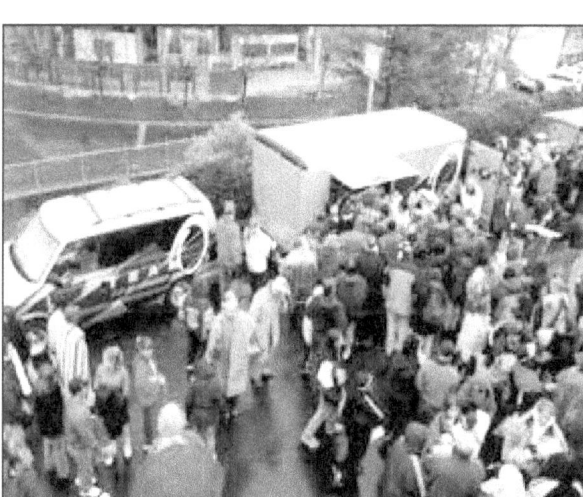

Believers are obviously valuable, but not everybody you reach can be a Believer. Few people are committed tobacco control advocates the first time that they hear about the issue. People change their opinions and level of commitment gradually. Programs attract Samplers, whom they try to convert to Allies. Some of those Allies eventually become Believers. Just a handful of those that you recruit are likely to become Believers.

There are many reasons to have people engaged in your program and many ways that they can make a difference. Once people get involved, you'll face issues related to organizing, effective advocacy tactics, and governance. Although those are important issues for the program at large, this chapter will only address the most salient marketing issue: How do you entice people to become more and more involved?

This question has been around for a long time. Active, organized grassroots support for tobacco control is often limited to the public health community. However, it doesn't have to be. Successful tobacco control programs have enlisted wide support on occasion by appealing to various groups, such as women's organizations, organizations that represent other specific populations, and, most notably, youth. Five of the most common ways that programs have engaged people in their effort on an ongoing basis are:

1. **Community coalitions.** Community members guide boards that may issue grants, implement community activities, or author community planning documents.

2. **Advocacy group.** Members and their supporters engage in statewide and community tobacco control activities.

3. **Internet communities.** A group of tobacco advocates can network and share ideas through a Web site or an e-mail list (listserv).

4. **Professional groups.** Such groups engage or target influential professionals, such as scriptwriters or physicians, to change how their professional group deals with tobacco.

5. **Partnerships.** The tobacco control program creates an ongoing relationship with another organization that may support tobacco control, or some aspect of it, but may not have tobacco control as one of its main goals. The program also engages the organization's members in furthering tobacco control goals.

There are almost as many ways to create these relationships as there are established groups. A lot will depend on where you're starting. Does a group already exist? Is the group well positioned to broaden its numbers? What kind of presence does the government agency overseeing the tobacco control program already have at the community level? Regardless of where you start, those with experience in grassroots marketing say that three principles should be followed in nearly every case:

1. **Be clear about the purpose of the relationship.** People will want to know where they fit with the overall goals of the program. The clearer that you are about the role you need them to play, the more informed they will be about whether they want to play that role.

2. **Show your partners that they will be doing meaningful work.** If people think that they're contributing to something they believe will make a difference, they're more likely to stay involved. This means that you need to allow for their contributions. Your participants need to be treated as partners who can help mold the effort, rather than servants simply being asked to undertake some tasks. Once you engage them, you'll also need to show them often that they're making important progress toward the goal. Your positive feedback will help to keep them motivated to do sometimes difficult and time-consuming work.

3. **Make it easy.** Try to minimize the barriers to getting involved, such as long or numerous meetings. Focus on what people want to do, not just on what you need them to do. Also, find out more about them—their strengths, experiences, and interests—to make the best match with the work to be done. For example, the former Coalition for a Healthy and Responsible Georgia (CHARGe) devoted 15 to 20 minutes during each of its coalition meetings to writing letters to legislators, newspaper editors, and other influentials to educate them about the tobacco settlement issue. They provided all of the necessary templates and materials, including preaddressed, postage-paid envelopes, so that it would be as easy as possible for coalition members to take action.

Using Community Partners To Reach Your Audience

Leveraging the interest and enthusiasm of community partners (which may include people at both the Ally and Believer levels of commitment) is an inexpensive way to boost the reach and frequency of your messages. But remember that the people you want to change are probably not the same people who will be involved in your program. Youth smokers, for example, are typically not joiners: They don't want to be part of an antitobacco group or any organized group. So although your partners aren't necessarily the people that you're trying to reach, they should be people who can talk to your audience—both directly and through the attention that their events attract—without turning them off.

However, recall that using community partners is not the same as paid advertising. You lose some control over the message and how it's presented. This can be minimized through training, but will always be a consideration. You are relying on your partners' credibility, not just your own. This can be positive. For example, some people will believe the American Cancer Society more than they'll believe the state health department. However, it also raises difficult issues. For example, youth who become antitobacco advocates aren't always the trendsetters in school. What if a teen who's widely regarded by his peers as "uncool" or a "goody two-shoes" is the main spokesperson in his school saying smoking isn't cool? The message may lack credibility. This is another reason that balancing the desires of your grassroots advocates with the

Case Study: Reaching Georgia Legislators

To encourage more legislators to support the allocation of tobacco settlement funds to tobacco control, the former Coalition for a Healthy and Responsible Georgia (CHARGe) organized and executed several efforts to involve advocates and community members at a grassroots level. First, they held community forums to educate individuals at the local level about the importance of allocating one-third of tobacco settlement dollars to tobacco prevention and control efforts. At those educational forums, they provided participants with sample letters to the editor, sample letters to legislators, fact sheets, talking points, and other materials to make it easy for participants to take action. A few months later, the American Cancer Society, the American Heart Association, and the American Lung Association, in partnership with the Fletcher Martin Ewing ad agency, developed a trifold brochure that summarized for local advocates the key benefits of allocating settlement funds to tobacco prevention and control, and included a tear-card that advocates could send to their local legislators about the issue. In addition, CHARGe and the Georgia Health Department's Tobacco Use Prevention Program developed a companion brochure that educated Georgians on the burden of tobacco in Georgia. (For more information, see Appendix 10.1: Georgia Burden of Tobacco Brochure.)

goals of your program is so important. In the example above, this teen could be steered into activities where he could be the most effective—perhaps making a presentation to the school board instead of lecturing his peers.

The main guideline here is that you must consider how your audience views your partners. Your partners may have credibility with your audience on some issues, but not on others. In Florida, teachers were encouraged to present media literacy modules that help teens deconstruct advertising. However, teachers were asked not to distribute any "truth"-branded materials because this antitobacco brand was supposed to be young and rebellious. It would have been much cheaper to promote the "truth" brand through the schools than through TV and events, but Florida passed up this cost-effective dissemination channel because it lacked the right kind of credibility to reposition tobacco control as hip and young.

The choices aren't always clear. Florida went so far as to brand its youth advocacy group as "Students Working Against Tobacco" (SWAT), instead of the much more widely recognized "truth." This was a way to put distance between the state's real youth advocates (who may or may not be seen by their peers as cool) and the state's hip, advertising-driven antitobacco brand. On the other hand, Minnesota branded both its teen advertising and its youth advocacy group as Target Market (TM), to invest more marketing muscle in creating activism and to save the cost of creating two brands. Both states have had documented success.

When using partners as a dissemination channel, a program manager also must match the right message with the right partner. Again, partners should only disseminate messages that will seem credible coming from them. Police, for example, may be good messengers on issues of law (such as enforcing smokefree restaurant policies or laws on youth access to tobacco), but less credible with youth on the practices of other youth. ("How would a police officer know how many of us smoke?" a teen might wonder. "Who is going to tell him?") This is true, regardless of whether the partner actually is an authority on the subject. The key question is whether the audience *perceives* him or her as an authority.

Partners can use dozens of tactics to disseminate messages. Four of the most common tactics are:

1. **Media events.** Partners often hold media events that, while not explicitly targeting potential tobacco users, are designed to send them a message. Many of the anti-industry events are staged with this in mind. Few partners expect the industry to change, but anti-industry events can highlight a message to smokers that the industry is trying to manipulate them.

2. **Counter-advertising.** Community groups rarely have enough money to buy a significant amount of media space or time. Sometimes they can develop a partnership with a local TV station or newspaper to place antitobacco advertising at low or no cost. It is also possible to develop a partnership with a radio disc jockey who is willing to read live

announcer radio ads, at no cost to the program.

3. **Speaking.** Partners can be very credible spokespeople when addressing community groups or their peers (especially younger peers). Several states have created programs where high school-age antitobacco advocates speak to students in elementary or middle schools. In Contra Costa County, California, coalition members persuasively presented qualitative research findings regarding community members' preferences for smokefree restaurants to local officials during hearings regarding smokefree restaurant ordinances.

4. **Advocacy.** As mentioned previously, advocacy activities can serve a number of purposes beyond a change in policy. One is positioning the issue with the target audience. Advocating for smokefree restaurants, for example, is a way to disseminate messages about secondhand tobacco smoke. For example, SmokeLess States Coalitions throughout the country initiated a "tobacco tax challenge" to the state governors, challenging them to help save lives (and increase state funds) by raising their tobacco taxes.

What makes a dissemination effort by your partners effective? Program managers suggest several guidelines for making it work:

- **Involve your partners early.** People who agree with your goal may not support your campaign if they feel like outsiders. If they don't understand your strategy, they could inadvertently promote messages that may undermine your effort. (If your strategy is to make not smoking rebellious, it would probably be counterproductive to warn teens that youth caught smoking will be punished.) Help them understand what you're trying to achieve (goal, key audiences, and message strategies) and the important role that you want them to play. Give them as much information as they need or want to do a good job and to sense the urgency of the issue.

- **Keep your partners in the loop.** When you surprise your partners, you run the risk of lost opportunities as well as hurt feelings. You probably don't know all of the ways that your partners could assist you in your marketing effort. By keeping them in the loop, you can be apprised of opportunities to leverage your investment.

- **Match the right message with the right partner.** As mentioned, no one is credible with every audience on every subject. Encourage your partners to focus on the messages that they're in the best position to deliver. They don't simply need to be able to reach the audience efficiently—they also need to be effective in what they say and how they say it. That means that they need to convey messages on which they are credible.

- **Provide training.** If you want your partners to be on message, you will have to train them as spokespeople for your campaign. Provide talking points and tips on how to talk to reporters, and let them practice if you can.

Evaluating Your Grassroots Marketing Efforts

To maximize the effectiveness of your grassroots marketing efforts, you'll need to evaluate what you're doing. Evaluation will not only

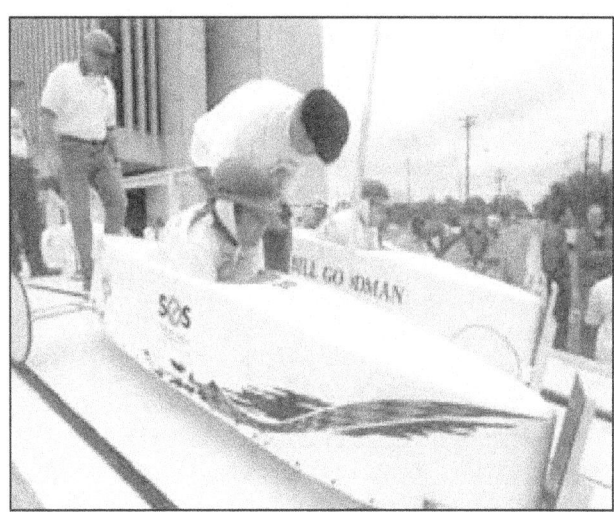

help you report to stakeholders about what you're doing, but it will also give you valuable insight about how to improve your approach. Adjusting your approach based on evaluation results can help you get more types of people involved and deepen their commitment and involvement.

Evaluation can help you answer questions such as the following:

- How is the funding for grassroots marketing being used?

- Was your approach implemented as planned?

- Did you reach your target audience, and did audience members find your approach to be beneficial, fun, accessible, and convenient?

- Did you reach a broad range of community partners? Were the partners credible to audience members and willing to deliver the antitobacco message to them?

- What tactics were most effective in reaching these partners? What tactics did partners use for disseminating antitobacco messages, and how effective were they in reaching the target audience?

- Did your effort help increase the audience's level of commitment or involvement?

- How can you use the results of the evaluation to improve your grassroots approach?

How to Evaluate Your Grassroots Marketing Efforts

You may want to review Chapter 5: Evaluating the Success of Your Counter-Marketing Program, which addresses the evaluation process in depth. Be pragmatic in developing your evaluation, and use an approach based on how the results will be used. Once you have determined whom the evaluation is for and what information they will need, you can develop the best questions to find out what you need to know, determine how to get the answers to those questions, and then provide the information to those who need it in a way that they can use. To do this, you'll want to involve those intended users in shaping the evaluation from the start. At a minimum, you'll want to assess both your process (process evaluation) and the outcome of your efforts (outcome evaluation). To conduct a process evaluation, you can use implementation logs to systematically monitor and track what you're doing and to assess whether you're meeting your process objectives. If your plan designates that certain tactics will be used to reach a certain number of targeted partners, an outreach log can be used to document how many people were reached in an outreach activity and what tactics were used. Data across outreach events can be summarized to measure your progress in meeting these process objectives.

To conduct an outcome evaluation, you'll need to determine what realistic outcomes you hope to achieve. Once again, these outcomes should be linked directly to your program's goals and objectives. Although the monitoring and tracking system can help you to determine whether you reached the expected number of targeted partners and what tactics were most effective in recruiting them, it won't tell you how your intervention affected these participants.

One outcome you'll probably want to achieve is an increase in the targeted partners' involvement in, and commitment to, the counter-marketing program. To learn whether this occurred, you must develop and use valid and reliable measures of commitment and involvement. For example, if you hope that your efforts will move a certain percentage of partners from being Allies to Believers, you'll need to clearly define what constitutes an Ally and a Believer. These definitions then should be used to accurately assess whether audience members have made this change.

Short surveys administered before the grassroots activity takes place (presurvey or baseline survey) and after it concludes (postsurvey) can determine participants' increased commitment to the issue and their intention to become more involved in the campaign. You could also follow up with a representative sample of the participants to see whether they have become more involved or committed.

Another outcome you'll want to achieve is making the Allies and Believers credible spokespeople. You can measure this through surveys among individuals aware of the grassroots work. For example, you can ask them whether they heard a speech by a representative of the organization (e.g., SWAT) or whether they talked with a member of the organization. Then you can ask them about their impressions of these Allies and Believers, what they learned from them, and other questions that would provide useful information.

Using Evaluation Results for Decision Making

If your evaluation results indicate that certain partners are more effective than others, this may tell you something about their credibility and help you decide which ones to work with in the future. If the results show that certain tactics or messages were more effective than others in involving the target audience or that they were more appealing to Allies than Believers, this information can help you better plan how to involve people initially and increase participants' involvement. After each round of grassroots activities, you'll see what worked and what didn't so that your next opportunity will be more fruitful. By evaluating your efforts regularly, you'll learn more about how to engage your partners and target audience, how to solicit their initial involvement in the counter-marketing program, and how to increase their commitment.

> ### *Points To Remember*
>
> In grassroots marketing, the bottom line is engagement. You're not just persuading people, you're getting them involved. This activity can be much more challenging than airing advertising or staging a press event. You're working with volunteers, not paid contractors, so they can bow out if they're not feeling motivated, rewarded, or satisfied. However, the potential benefits are enormous. An ad may run for several months, but true Believers are around for a long time.

Bibliography

Centers for Disease Control and Prevention. *Best Practices for Comprehensive Tobacco Control Programs–August 1999*. Atlanta, GA: U.S. Department of Health and Human Services, Centers for Disease Control and Prevention, National Center for Chronic Disease Prevention and Health Promotion, Office on Smoking and Health, August 1999. Reprinted with corrections.

Godin S. *Permission Marketing: Turning Strangers into Friends, and Friends into Customers*. New York, NY: Simon and Schuster, 1999.

Hall GE, Hord SM. *Implementing Change: Patterns, Principles, and Potholes*. Boston, MA: Allyn and Bacon, 2001.

McKenzie-Mohr D, Smith W. *Fostering Sustainable Behavior: An Introduction to Community-Based Social Marketing*. Gabriola Island, BC, Canada: New Society Publishers, 1999.

Chapter 11
Media Literacy

Media literacy is like the dog in "The Wizard of Oz" who pulls back the curtain to reveal the man behind the Wizard image.

— Frank Baker, media literacy expert

In This Chapter

- Media Literacy and Youth
- Essential Ingredients of Media Literacy
- How Media Literacy Complements Counter-Marketing
- Implementing a Media Literacy Program
- Evaluating Your Efforts
- Resources

Media literacy helps people ask questions about what they watch, see, hear, and read. It helps them critically assess how the mass media normalize, glamorize, and create role models for unhealthy lifestyles and behaviors, such as smoking. Media literacy involves examining the techniques, technologies, and institutions involved in media production; critically analyzing media messages; and recognizing the role that audiences play in attaching a meaning to those messages. The idea behind media literacy is that teaching people to recognize how a message tries to influence them will lessen the impact of that message. On a broader level, media literacy can be viewed as a form of protection or "inoculation" against unhealthy behaviors shown in the media.

This chapter gives an overview of media literacy and how it fits into a counter-marketing campaign. An extensive resources section at the end of this chapter lists media literacy curricula and other planning aids.

Media Literacy and Youth

Although some media literacy efforts target adults, most focus on young people and teens—and with good reason. Consider the following data:

- Adolescents spend 24 hours per week watching television—twice as much time as they spend in school over the course of one year (Kaiser Family Foundation 1999; Strasburger et al. 2000).

- Thirty-seven percent of children ages 6 to 11 and 55.8 percent of teens ages 12 to 17 have TV sets in their bedrooms (Kaiser Family Foundation 1999; Strasburger et al. 2000).

- Eighty-two percent of adolescents use the Internet (Kaiser Family Foundation 1999; Strasburger et al. 2000).

- Adolescents listen to about 40 hours of popular music per week (Kaiser Family Foundation 1999; Strasburger et al. 2000).

- Studies show that many parents don't see their children's media habits as a cause for concern.

Youth love learning about media. Their culture and much of their identities are immersed in media. Teaching media literacy is an excellent way to attract their attention and to build their interest in health and smoking issues.

Couple these facts with the tobacco industry's advertising and marketing practices:

- In 2000, the industry spent $9.57 billion to advertise and market tobacco products (Federal Trade Commission 2002).

- Although no cigarette advertising appears on TV and radio, tobacco images are pervasive. They appear in movies, on clothing, at sporting events, and in other places. One study from Dartmouth College and Dartmouth Medical School showed that smoking in movies is linked to adolescents trying their first cigarette (Sargent et al. 2001).

- A landmark study in the 1980s showed that as many young children recognized Joe Camel as they did Mickey Mouse (Fischer et al. 1991).

- Camel's market share among underage smokers rose from 0.5 percent to 32.8 percent after the Joe Camel campaign was introduced (DiFranza et al. 1991).

> "It is a well known fact that teenagers like sweet products. Honey might be considered."
> – KOOL cigarettes memo

Consequently, media literacy has developed a large following among U.S. educators and health educators interested in youth. All 50 states have some requirement for media literacy in their education standards (see http://www.med.sc.edu:1081/statelit.htm). Furthermore, many tested curricula are available to teach about media literacy on tobacco and alcohol use.

Media literacy programs have shown some success. For example, research shows that media literacy programs addressing alcohol ads can help children become more informed; can diminish the perception that "everybody" is using alcohol; can encourage children to be more critical of the alcohol industry's advertising techniques; and can reduce intentions to use alcohol over the short term (Austin 1997; Slater 1996). The programs may even help to improve long-term cognitive resistance to

Designing and Implementing an Effective Tobacco Counter-Marketing Campaign

What Media Literacy Can and Can't Do

Can
- Help change attitudes
- Teach people to recognize how messages are designed to influence them
- Contribute to changing long-term behavior

Can't
- Change long-term behavior in the absence of other program elements
- Replace classes or programs that explain tobacco's impact on health

alcohol ads (Slater 1996). Qualitative research and the experiences of media literacy experts indicate that, if executed well, these programs can change people's knowledge, attitudes, and/or behaviors.

Essential Ingredients of Media Literacy

Media literacy has four main concepts. All media:

- Are constructed
- Have codes and conventions
- Convey value messages
- Have financial interests

Media literacy includes these activities:

- Critically analyzing media messages
- Evaluating the source of information
- Discussing issues of bias and credibility
- Raising awareness about how media techniques (such as the use of color, sound, editing, or symbolism) influence people's beliefs, attitudes, and behaviors
- Producing messages using different forms of media

Media literacy has four stages:

1. The first stage is *becoming aware* of why it's important to manage the amount of time spent with TV, videos, electronic games, the Internet, films, and various print media.

2. The second stage is *learning specific skills* of critical viewing, such as analyzing and questioning what's in the "frame" (the perspective brought to the subject), how it's constructed, and what may have been left out.

3. The third stage is *exploring deeper issues* of who produces the media we experience and why. Questions to explore include: Who profits? Who loses? Who decides?

Chapter 11: Media Literacy

> ### *Key Questions in Analyzing Media Messages*
>
> - What story is being told?
> - From whose perspective is it presented?
> - How is it captured?
> - How is it edited?
> - What type of music is used?
> - Whose voice do we hear?
> - What is the message?
> - Who created the message and why are they sending it?
> - Who is speaking?
> - Whose viewpoint is not heard?
> - Which lifestyles, values, and points of view are represented in the message?
> - Who owns the medium?
> - What is our role as spectators?

4. The fourth stage is *creating and producing one's own media messages* to counter the intended message. For example, a cigarette ad could be recast to reflect tobacco's effects on health; the ad could then be used against the industry. At this stage, the participant's role is that of an advocate.

How Media Literacy Complements Counter-Marketing

Media literacy programs can complement and reinforce a state's counter-marketing program. Educating people about advertisers' motives and about the techniques that advertisers use to influence attitudes and behaviors helps people to analyze and to decipher tobacco industry marketing efforts and also increases the effectiveness of counter-marketing efforts.

Media literacy programs are easy to integrate with other counter-marketing components. For example, most media literacy programs include a module in which youth develop messages in response to industry marketing. This part of the program can be promoted through public relations and incorporated into grassroots efforts to educate the entire target audience about how the tobacco industry has tried to influence youth.

Although media literacy programs can be an effective component within any counter-marketing effort, they're most likely to be effective when the counter-marketing programs use an industry manipulation or repositioning strategy. (See Chapter 7: Advertising.) Florida's "truth" campaign used media literacy strategies to motivate young people to actively participate in tobacco control activities. In fact, many of Florida's original ads are believed to have helped the viewing audience become more media literate by exposing the role of ad agencies and marketing groups in creating positive images of tobacco.

Media literacy often leads to media advocacy efforts. In many cases, once youth are sensitized to deceptive marketing messages and practices, they're eager to work to counter those messages. At the community level, many community advocates use media literacy techniques to educate the public about the influence of tobacco ads in convenience stores and at sporting events.

Media literacy is also an effective tool for educating legislators and health policy decision makers. Because it's based on educational theories and addresses issues beyond tobacco control, media literacy can be viewed as a less charged critique of industry practices. It can be a useful way to educate policy makers about why the tobacco control movement needs effective policies for youth marketing, youth access, and clean indoor air.

It may be difficult to convey the direct impact a well-crafted media literacy program can have on youth. The best way to convince your state tobacco control advocates of the power of media literacy is to invite them to attend a media literacy session or to conduct a session designed especially for them.

Implementing a Media Literacy Program

Once you decide that media literacy supports your counter-marketing program's goals, you can begin your search for the right strategies and activities. Many media literacy programs and curricula are available; do some research to find the ones that will work best with your program. (See Programs and Resources section at the end of this chapter.) Here are the general steps for implementing your program:

- **Talk to other state tobacco control program staff about how media literacy fits into their counter-marketing programs.** Many states have used locally developed and tested programs and teaching tools. Ask them about their experiences with media literacy programs and experts.

- **Develop a strategy for media literacy in your counter-marketing plan.** Apply strategies that work with your target audiences. Media literacy is an obvious match for youth prevention programs. If your focus is on industry manipulation, you can use media literacy strategies with adults to deconstruct the tobacco industry's public relations ads and youth smoking prevention messages. Make sure that you have the resources, staff, and time to invest in media literacy as a program strategy. In addition, you'll

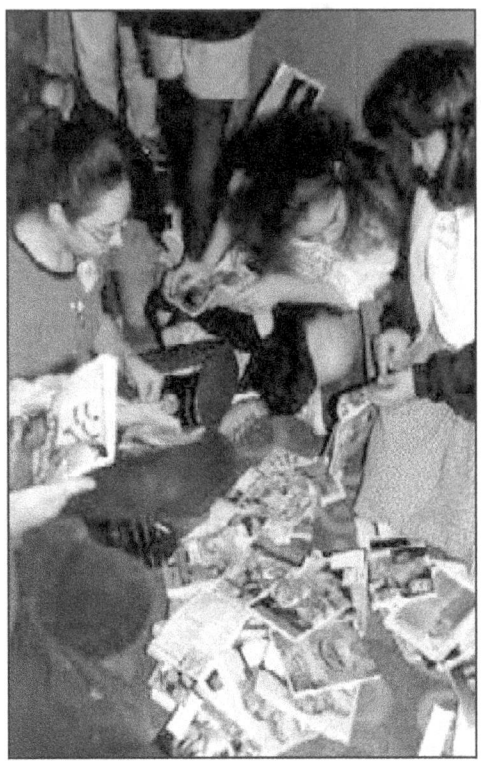

need to find one or more experts who can implement media literacy programs in your state. (See the Resources list at the end of this chapter.)

- **Learn about media literacy programs and resources.** The Centers for Disease Control and Prevention's Office on Smoking and Health, the American Academy of Pediatrics, the National Education Association's Health Information Network, and the Center for Substance Abuse Prevention jointly developed *MediaSharp: Analyzing Tobacco and Alcohol Messages,* a tool kit for educators, youth group leaders, pediatricians, and others who work with youth ages 11 through 14. The kit includes worksheets, suggested activities, references and resources, and a video module to use across the learning modules. In addition, several Web sites offer information about media literacy organizations and resources for media literacy. Experts around the country also can help you design a state program. (See the Resources list at the end of this chapter.)

- **Track who is using the program and how it is working in different settings.** Once you've chosen a program and implemented it, be sure to evaluate your efforts. Evaluation will enable you to identify and correct any problems with the program.

Here are several tips from media literacy experts for launching your effort:

- **Include links to media literacy Web sites on your state tobacco control site.** These links will make media literacy tools readily available for teachers, health educators, and others who may be interested in working on tobacco control.

- **Visit state and local departments of education, health, or alcohol and other drug services.**

  – Learn about your state's education standards on media literacy.

  – Determine the department's interest in tobacco media literacy and find out who is addressing the issue.

- Make tobacco media literacy resources and materials available to the department.

- Work with the department to create professional development opportunities in media literacy.

- Provide access to teaching tools and resources, and offer to train teachers, health educators, or other staff.

- Introduce media literacy programs and teaching tools at state and local health and education conferences.

- Find state media literacy experts to speak to students, parents, or teachers or at teacher training programs.

- Train people to present media literacy programs at schools and other youth gatherings.

- **Identify youth organizations, religious groups, community hospitals, pediatricians, and other community groups open to addressing the issue of media literacy with their members.** If your counter-marketing program addresses youth prevention, this can be an important addition to your media efforts.

  - Present information on media literacy to the organization leaders.

  - Determine whether they're interested in offering media literacy programs.

  - Make resources and teaching tools available.

  - Offer to train staff from the organizations or offer to provide staff to conduct the programs for them.

  - Encourage organizations to publish or display artwork, ads, or other media literacy products developed by youth.

- **Approach local commercial and public television stations, education writers at newspapers, and cable stations with distance-learning access channels.**

  - Offer experts to talk about the concepts behind media literacy.

  - Showcase classes or organizations that are involving youth in media literacy programs.

  - Broadcast ads or other media messages developed by young people.

  - Develop a distance-learning program on media literacy for a cable channel.

  - Propose media literacy articles for newspapers with youth pages.

- **Involve parents.** Help parents learn about media literacy programs so that they can reinforce and sustain media literacy at home. Inform them about school or community programs through parent resource groups such as the Parent Teacher Association.

Evaluating Your Efforts

Evaluating your media literacy efforts will help you report to stakeholders and will give you valuable insights on improving your approach. Fine-tuning your approach using evaluation results can help you increase the public's ability to analyze tobacco advertising, its motivation to counter the tobacco industry's goals, and its involvement in the counter-marketing program. Some smokers may tell you that what they learn in media literacy justifies their addiction (i.e., they're victims of industry manipulation). If this happens, don't think that your program is having an adverse effect; instead, consider this argument a "teachable moment." You may need to present additional information to these individuals, including information on health effects and cessation services.

Evaluation will help you answer these types of questions:

- How is the funding for media literacy being used?

- Was your media literacy program implemented the way it was designed?

- Was the audience attentive and engaged throughout?

- Were there significant changes in the audience's awareness, attitudes, perceptions, intentions, and behaviors?

- How can you use the evaluation results to adjust your media literacy efforts and be more successful?

How To Evaluate Your Media Literacy Efforts

You may want to review Chapter 5: Evaluating the Success of Your Counter-Marketing Program, which addresses evaluation in depth. Base your approach to evaluation on how the results will be used and by whom. Once you have determined how the evaluation results will be used, you can develop the most effective questions, plan a strategy for getting answers, and then provide the information to those who need it in a format that they can use. Involve the intended users and allow them to provide input from the start about the type(s) of information that they need from the evaluation.

> **KIDS LOVE CARTOON CHARACTERS. UNFORTUNATELY, SO DOES THE TOBACCO INDUSTRY.**

To help manage the implementation of your media literacy efforts—and to respond to inquiries from your stakeholders—you must monitor and track your activities. As discussed in Chapter 5, you'll need to complete or obtain logs and other documentation tools regularly to track the activities linked to your plan's goals and objectives. For example, if one objective is to teach a certain number of targeted youth about specific content areas and skills within a given time frame, a log can allow you to document how many youth were reached, what areas and skills were addressed during each session, and when the instruction took place.

Most importantly, you'll want to assess outcomes to determine the effectiveness of your media literacy efforts. This assessment involves measuring the impact on program participants, including changes in:

- Awareness of the role of the media
- Attitudes toward and perceptions of the tobacco industry, its advertising, and the harm both perpetuate
- Critical viewing skills
- Ability to develop their own counter-marketing messages
- Intentions to talk with others about what they have learned

If you conduct an outcome evaluation, use the strongest design possible. A pretest and posttest measurement that uses a comparison or a control group that didn't receive the media literacy education is preferable. A participant survey is one important way to measure outcomes. You may also want to review items from other surveys that evaluated the outcomes of similar programs and to involve one or more experts in the survey development and data analysis.

Using Evaluation Results for Decision Making

The results of your outcome evaluation may show that some outcomes were achieved and others weren't. To understand these results, check your monitoring and tracking data to see whether your media literacy activities were implemented according to plan. If the activities and content linked to certain outcomes weren't taught appropriately or at all, you and your instructors will need to pay closer attention to program design and implementation.

If your monitoring and tracking data show that your activities were implemented as planned, it may be helpful to conduct interviews or focus groups with members of your target audience to understand why certain outcomes weren't achieved. If the focus group is designed and conducted effectively, these qualitative findings may help identify and correct problems with your media literacy efforts, such as low credibility of instructors, inappropriate learning techniques, program content that doesn't resonate with the audience, or lack of time to practice relevant skills. By evaluating your efforts regularly, you'll learn more about how to best engage your target audience, how to increase their knowledge, and how to motivate them to get involved in the tobacco counter-marketing program. Then you'll be able to make adjustments so that each round of media literacy efforts becomes more successful.

> ### Points To Remember
>
> - Make sure that media literacy fits into your overall counter-marketing strategy.
>
> - Learn about media literacy programs and resources. Talk to program staff from states conducting media literacy efforts.
>
> - Identify which media literacy programs and resources match your audience and strategy.
>
> - Determine which organizations can help you implement a media literacy program. Offer them tools and training.
>
> - Track who is using the program and how it's working.

Resources

Health Education

Centers for Disease Control and Prevention. Guidelines for school health programs to prevent tobacco use and addiction. *Morbidity and Mortality Weekly Report Recommendation Report* 1994;43(RR-2):1–18.

Shelov S, Baron M, Beard L, Hogan M, et al. Children, adolescents and advertising. *Pediatrics* 1995;95:295–7.

U.S. Department of Health and Human Services. *Preventing Tobacco Use Among Young People: A Report of the Surgeon General.* Atlanta, GA: USDHHS, Public Health Service, Centers for Disease Control and Prevention, National Center for Chronic Disease Prevention and Health Promotion, Office on Smoking and Health; 1994. Reprinted with corrections, July 1994.

Programs and Resources

- MediaSharp is an interactive, multimedia program designed to help young people critically assess how the media normalize, glamorize, and create role models for unhealthy lifestyles and behaviors. It focuses on analyzing tobacco and alcohol messages delivered through entertainment, news, and marketing. The MediaSharp kit includes a video, a leader's guide, handouts, exercises, and an extensive list of media literacy resources; it can be ordered free from the Centers for Disease Control and Prevention/Office on Smoking and Health Web site (http://www.cdc.gov/tobacco).

- Smoke Screeners is an educational program that helps young people learn media literacy skills by improving their ability to critically analyze messages about tobacco use in movies and on television. The program includes a moderator's guide and video, and it can be used in a classroom or in a youth group setting. Created as part of the youth initiative of the Massachusetts Department of Public Health's antismoking campaign, this program is now a national effort. Smoke Screeners is free and can be ordered from the Centers for Disease Control and Prevention/Office on Smoking and Health Web site (http://www.cdc.gov/tobacco).

- The Center for Media Literacy (http://www.medialit.org) is the leading organization for media literacy in the United States. The center has an extensive catalogue of recommended books, videos, and curriculum resources.

- The Alliance for a Media Literate America (http://www.nmec.org) is a professional development collaboration that organizes and hosts the annual National Media Education Conference for teachers, administrators, and community leaders.

- South Carolina Educational Television's Media Literacy Program Web site (http://www.med.sc.edu/medialit) provides numerous teaching tools for tobacco media literacy.

- The New Mexico Media Literacy Project (http://www.aa.edu), sponsored by the Albuquerque Academy, offers a wealth of information for teaching media literacy skills to youth.

- Hip Hop! Influence Within Youth Popular Culture: A Catalyst for Reaching America's Youth with Substance Abuse Messages is a report by Dr. Thandi Hicks-Harper that can help readers to understand hip hop in a prevention context (http://www.hiphop4kids.com).

Research Literature

American Academy of Pediatrics. Media education. *Pediatrics* 1999;104:341–3.

Brunner C, Talley W. *The New Media Literacy Handbook: An Educator's Guide to Bringing New Media into the Classroom.* New York, NY: Anchor Books/Doubleday, 1999.

Hobbs R. Literacy in the information age. In: Flood J, Lapp D, Brice Heath S, eds. *Handbook of Research on Teaching Literacy Through the Communicative and Visual Arts.* International Reading Association. New York, NY: Macmillan, 1998. pp. 7–14.

Hobbs R. Media literacy in Massachusetts. In: Hart A, ed., *Teaching the Media: International Perspectives.* Mahwah, NJ: Lawrence Erlbaum Associates, 1998. pp. 127–440.

Hobbs R. The seven great debates in the media literacy movement. *Journal of Communication* 1998;48(2):9–29.

Hobbs R. Classroom strategies for exploring realism and authenticity in media messages. *Reading Online* (International Reading Association) 2001;4(9). Available at: http://www.readingonline.org/newliteracies/lit_index.asp?HREF=hobbs/index.html. Accessed June 20, 2003.

Hobbs R. Improving reading comprehension by using media literacy activities. *Voices from the Middle* (National Council of Teachers of English) 2001;8(4):44–50.

Hobbs R, Frost R. Instructional practices in media literacy education and their impact on students' learning. *New Jersey Journal of Communication* 1999;6(2):123–48.

Krueger E, Christel MT. Seeing and Believing: *How to Teach Media Literacy in the English Classroom*. Portsmouth, NH: Boynton/Cook Publishers, 2001.

Kubey R, Baker F. Has media literacy found a curricular foothold? *Education Week* 1999;19(9):56. Available at: www.edweek.org/ew/newstory.cfm?slug=09ubey2.h19. For current links to all 50 states, see http://www.med.sc.edu:1081/statelit.html. Accessed June 20, 2003.

Project Look Sharp. *12 Basic Principles for Incorporating Media Literacy into Any Curriculum*. Ithaca, NY: Ithaca College, 1999.

Silverblatt A. *Media Literacy: Keys to Interpreting Media Messages*, 2nd ed. Westport, CT: Praeger, 2001.

Silverblatt A, Ferry J, Finan B. *Approaches to Media Literacy: A Handbook*. Armonk, NY: M.E. Sharpe, 1999.

Tyner K. *Literacy in a Digital World: Teaching and Learning in the Age of Information*. Mahwah, NJ: Lawrence Erlbaum Associates, 1998.

Teaching and Learning Resources

American Cancer Society. *National Health Education Standards: Achieving Health Literacy*. Atlanta, GA: American Cancer Society, 1995.

DeGaetano G, Bander K. *Screen Smarts: A Family Guide to Media Literacy*. New York, NY: Houghton Mifflin,1996.

Hobbs R. To your health. *Cable in the Classroom* 1995;Oct:12–13.

Hobbs R. *Know TV: Changing What, Why and How You Watch*. Bethesda, MD: Discovery Communications, 1996.

Hobbs R. Start early to help children combat alcohol-saturated TV. *American Academy of Pediatrics News* 1998;14(3):20–1.

Hobbs R. *Media Literacy.* New York, NY: Newsweek Education, 2000.

Johnson LL. *Media, Education and Change.* New York, NY: Peter Lang Publishing, 2001.

Manzo KK. Schools begin to infuse media literacy into the 3 R's. *Education Week* 2000;Dec:6–7. Available at: http://www.edweek.org/ew/ewstory.cfm?slug=14media.h20&. Accessed July 3, 2002.

Thoman E. Skills & strategies for media education. *Educational Leadership* 1999;56(5):50.

Walsh B. *Understanding Media Literacy.* Center for Media Literacy, 2000.

Zollo P. *Wise Up to Teens: Insights Into Marketing and Advertising to Teenagers.* Ithaca, NY: New Strategist Publications, 1995.

Videos

Centers for Disease Control and Prevention, Office on Smoking and Health; Massachusetts Department of Public Health. *Smoke Screeners.* 1999. To order, call 1-800-CDC-1311.

DeBenedittis P. *Rebelling Against Tobacco Ads.* 2000. Available at: http://www.medialiteracy.net/purchase.

Hobbs R. *Tuning In to Media: Literacy for the Information Age.* 1994. Available at: http://gpn.unl.edu/cml/product_.index_alph.aspMangan M. *Corporate Deceit: Big Tobacco's Target* (CD-ROM). 2001. Available at: http://www.medialiteracy.net/purchase

National Institute for Media & The Family. *Smoke & Mirrors.* 1999. Available at: http://www.mediafamily.org/store/tools.shtml

New Mexico Media Literacy Project. *Just Do Media Literacy* (companion teacher guide included). 1997. Available at: http://www.nmmlp.org/products.htm

New Mexico Media Literacy Project. *Media Literacy for Health* (CD-ROM, K–12 curriculum). 2001. Available at: http://www.nmmlp.org/products.htm

Substance Abuse and Mental Health Services Administration, Center for Substance Abuse Prevention; Centers for Disease Control and Prevention, Office on Smoking and Health; American Academy of Pediatrics; National Education Association Health Information Network. *MediaSharp: Analyzing Tobacco and Alcohol Messages.* 1998. Available at: http://www.cdc.gov/tobacco/mediashrp.htm.

Web Sites and Internet Resources

Alliance for a Media Literate America: http://www.nmec.org.

American Academy of Pediatrics, *Understanding the Impact of Media on Children and Teens:* http://www.aap.org/family/mediaimpact.htm.

Center for Media Literacy: http://www.medialit.org.

Countering the Influence of Alcohol and Tobacco Advertising: http://www.drugs.indiana.edu/prevention/advert.html.

Deconstructing Media Messages: http://www.etr.org/recapp/practice/youthskills200106.htm.

Media Education Foundation: http://www.mediaed.org/

Media Literacy Clearinghouse: http://www.med.sc.edu/medialit.

Media Literacy for Prevention, Critical Thinking and Self-Esteem (Web site of media literacy expert Dr. Peter DeBenedittis): http://www.medialiteracy.net.

Media Literacy Review, Media Literacy Online Project, College of Education, University of Oregon: http://interact.uoregon.edu/medialit/mlr/home/index.html.

Media Literacy and Substance Abuse Virtual Library: http://www.health.org/features/medlit/library.htm.

New Mexico Media Literacy Project: http://www.nmmlp.org.

Bibliography

Austin EW, Johnson KK. Effects of general and alcohol-specific media literacy training on children's decision making about alcohol. *Journal of Health Communication* 1997; 2:17–42.

DiFranza JR, Richard JW, Paulman PM, et al. RJR Nabisco's cartoon camel promotes Camel cigarettes to children. *Journal of the American Medical Association* 1991;266(22):3149–53.

Federal Trade Commission. *FTC Cigarette Report for 2000.* Washington, DC: FTC, 2002.

Fischer PM, Schwartz MP, Richards JW Jr, et al. Brand logo recognition by children aged 3 to 6 years. Mickey Mouse and Old Joe the Camel. *Journal of the American Medical Association* 1991;266(22):3145–8.

Kaiser Family Foundation. *Kids & media @ the new millennium.* Washington, DC: Kaiser Family Foundation; 1999.

Sargent JD, Beach ML, Dalton MA, et al. Effect of seeing tobacco use in films on trying smoking among adolescents: a cross-sectional study. *British Medical Journal* 2001;323(7326):1394–7.

Slater MD, Beauvais F, Rouner D, Van Leuven J, Murphy K, Domenech-Rodriguez MM, et al. Adolescent counter arguing of TV beer advertisements; evidence for effectiveness of alcohol education and critical viewing discussion. *Journal of Drug Education* 1996;26(2):143–58.

Strasburger VC, Donnerstein E. Children, adolescents, and the media in the 21st century. *Adolescent Medicine* 2000;11(1):51–68.

Resources and Tools

Federal Government Agencies

Agency for Healthcare Research and Quality (AHRQ)

The Agency for Healthcare Research and Quality (AHRQ), a part of the U.S. Department of Health and Human Services, is the lead agency charged with supporting research designed to improve the quality of health care, to reduce its cost, to improve patient safety, to decrease medical errors, and to broaden access to essential services. The agency provides materials on smoking cessation for health professionals and consumers.

AHRQ Publications Clearinghouse
P.O. Box 8547
Silver Spring, MD 20907-8547
800-358-9295
www.ahrq.gov

Centers for Disease Control and Prevention's Office on Smoking and Health (CDC/OSH)

The Centers for Disease Control and Prevention (CDC) is the lead federal agency for protecting the health and safety of all U.S. citizens at home and abroad, for providing credible information to enhance health decisions, and for promoting health through strong partnerships. CDC develops and implements disease prevention and control, environmental health, and health promotion and education activities to improve the public's health.

The Office on Smoking and Health (OSH) is a division of the National Center for Chronic Disease Prevention and Health Promotion (NCCDPHP), one of the centers within the CDC. OSH is responsible for leading and coordinating strategic efforts to prevent tobacco use among youth, to promote smoking cessation, and to protect nonsmokers from secondhand tobacco smoke. OSH's Web site, the Tobacco Information and Prevention Source (TIPS), provides a range of materials on tobacco control and prevention.

Office on Smoking and Health
National Center for Chronic Disease Prevention and Health Promotion
Centers for Disease Control and Prevention
4770 Buford Highway NE, MS K-50
Atlanta, GA 30341-3717
800-CDC-1311 (toll free) / 770-488-5705 (phone)
tobaccoinfo@cdc.gov (e-mail)
www.cdc.gov/tobacco

Centers for Disease Control and Prevention's Office on Smoking and Health National Networks

To help eliminate tobacco-related disparities among priority populations, the Office on Smoking and Health (OSH) has established national networks to plan, initiate, coordinate, and evaluate tobacco control activities. The networks include the following:

- Northwest Portland Area Indian Health Board (NPAIHB)
  www.npaihb.org

- Association of Asian Pacific Community Health Organizations (AAPCHO)
  www.aapcho.org

- The National Association of Lesbian, Gay, Bisexual and Transgender Community Centers (NALGBTCC)
  www.lgbtcenters.org

- The National Alliance for Hispanic Health
  www.hispanichealth.org

- National Latino Council on Alcohol and Tobacco Prevention
  www.nlcatp.org

- The BACCHUS and GAMMA Peer Education Network
  www.bacchusgamma.org

- Health Education Council
  www.healthedcouncil.org

- Employee and Family Resources, Inc.
  www.efr.org

Centers for Disease Control and Prevention's Office on Smoking and Health Tribal Support Centers

The Office on Smoking and Health (OSH) has established tribal support centers to develop or improve tobacco-related regional resource networks and outreach to tribes. The centers provide and support training and technical assistance, data collection, materials development, partnership building, and programs. The centers include the following:

- Aberdeen Area Tribal Chairmen Health Board (AATCHB)
  www.aatchb.org

- Alaska Native Health Board (ANHB)
  www.anhb.org

- California Rural Indian Health Board (CRIHB)
  www.crihb.org

- Intertribal Council of Arizona (ITCA)
  www.itcaonline.com

- Inter-Tribal Council of Michigan, Inc.
  www.itcmi.org

- Muscogee Creek Nation of Oklahoma
  www.ocevnet.org/creek/index.html

- Northwest Portland Area Indian Health Board (NPAIHB)
  www.npaihb.org

Center for Substance Abuse Prevention (CSAP) National Clearinghouse on Alcohol and Drug Information

The Center for Substance Abuse Prevention (CSAP) provides national leadership in the development of policies, programs, and services to prevent the onset of illicit drug use, to prevent underage alcohol and tobacco use, and to reduce the negative consequences of using substances. CSAP is one of three centers in the Substance Abuse and Mental Health Services Administration (SAMHSA) in the U.S. Department of Health and Human Services. CSAP funds the National Clearinghouse on Alcohol and Drug Information, which disseminates materials for professionals and the public on alcohol, tobacco, and other drugs. Information is available in various forms, including videos, fact sheets, posters, and pamphlets.

Center for Substance Abuse Prevention
National Clearinghouse on Alcohol and Drug Information
P.O. Box 2345
Rockville, MD 20847-2345
800-SAY-NO-TO (toll-free) / 301-468-6433 (fax)
www.samhsa.gov/centers/clearinghouse/clearinghouses.html
www.health.org

Environmental Protection Agency (EPA)

The Environmental Protection Agency (EPA) serves as the federal lead agency on environmental issues. Its Indoor Air Quality Information Clearinghouse offers publications and information on the harmful effects of secondhand smoke and indoor air pollution.

Environmental Protection Agency
Indoor Air Quality Information Clearinghouse
P.O. Box 37133
Washington, DC 20013-7133
800-438-4318 (toll-free) / 703-356-5386 (fax)
iaqinfo@aol.com (e-mail)
www.epa.gov/iaq

Federal Trade Commission (FTC)

The Federal Trade Commission (FTC) is the U.S. government's main authority on trade issues. It provides publications and information related to trade policies and tobacco advertising, including health warning labels, and produces a report that contains data on the tar, nicotine, and carbon monoxide in domestic cigarettes.

Federal Trade Commission
Consumer Response
600 Pennsylvania Avenue NW
Washington, DC 20580
202-326-2222 (phone) / 202-326-3090 (tobacco-related questions)
www.ftc.gov

Food and Drug Administration (FDA)

The Food and Drug Administration (FDA) responds to consumer requests for information and publications and provides information about regulations restricting the sale and distribution of cigarettes and smokeless tobacco to protect children and adolescents.

Food and Drug Administration
5600 Fishers Lane
Rockville, MD 20857
888-INFO-FDA (toll-free)
www.fda.gov

Indian Health Service (IHS)

The Indian Health Service (IHS) provides a comprehensive health services delivery system for American Indians and Alaska Natives, with the opportunity for maximum tribal involvement in developing and managing programs to meet their health needs. The IHS facilitates and assists in coordinating health planning and in obtaining and using health resources available through federal, state, and local programs.

Indian Health Service
Public Affairs Staff
801 Thompson Avenue, Suite 400
Rockville, MD 20852-1627
301-443-3593 (phone)
www.ihs.gov

National Cancer Institute (NCI)

The National Cancer Institute (NCI) supports research on counter-marketing and other tobacco control interventions and produces publications on smoking. It also provides telephone counseling services for smoking cessation. Programs and materials are available to health professionals and the public.

National Cancer Institute
Office of Cancer Communications
6116 Executive Boulevard, Suite 3036A, MSC-8322
Bethesda, MD 20892-8322
800-4-CANCER (toll-free)
www.nci.nih.gov
www.smokefree.gov (for smoking cessation information and tools)

National Center for Health Statistics (NCHS)

The CDC's National Center for Health Statistics (NCHS) answers requests for catalogs, electronic data products, and single copies of publications, such as Advance Data reports and Monthly Vital Statistics reports. Ordering information is available for publications and electronic products sold through the Government Printing Office and the National Technical Information Service. Specific statistical data collected by the NCHS are also available.

National Center for Health Statistics
Division of Data Services
3311 Toledo Road
Hyattsville, MD 20782
301-458-4636 (phone)
www.cdc.gov/nchs

National Heart, Lung, and Blood Institute (NHLBI)

The National Heart, Lung, and Blood Institute (NHLBI) provides information and materials on risk factors for cardiovascular disease. It disseminates public education materials and programmatic and scientific information.

National Heart, Lung, and Blood Institute
Health Information Center
P.O. Box 30105
Bethesda, MD 20824-0105
301-592-8573 (phone) / 301-592-8563 (fax)
www.nhlbi.nih.gov

National Institute on Drug Abuse (NIDA)

The National Institute on Drug Abuse (NIDA) provides information on nicotine addiction, its health hazards, and its treatment. It fulfills requests for catalogs and publications. It also publishes *NIDA Notes*, which covers topics such as nicotine addiction and smokeless tobacco use. The institute's Web site has news releases and links to other resources.

National Institute on Drug Abuse
6001 Executive Boulevard, Room 5213
Bethesda, MD 20892-9561
301-443-1124 (phone) / 301-443-7397 (fax)
www.drugabuse.gov

National Institute for Occupational Safety and Health (NIOSH)

The National Institute for Occupational Safety and Health (NIOSH) provides information on chemical and physical hazards in the workplace, training courses, publications, and the health hazard evaluation program. It distributes a subject-indexed catalog of its materials. NIOSH also maintains an automated database on occupational safety and health, and its library is open to the public.

National Institute for Occupational Safety and Health
Information Retrieval and Analysis Team
4676 Columbia Parkway, MSC-13
Cincinnati, OH 45226
800-35-NIOSH (toll-free) / 513-533-8573 (publications fax)
www.cdc.gov/niosh/homepage.html

National Technical Information Service (NTIS)

The National Technical Information Service (NTIS) offers a variety of information, including reports by U.S. government research and development agencies, databases produced by federal agencies, and descriptions of ongoing research sponsored by the U.S. government. NTIS has absorbed the National Audiovisual Center (NAC) and offers materials previously available from the NAC.

National Technical Information Service
5285 Port Royal Road
Springfield, VA 22161
800-553-6847 (toll free) / 703-605-6000 (regular and rush services) / 703-605-6900 (fax)
www.ntis.gov

Occupational Safety and Health Administration (OSHA)

The Occupational Safety and Health Administration (OSHA) develops and promulgates occupational safety and health standards, develops and issues regulations, conducts investigations and inspections to determine the status of compliance with safety and health standards and regulations, and issues citations and proposes penalties for noncompliance with safety and health standards and regulations.

Occupational Safety and Health Administration
U.S. Department of Labor
200 Constitution Avenue, NW
Washington, DC 20210
800-321-OSHA (toll-free)
www.osha.gov

Substance Abuse and Mental Health Services Administration (SAMHSA)

The Substance Abuse and Mental Health Services Administration (SAMHSA) is the federal agency charged with improving the quality and availability of prevention, treatment, and rehabilitative services to reduce the health and social costs of substance abuse and mental illnesses. SAMHSA funds a number of projects, including information clearinghouses and data collection efforts, to monitor the prevalence of substance use and mental health issues.

Substance Abuse and Mental Health Services Administration
5600 Fishers Lane
Rockville, MD 20857
info@samhsa.gov (e-mail)
www.samhsa.gov

U.S. Department of Agriculture (USDA)

The Department of Agriculture (USDA) provides information on tobacco price support programs and other tobacco-related agricultural issues.

U.S. Department of Agriculture
Tobacco Division
Stop 0514 (for Express Mail, use Room 5750)
1400 Independence Avenue SW
Washington, DC 20250-0514
202-720-4318 (phone) / 202-690-2298 (fax)
www.usda.gov

U.S. Department of Health and Human Services (USDHHS): Office of Minority Health's Initiative To Eliminate Racial and Ethnic Disparities in Health

This Department of Health and Human Services (USDHHS) initiative supports the goal of eliminating disparities in six areas of health status among U.S. racial and ethnic minority populations by 2010. The initiative's Web site provides background on the initiative, news, a calendar of events, and links to publications and Web resources developed by USDHHS agencies to support the initiative.

Office of Minority Health
Tower Building, Suite 600
1101 Wootton Parkway
Rockville, MD 20852
301-443-9923 (phone) / 301-443-8280 (fax)
raceandhealth@osophs.dhhs.gov (e-mail)
www.raceandhealth.hhs.gov

U.S. Department of the Treasury: Bureau of Alcohol, Tobacco, Firearms and Explosives (ATF)

The Bureau of Alcohol, Tobacco, Firearms and Explosives (ATF) is a law enforcement organization within the Treasury Department that provides general information on current tax rates and tax revenues pertaining to tobacco.

U.S. Department of the Treasury
Bureau of Alcohol, Tobacco, Firearms and Explosives
Regulations Division–Office of Alcohol and Tobacco
650 Massachusetts Avenue NW, Room 5000
Washington, DC 20226
202-927-8210 (phone)
www.atf.treas.gov

Volunteer and Professional Organizations

Action on Smoking and Health (ASH)

Action on Smoking and Health (ASH) produces materials on a variety of smoking and health topics, with an emphasis on legal action to protect nonsmokers' health.

Action on Smoking and Health
2013 H Street NW
Washington, DC 20006
202-659-4310 (phone) / 202-833-3921 (fax)
www.ash.org

The Advocacy Institute

The Advocacy Institute works to counter the influence of the tobacco industry and provides strategic consulting and advocacy support on policy issues related to tobacco control.

The Advocacy Institute
1629 K Street NW, Suite 200
Washington, DC 20006-1629
202-777-7575 (phone) / 202-777-7577 (fax)
www.advocacy.org/tobacco.htm

American Cancer Society (ACS)

The American Cancer Society (ACS) provides smoking education, prevention, and cessation programs and distributes pamphlets, posters, and exhibits on smoking. Check your telephone book for the ACS chapter in your area or contact the national office below for more information.

American Cancer Society
1599 Clifton Road NE
Atlanta, GA 30329
800-ACS-2345 (toll-free)
www.cancer.org

American Council on Science and Health

The American Council on Science and Health provides scientific evaluations on tobacco-related topics.

American Council on Science and Health
1995 Broadway, Second Floor
New York, NY 10023-5860
212-362-7044 (phone) / 212-362-4919 (fax)
www.acsh.org/tobacco/index.html

American Dental Association (ADA)

The dentists' association's Web site contains American Dental Association (ADA) letters, which address these topics: excise taxes on tobacco products, tobacco settlement legislation, reduction of tobacco use, smokeless tobacco, the Warning Label Act, and advocacy.

American Dental Association
211 East Chicago Avenue
Chicago, IL 60611
312-440-2500 (phone) / 312-440-7494 (fax)
www.ada.org

American Dental Education Association (ADEA)

The American Dental Education Association (ADEA) (formerly the American Dental Schools Association) offers a Tobacco-Free Initiatives Special Interest Group, an informal affiliation of dental and allied dental faculty interested in the promotion of tobacco cessation activities in dental education. The group represents ADEA interests in collaborative projects of the National Cancer Institute and the American Cancer Society. The group offers programs that help participants discuss, design, implement, and evaluate tobacco cessation programs in dental settings.

American Dental Education Association
1625 Massachusetts Avenue NW, Suite 600
Washington, DC 20036-2212
202-667-9433 (phone) / 202-667-0642 (fax)
www.adea.org

American Heart Association

The American Heart Association promotes smoking intervention programs at schools, workplaces, and health care sites. Check your phone book for an association chapter in your area or contact the national office below for further information.

American Heart Association
National Center
7272 Greenville Avenue
Dallas, TX 75231
800-AHA-USA-1 (toll-free)
www.americanheart.org

American Legacy Foundation

The American Legacy Foundation was established to reduce tobacco use in the United States as outlined in the Master Settlement Agreement. Its Web site provides information about the antitobacco movement and ways that the Master Settlement Agreement's funding is being used. There are also updates about public education efforts, including the national "truth" campaign, and stories that people share about their personal struggles with tobacco.

American Legacy Foundation
1001 G Street NW, Suite 800
Washington, DC 20001
202-454-5555 (phone) / 202-454-5599 (fax)
www.americanlegacy.org

American Lung Association (ALA)

The American Lung Association (ALA) conducts programs addressing smoking cessation, prevention, and protection of nonsmokers' health and provides a variety of educational materials for the public and health professionals. Check your telephone book for an association chapter in your area or contact the national office below for further information.

American Lung Association
61 Broadway, Sixth Floor
New York, NY 10006
212-315-8700 (phone) / 800-LUNG-USA (toll-free)
www.lungusa.org

American Medical Association (AMA)

The Web site of the American Medical Association (AMA) offers articles from the *Journal of the American Medical Association, American Medical News, Archives of Internal Medicine,* and other publications on tobacco-related issues. Some articles require a subscription or an association membership to view.

American Medical Association
515 North State Street
Chicago, IL 60610
312-464-5000 (phone) / 312-464-4184 (fax)
www.ama-assn.org

American Medical Association/SmokeLess States

SmokeLess States is the largest non-government-funded national effort in tobacco prevention and control. The 30 grantees concentrate their efforts in three general areas: 1) promoting public awareness of the dangers of tobacco use, 2) educating the public about policy options related to tobacco, and 3) enhancing local prevention and treatment programs.

American Medical Association/SmokeLess States
515 North State Street
Chicago, IL 60610
312-464-5000 (phone) / 312-464-4184 (fax)
www.ama-assn.org/ama/pub/category/3229.html

Americans for Nonsmokers' Rights (ANR)

Americans for Nonsmokers' Rights (ANR) provides information to organizations and individuals to help pass ordinances, to implement workplace regulations, and to develop smoking policies in the workplace. Its Web site features a section covering "Tobacco's dirty tricks."

Americans for Nonsmokers' Rights
2530 San Pablo Avenue, Suite J
Berkeley, CA 94702
510-841-3032 (phone) / 510-841-3071 (fax)
www.no-smoke.org

Asian Pacific Partnerships for Empowerment and Leadership (APPEAL)

Asian Pacific Partnerships for Empowerment and Leadership (APPEAL) works to prevent tobacco use among the Asian American and Pacific Islander community through five priority areas: network development, capacity building, education, advocacy, and leadership development.

APPEAL c/o AAPCHO (Association of Asian Pacific Community Health Organizations)
439 23rd Street
Oakland, CA 94612
510-272-9536 (phone) / 510-272-0817 (fax)
www.appealforcommunities.org

Association of State and Territorial Health Officials (ASTHO)

The Association of State and Territorial Health Officials (ASTHO) is the national nonprofit organization representing state and U.S. territorial public health agencies. The association has a Tobacco Control Program that develops and promotes policies that enhance the health agencies' ability to address tobacco use prevention and control. ASTHO offers information on the tobacco settlement, state tobacco settlement updates, newsletters, reprints from ASTHO reports, and resource links.

Association of State and Territorial Health Officials
1275 K Street NW, Suite 800
Washington, DC 20005-4006
202-371-9090 (phone) / 202-371-9797 (fax)
www.astho.org

BACCHUS and GAMMA Peer Education Network

The BACCHUS and GAMMA Peer Education Network is an international association of college- and university-based peer education programs dedicated to alcohol abuse prevention and related student health and safety issues (including tobacco use).

The BACCHUS and GAMMA Peer Education Network
P.O. Box 100430
Denver, CO 80250-0430
303-871-0901 (phone) / 303-871-0907 (fax)
admin@bacchusgamma.org (e-mail)
www.bacchusgamma.org

Campaign for Tobacco-Free Kids

The Campaign for Tobacco-Free Kids is one of the nation's largest nongovernmental initiatives ever launched to protect children from tobacco addiction and exposure to secondhand smoke.

Campaign for Tobacco-Free Kids
1400 I Street NW, Suite 1200
Washington, DC 20005
202-296-5469 (phone) / 202-296-5427 (fax)
info@tobaccofreekids.org (e-mail)
www.tobaccofreekids.org

Center for Media Literacy

The Center for Media Literacy is the leading organization for media literacy in the United States. It has an extensive catalog of recommended books, videos, and curriculum resources.

Center for Media Literacy
3101 Ocean Park Boulevard, Suite 200
Santa Monica, CA 90405
310-581-0260 (phone) / 310-581-0270 (fax)
cml@medialit.org (e-mail)
www.medialit.org

Center for Social Gerontology: Tobacco & Adult Minorities

The Center for Social Gerontology's Web site provides information on tobacco use and its effects on old and young adults from communities of color. Because people in communities of color have been specifically targeted by the tobacco industry, this site has information on lawsuits and legislative action against the tobacco industry and information related to the recent state tobacco settlements.

Tobacco & Adult Minorities
The Center for Social Gerontology
2307 Shelby Avenue
Ann Arbor, MI 48103
734-665-1126 (phone) / 734-665-2071 (fax)
tcsg@tcsg.org (e-mail)
www.tcsg.org/tobacco/minorities/minorities.htm

Chronic Disease Directors: Association of State and Territorial Chronic Disease Program Directors

The Chronic Disease Directors (CDD) represents the chronic disease interests of the state and territorial health agencies and the District of Columbia. (Tobacco use is a common risk factor that contributes to one or more chronic diseases.) State health agencies play a major role in educating the public about risks and choices, and in creating better access to preventive and diagnostic health services.

Association of State and Territorial Chronic Disease Program Directors
Chronic Disease Directors
8201 Greensboro Drive, Suite 300
McLean, VA 22102
703-610-9033 (phone) / 703-610-9005 (fax)
info@chronicdisease.org (e-mail)
www.chronicdisease.org

Doctors Ought to Care (DOC)

Doctors Ought to Care (DOC) mobilizes doctors and health organizations to speak out against tobacco and to publicize its effects. DOC provides school curricula, smoking intervention information, and tobacco counter-advertising for use in clinics, classrooms, and communities.

Doctors Ought to Care
5615 Kirby Drive, Suite 440
Houston, TX 77005
713-528-1487 (phone) / 713-528-2146 (fax)
www.bcm.tmc.edu/doc

The Foundation for a Smokefree America

Created by Patrick Reynolds, grandson of tobacco company founder R.J. Reynolds, the foundation is a non-profit organization that educates people of all ages about smoking and tobacco use. The foundation's Web site provides antitobacco messages to youth and adults, antismoking videos, live talks, ads, photos, and art.

The Foundation for a Smokefree America
P.O. Box 492028
Los Angeles, CA 90049-8028
800-541-7741 (toll-free) / 310-471-4270 (phone) / 310-471-0335 (fax)
www.tobaccofree.org

Global Partnerships for Tobacco Control: Essential Action

The Global Partnerships for Tobacco Control's Essential Action program helps to support and strengthen international tobacco control activities at the grassroots level. The program pairs groups in the United States and Canada with groups in Asia, Africa, Latin America, Central and Eastern Europe, and the former Soviet Union and helps them initiate meaningful shared activities.

Global Partnerships for Tobacco Control
P.O. Box 19405
Washington, DC 20036
202-387-8030 (phone) / 202-234-5176 (fax)
tobacco@essential.org (e-mail)
www.essentialaction.org/tobacco

Healthy People 2010

Healthy People 2010 is the federal blueprint for public health for the next 7 years. The set of health objectives can be used by individuals, states, communities, professional organizations, and others in developing programs to improve health. Healthy People 2010's two main goals are: 1) to help individuals of all ages increase their life expectancy and improve their quality of life, and 2) to eliminate health disparities among different segments of the population. Each of the 28 focus-area chapters contains a concise goal statement that frames the overall purpose of the focus area.

www.health.gov/healthypeople/About/goals.htm

Healthy People 2010 Companion Document for Lesbian, Gay, Bisexual, and Transgender (LGBT) Health

Published by the Gay and Lesbian Medical Association, this document is a comprehensive look at the Lesbian, Gay, Bisexual, and Transgender (LGBT) community and is intended for health care consumers, providers, researchers, educators, government agencies, schools, clinics, advocates, and health professionals in all settings. The document focuses on about 120 objectives and 12 focus areas from Healthy People 2010.

www.glma.org/policy/hp2010/index.html

Join Together Online (JTO)

Join Together Online (JTO) is a national Web resource for communities fighting substance abuse. JTO offers tobacco facts, the latest news on tobacco, and links to tobacco control resources. The site also has a Tobacco Information Packet, a technical assistance packet that includes a list of national organizations, publications, community stories, and community leaders with expertise in tobacco.

Join Together Online
One Appleton Street, Fourth Floor
Boston, MA 02116-5223
617-437-1500 (phone) / 617-437-9394 (fax)
info@jointogether.org (e-mail)
www.jointogether.org/sa

Media Literacy for Prevention, Critical Thinking, Self Esteem

Media Literacy for Prevention, Critical Thinking, Self Esteem provides a Web site that presents the work of Dr. Peter DeBenedittis and provides articles and tools for teaching media literacy.

www.medialiteracy.net

National Alliance for Hispanic Health

The National Alliance for Hispanic Health is the oldest and largest network of health and human service providers, serving more than 10 million Hispanic consumers throughout the United States. The alliance's Hispanic youth tobacco policy and leadership initiative, Nuestras Voces, is an effort to give a policy voice to Hispanic youth in the tobacco control movement. Nuestras Voces brings together Hispanic community-based organizations in five sites to implement local action plans against the strategic marketing of tobacco products to Hispanic youth.

National Alliance for Hispanic Health
1501 16th Street NW
Washington, DC 20036
202-387-5000 (phone) / 202-797-4353 (fax)
alliance@hispanichealth.org (e-mail)
www.hispanichealth.org

National Association of Attorneys General (NAAG)

The National Association of Attorneys General (NAAG) promotes coordination, cooperation, and communication among U.S. attorneys general. NAAG's Web site offers information on the Master Settlement Agreement, including the full text of the agreement, information on state and industry participants, and other information on tobacco settlement issues.

National Association of Attorneys General
750 First Street NE, Suite 1100
Washington, DC 20002
202-326-6000 (phone) / 202-408-7014 (fax)
www.naag.org

National Association of County and City Health Officials (NACCHO)

The National Association of County and City Health Officials (NACCHO) provides education, information, research, and technical assistance to local health departments and facilitates partnerships among local, state, and federal agencies to promote and strengthen public health. NACCHO's Tobacco Prevention and Control Project aims to strengthen local health departments' ability to engage in tobacco use prevention and control. NACCHO's Web site offers a number of tobacco control resources and links, including "Program and Funding Guidelines for Comprehensive Local Tobacco Control Programs."

National Association of County and City Health Officials
1100 17th Street NW, Second Floor
Washington, DC 20036
202-783-5550 (phone) / 202-783-1583 (fax)
www.naccho.org

National Association of Lesbian and Gay Addiction Professionals (NALGAP)

The National Association of Lesbian and Gay Addiction Professionals (NALGAP) works to prevent and treat alcoholism, substance abuse, and other addictions in the lesbian, gay, bisexual, and transgender (LGBT) communities. NALGAP's mission is to confront prejudice in the delivery of services to LGBT people and to advocate for LGBT-affirming programs and services. NALGAP provides information, training, networking, advocacy, and support for addiction professionals, individuals in recovery, and others concerned about LGBT health.

National Association of Lesbian and Gay Addiction Professionals
901 North Washington Street, Suite 600
Alexandria, VA 22314
703-465-0539 (phone) / 703-741-6989 (fax)
www.nalgap.org

National Association of Lesbian, Gay, Bisexual, and Transgender Community Centers (NALGBTCC)

The National Association of Lesbian, Gay, Bisexual, and Transgender Community Centers (NALGBTCC) works to sustain and empower its 107 member community centers in 36 states, while encouraging the creation of new centers. The association supports a CDC Tobacco Prevention and Control Initiative.

www.lgbtcenters.org

National Association of Local Boards of Health (NALBOH)

The National Association of Local Boards of Health (NALBOH) is a nonprofit organization that represents the interests of local boards of health. NALBOH published a national survey of the legal authority for tobacco control of local boards of health and other local, state, and federal governmental agencies. NALBOH's Web site provides tobacco control and prevention resources.

National Association of Local Boards of Health
1840 East Gypsy Lane
Bowling Green, OH 43402
419-353-7714 (phone) / 419-352-6278 (fax)
nalboh@nalboh.org (e-mail)
www.nalboh.org

National Coalition for Women Against Tobacco

The National Coalition for Women Against Tobacco, which was founded by the American Medical Women's Association, aims to increase awareness of the dangers of tobacco use and exposure and to provide leadership in helping the global community of women and girls to lead tobacco-free lives.

www.womenagainst.org

National Governors Association (NGA)

The Center for Best Practices of the National Governors Association (NGA) focuses on state innovations and best practices on a range of issues, including tobacco control. The NGA publishes an annual issue of briefs on the spending initiatives from tobacco settlement revenues, tracks spending decisions and legislation related to the Master Settlement Agreement, and provides information and technical assistance to states as they develop and reexamine spending decisions. The NGA Web site offers information on the tobacco settlement, including initiatives in each state.

National Governors Association
Hall of States
444 North Capitol Street NW, Suite 267
Washington, DC 20001-1512
202-624-5300 (phone) / 202-624-5313 (fax)
www.nga.org

National Indian Health Board (NIHB)

The National Indian Health Board (NIHB) represents tribal governments that operate their own health care delivery systems or receive health care directly from the Indian Health Service (IHS). The NIHB conducts research, policy analysis, program assessment and development, national and regional meeting planning, project management, and training and technical assistance programs. These services are provided to tribes, area health boards, tribal organizations, federal agencies, and private foundations. The NIHB presents the tribal perspective while monitoring federal legislation and networking with other national health care organizations.

National Indian Health Board
101 Constitution Avenue, NW, Suite 8-B09
Washington, DC 20001
202-742-4262 (phone) / 202-742-4285 (fax)
www.nihb.org

National Indian Health Board
Albuquerque Area Office, 2301 Renard Place SE, Suite 101
Albuquerque, NM 87106
505-764-0036 (phone) / 505-764-0466 (fax)

National Latino Council on Alcohol and Tobacco Prevention (LCAT)

The National Latino Council on Alcohol and Tobacco Prevention (LCAT) works to reduce the harm caused by alcohol and tobacco use in the Latino community, using research, policy analysis, education, training, and information dissemination.

National Latino Council on Alcohol and Tobacco Prevention
1875 Connecticut Avenue NW, Suite 732
Washington, DC 20009
202-265-8054 (phone) / 202-265-8056 (fax)
lcat@nlcatp.org (e-mail)
www.nlcatp.org

National Latina/o Lesbian, Gay, Bisexual, and Transgender Organization

The National Latina/o Lesbian, Gay, Bisexual, and Transgender Organization organizes Latina/o lesbian, gay, bisexual, and transgender (LGBT) communities on the local, regional, national, and international levels. The organization addresses the need to overcome social, health, and political barriers faced because of sexual orientation, gender identity, and ethnic background.

National Latina/o Lesbian, Gay, Bisexual, and Transgender Organization
1420 K Street NW, Suite 200
Washington, DC 20005
202-408-5380 (phone) / 202-408-8478 (fax)
www.llego.org

National Network of Libraries of Medicine

The National Network of Libraries of Medicine is responsible for eight regional medical libraries, each with a large geographic area. These regional libraries maintain information about local libraries that provide health information and database searches.

National Network of Libraries of Medicine
800-338-7657 (toll-free)

National Oral Health Information Clearinghouse (NOHIC)

The National Oral Health Information Clearinghouse (NOHIC), a service of the National Institutes of Health's National Institute of Dental and Craniofacial Research, develops and distributes information and educational materials on special care topics. It maintains a bibliographic database on oral health information and materials and provides information services. Trained staff respond to specific interests and questions in the area of special care.

National Oral Health Information Clearinghouse
ATTN: SH
1 NOHIC Way
Bethesda, MD 20892-3500
301-402-7364 (phone) / 301-907-8830 (fax)
nohic@nidcr.nih.gov (e-mail)
www.nohic.nidcr.nih.gov

Office of Minority Health Resource Center

The Office of Minority Health Resource Center responds to information requests from health professionals and consumers on minority health issues and locates sources of technical assistance. It also provides referrals to relevant organizations and distributes materials. Spanish-speaking operators are available.

Office of Minority Health Resource Center
P.O. Box 37337
Washington, DC 20013-7337
800-444-6472 (toll-free) / 301-251-2160 (fax)
www.omhrc.gov

The Onyx Group

The Onyx Group is a consulting firm that provides marketing communications, qualitative research, strategic planning, diversity services, program development, and training, with particular emphasis on tobacco control, health promotion, coalition building, youth services, and education. The firm develops culturally competent products and media for target markets, including communities of color, women, youth, older adults, and rural, urban, and other underserved populations.

The Onyx Group
P.O. Box 60
Bala Cynwyd, PA 19004
610-617-9971 (phone) / 610-617-9972 (fax)
onyxcom1@aol.com (e-mail)
www.onyx-group.com

Oral Health America Foundation

The Oral Health America Foundation develops resources for the improvement and promotion of the nation's oral health. Its National Spit Tobacco Education Program (NSTEP) informs the public that the use of spit (smokeless) tobacco is not a safe alternative to smoking and can lead to oral cancer. The foundation offers literature on spit tobacco and information on cessation for health care professionals and the public.

Oral Health America Foundation
410 North Michigan Avenue, Suite 352
Chicago, IL 60611-4211
312-836-9900 (phone) / 312-836-9986 (fax)
www.oralhealthamerica.org

Robert Wood Johnson Foundation (RWJF)

The Robert Wood Johnson Foundation (RWJF) works to improve the health and health care of all Americans. It concentrates on awarding grants in three areas: 1) ensuring that all Americans have access to basic health care at reasonable cost, 2) improving care and support for people with chronic health conditions, and 3) promoting health and preventing disease by reducing the harm caused by substance abuse, tobacco, alcohol, and illicit drugs.

Robert Wood Johnson Foundation
P.O. Box 2316
Route 1 and College Road East
Princeton, NJ 08543-2316
888-631-9989 (toll-free)/ 609-627-6401 (fax)
www.rwjf.org

Society for Research on Nicotine and Tobacco (SRNT)

The Society for Research on Nicotine and Tobacco (SRNT) sponsors scientific meetings and publications fostering the exchange of information on the biological, behavioral, social, and economic effects of nicotine. It supports scientific research on public health efforts for the prevention and treatment of tobacco use. SRNT provides the means by which various legislative, governmental, regulatory, and other public agencies and the drug industry can obtain expert advice and consultation on critical issues concerning tobacco use, nicotine dependence, and therapeutic uses of nicotine. The society's publications include newsletters, *Nicotine and Tobacco Research*, and abstracts from its annual meetings.

Society for Research on Nicotine and Tobacco
7600 Terrace Avenue, Suite 203
Middleton, WI 53562
608-836-3787 (phone) / 608-831-5485 (fax)
info@srnt.org (e-mail)
www.srnt.org

The Tobacco Control Resource Center, Inc., & The Tobacco Products Liability Project

The Tobacco Products Liability Project, which was founded by doctors, academics, and lawyers, encourages and coordinates product liability suits against the tobacco industry, as well as legislative and regulatory initiatives to control the sale and use of tobacco as a public health strategy. The project provides legal assistance to states and municipalities attempting to pass tobacco control measures.

The Tobacco Control Resource Center, Inc.
Northeastern University School of Law
400 Huntington Avenue
Boston, MA 02115
617-373-2026 (phone) / 617-373-3672 (fax)
info@tplp.org (e-mail)
www.tobacco.neu.edu

Tobacco Industry Documents

The CDC's Web site includes a section that facilitates access to tobacco industry documents. It provides links to and descriptions of other Internet sites with tobacco industry documents, as well as search access to three tobacco industry indexes.

www.cdc.gov/tobacco/industrydocs/index.htm

University of California, San Francisco, Tobacco Control Archives

The Tobacco Control Archives is a central, organized source of tobacco-related information. Its purpose is to collect, preserve, and provide access to papers, unpublished documents, and electronic resources relevant to tobacco control issues, primarily in California. The University of California, San Francisco (UCSF), also houses the Legacy Tobacco Documents Library, a digital library of internal tobacco industry documents from tobacco company files and two additional collections from the Tobacco Control Archives.

The Library and Center for Knowledge Management
University of California, San Francisco
tobacco-info@library.ucsf.edu (e-mail)
www.library.ucsf.edu/tobacco
www.legacy.library.ucsf.edu (Legacy Tobacco Documents Library)

University of North Carolina, School of Public Health, Minority Health Project

The Minority Health Project (MHP) is designed to improve the quality of available data on racial and ethnic populations, to increase the ability of minority health researchers to conduct statistical research and develop research proposals, and to foster a network of researchers in minority health. MHP conducts educational programs (including the Annual Summer Public Health Research Institute and Videoconference on Minority Health), provides information on research and sources of data on minority health, and maintains an extensive set of links to related Web sites.

Minority Health Project
Department of Maternal and Child Health
UNC School of Public Health
Campus Box 7445
Chapel Hill, NC 27599-7445
919-843-6934 (phone) / 919-966-6735 (fax)
Minority_Health@unc.edu (e-mail)
www.minority.unc.edu

National Clearinghouses

Media Campaign Resource Center (MCRC)

The CDC's Media Campaign Resource Center (MCRC) provides access to ads developed by a number of states and federal agencies as well as guidance and technical assistance on developing an ad campaign.

Media Campaign Resource Center
Office on Smoking and Health
Centers for Disease Control and Prevention
4770 Buford Highway NE, MS K-50
Atlanta, GA 30341-3717
770-488-5705, press 2 (phone)
mcrc@cdc.gov (e-mail)
www.cdc.gov/tobacco/mcrc

National Health Information Center (NHIC)

The National Health Information Center (NHIC) helps the public and health professionals find information on tobacco and other topics through an information and referral system and publications. It uses a database containing descriptions of health-related organizations to refer inquirers to the most appropriate resources. It also prepares and distributes publications and directories on health promotion and disease prevention topics.

National Health Information Center
P.O. Box 1133
Washington, DC 20013-1133
800-336-4797 (toll-free) / 301-565-4167 (phone) / 301-984-4256 (fax)
www.health.gov/nhic
www.healthfinder.gov

National Women's Health Information Center

The National Women's Health Information Center is supported by the Office on Women's Health (which is a part of the U.S. Department of Health and Human Services). Its Web site offers a variety of resources and information tailored for women.

www.4women.org

State Campaigns and Clearinghouses

Arizona

Tobacco Education and Prevention Program (TEPP)
www.tepp.org

Arizona Tobacco Information Network Clearinghouse
www.tepp.org/atin/clearinghouses/index.htm

California

For A Voice
www.foravoice.com

California Department of Health Services, Tobacco Control Section
www.dhs.cahwnet.gov/tobacco/index.htm

California Tobacco Education Media Campaign (TEMC)
www.dhs.ca.gov/tobacco/html/media.htm

Tobacco Education Clearinghouse of California (TECC)
P.O. Box 1830
Santa Cruz, CA 95061-1830
800-258-9090, ext. 234 (toll-free) / 831-438-3618 (fax)
www.etr.org/TECC

Delaware

Delaware Tobacco Prevention and Control Program
www.state.de.us/dhss/dph/impact.htm

Florida

Florida Online Tobacco Education Resources
www9.myflorida.com/tobacco/index.html

Florida Tobacco Control Clearinghouse
www.ftcc.fsu.edu

Students Working Against Tobacco
http://swatonline.proboards20.com/

Tools and Tactics for Fighting Big Tobacco
www.ftcc.fsu.edu/teensite/main-page.cfm

Truth
www.wholetruth.com

Georgia

UNITE Georgia
www.unitegeorgia.com

Georgia Alliance for Tobacco Prevention
www.gatobaccoprevention.org

Illinois

Reality Illinois
www.realityillinois.com

Indiana

Indiana Tobacco Prevention and Cessation Program
www.in.gov/itpc/statePartners.asp

White Lies
www.whitelies.tv

Iowa

Iowa Division of Tobacco Use Prevention and Control
www.idph.state.ia.us/tobacco

Kansas

Kansas Department of Health and Environment, Tobacco Use Prevention Program
www.kdhe.state.ks.us/tobacco

Tobacco Free Kansas Coalition
www.tobaccofreekansas.org

TASK
www.kstask.org

Kentucky

Kentucky Action
www.kyaction.com

Kentucky Health Action for Kids
www.khik.org/thecampaign.htm

Louisiana

Louisiana Tobacco Prevention Program
www.dhh.state.la.us/OPH/chrondis/Tobacco/Tobacco.htm

Maryland

Smokefree Maryland Coalition
www.smokefreemd.org/initiative

Smoking Stops Here
www.SmokingStopsHere.com

Massachusetts

Get Outraged
www.getoutraged.com

Massachusetts Tobacco Control Program
www.state.ma.us/dph/mtcp/home.htm

Massachusetts Tobacco Media Education Campaign
www.state.ma.us/dph/mtcp/media.htm

Massachusetts Tobacco Education Clearinghouse
www.jsi.com/health/mtec/home.htm (Tobacco Education Materials Catalog)

Trytostop.org
www.trytostop.org

Minnesota

Minnesota Partnership for Action Against Tobacco
www.mpaat.org

Minnesota Department of Health, Tobacco Prevention and Control Program
www.health.state.mn.us/divs/fh/assist/tpc.html

Minnesota Youth Tobacco Prevention Initiative
www.mntobacco.net

Target Market
www.tmvoice.com

Mississippi

Question It
www.questionit.com

Partnership for a Healthy Mississippi
www.healthy-miss.org

Missouri

Missouri Comprehensive Tobacco Use Prevention Program
www.dhss.state.mo.us/MTCPUpdate

Montana

Tobacco Media Campaign: Montana Tobacco Use Prevention Program (MTUPP)
www.dphhs.state.mt.us/hpsd/pubheal/disease/tobacco/media.htm

New Jersey

Reaching Everyone by Exposing Lies (REBEL)
www.njrebel.com

New Mexico

New Mexico Tobacco Use Prevention and Control (TUPAC) Program
www.health.state.nm.us/TheStink/pop_up.html

New York

New York City Department of Health and Mental Hygiene, Tobacco Control Program
www.ci.nyc.ny.us/html/doh/html/smoke/smoke.html

New York State Smoker's Quitsite
www.nysmokefree.com

North Carolina

North Carolina Tobacco Prevention and Control Branch
www.communityhealth.dhhs.state.nc.us/tobacco.htm

Ohio

Stand
www.standonline.org

Oklahoma

Students Working Against Tobacco
www.okswat.com

Oregon

Oregon Tobacco Prevention and Education
www.dhs.state.or.us/publichealth/tobacco/index.cfm

Oregon Tobacco Quitline
www.oregonquitline.org

Pennsylvania

Coalition for a Tobacco Free Pennsylvania
www.tobaccofreepa.org

Texas

Duck Texas
www.ducktexas.com

Utah

Tobacco Free Utah
www.tobaccofreeutah.org

Virginia

ydoyouthink
www.ydoyouthink.com

Washington

Unfiltered TV
www.unfilteredtv.com

Washington State's Unfiltered: Online Reality Show
www.outrageavenue.com

Washington State Tobacco Prevention and Control Program
www.doh.wa.gov/Tobacco

Wisconsin

Had Enough?
www.hadenoughwisconsin.com

Tobacco Control Resource Center for Wisconsin
1552 University Avenue
Madison, WI 53726
800-248-9244 (toll-free) / 608-262-6346 (fax)
tcrcw@tobwis.org (e-mail)
www.tobwis.org

Electronic Mailing Lists

Entertainment Media List
The entertainment media list provides information, sharing, and event updates on the depiction of tobacco in film, TV, and music. To join, send an e-mail message to Melissa Havard at mcaplan@cdc.gov.

GLOBALink: The International Tobacco Control Network
GLOBALink: The International Tobacco Control Network, which is sponsored by the Europe Against Cancer Programme, supports the international tobacco community. It provides news bulletins, electronic conferences, access to tobacco control documents, reports, and e-mail service from more than 1,500 tobacco control professionals and advocates from more than 100 countries.

www.GLOBALink.org

Media Network

The Media Network joins media specialists from tobacco control programs in states and national organizations on monthly conference calls to share information about current media topics and to learn about tobacco counter-marketing from a variety of experts and guest speakers. Between calls, Media Network members receive electronic newsletters.

To join, send an e-mail message to Diane Beistle at DBeistle@cdc.gov.

SmokeScreen Action Network

This network provides a forum for antitobacco discussion locally and nationally. You may subscribe to the lists of your choice or start your own e-mail list (see below).

www.smokescreen.org

SmokeScreen E-Mail Lists

agingtob-talk@smokescreen.org

This list provides a private discussion among 135 participants about all topics related to tobacco and aging.

www.agingtob-talk@smokescreen.org

anr-announce@smokescreen.org

This public announcement list distributes announcements from Americans for Nonsmokers' Rights (ANR). It focuses on activities that support local clean indoor air ordinances and oppose preemption bills. The list is useful for exposing front groups.

www.anr-announce@smokescreen.org

atmc-talk@smokescreen.org

This list supports the Addressing Tobacco in Managed Care (ATMC) project, supported by the University of Wisconsin and the American Association of Health Plans, funded by the Robert Wood Johnson Foundation. The Health Alliance Plans in Detroit and the Prudential Center for Health Care Research in Atlanta partner with the American Association of Health Plans, to form the National Technical Assistance Office for ATMC.

www.atmc-talk@smokescreen.org

bg-announce@smokescreen.org

This private announcement list serves 3,839 participants. It keeps subscribers aware of federal developments, helps move the news, follows hot topics, supports creative interaction, and is useful in support of media advocacy activities.

www.bg-announce@smokescreen.org

doc-alert@smokescreen.org

Serving 648 subscribers, this forum provides a once-a-day mailing that reports on important finds from the 39 million formerly secret tobacco industry documents.

www.doc-alert@smokescreen.org

docdata-talk@smokescreen.org

This small, highly focused public discussion list is devoted to technical issues surrounding the organization and categorization of tobacco industry documents.

www.docdata-talk@smokescreen.org

doc-talk@smokescreen.org

This counterpart private discussion list engages 72 participants in active conversation about documents available online.

www.doc-talk@smokescreen.org

ets-talk@smokescreen.org

This forum, founded by the ANR, serves 167 participants with announcements, news, and developments surrounding secondhand smoke.

www.ets-talk@smokescreen.org

localets-talk@smokescreen.org

Created by ANR, this discussion list focuses on secondhand smoke issues, particularly local ordinance activity.

www.localets-talk@smokescreen.org

media-alert@smokescreen.org

This list notifies members of the media of late-breaking tobacco news and events.

www.media-alert@smokescreen.org

StanGlantz-L@smokescreen.org

Serving 1,494 participants, this list takes on a public announcement format. Stan Glantz, a professor of medicine at the University of California at San Francisco, uses this forum to instigate action (e.g., getting the voluntary associations in Florida to take a public stand against legislation to protect the tobacco industry from the Engle jury) and then announces the development to the public.

www.StanGlantz-L@smokescreen.org

talc-announcement@smokescreen.org

This private discussion list serves 199 participants with announcements from the Technical Assistance Legal Center, which provides free technical assistance to California communities seeking to restrict tobacco advertising and promotions, limit tobacco sales, or divest their pension funds from tobacco stocks.

www.talc-announcement@smokescreen.org

tp-talk@smokescreen.org

This private list is rich in policy strategy and is helpful for litigation support. Expert witnesses can access this forum before their testimonies, ask for help on esoteric topics, or get answers to specific questions. The Tobacco Products Liability Project is active and helpful on this list.

www.tp-talk@smokescreen.org

News Services

PR Newswire

This Web site's search engine lets you track tobacco companies' press releases.

http://biz.yahoo.com/prnews

Tobacco Documents Online

This collection of tobacco industry documents is searchable and constantly growing in capacity and capability.

www.tobaccodocuments.org

Tobacco.org

This Web site provides daily quotes on tobacco (pro and con), customizable news, and everything that you need to keep on top of the tobacco conglomerates. Its news database contains summaries of every article concerning tobacco published in four national papers: USA Today, Wall Street Journal, Washington Post, and New York Times.

www.tobacco.org

Tobaccoresolution.com

This Web site contains links to the tobacco companies' online collections of industry documents made available as a result of litigation.

www.tobaccoresolution.com

Glossary

Advertising threshold. The level of message exposure that is required to make an impact with your target audience.

Appeal. A message quality that can be tailored to one's target audience(s). This term refers to the motivation within the target audience that a message strives to encourage or ignite (e.g., appeal to the love of family, appeal to the desire to be accepted by peer group).

Attitudes. An individual's predispositions toward an issue, object, person, or group, which influence his or her response to be either positive or negative, favorable or unfavorable.

Audience. The number of people or households that are potentially exposed to a counter-marketing tactic (e.g., radio ad, grassroots event, newspaper article) or other intervention.

Audience profile. A formal description of the characteristics of the people who make up a target audience. Some typical characteristics useful in describing audiences include media habits (e.g., newspaper and magazine readership, television [TV] viewership, radio listenership, and Internet use), family size, residential location, education, income, lifestyle preferences, leisure activities, religious and political beliefs, level of acculturation, ethnicity, ancestral heritage, consumer purchases, and psychographics. An audience profile can help you to develop more effective media messages and interventions based on an improved understanding of the audience.

Audience segment(s). A group of people who share a set of common characteristics. On the basis of these similarities, one can develop program elements and communications activities that are likely to be successful with most members of the segment.

Audience segmentation. The process of dividing up or grouping a large target audience into smaller groups based on common characteristics related to behaviors or predictors of behavior. Audience segmentation will help you to target media messages and key strategies more precisely.

Barriers (or audience barriers). Hindrances to desired change. These may be factors external or internal to audience members themselves (e.g., lack of information about health effects of tobacco use, the belief that fate causes illness and one cannot alter fate, lack of access to cessation services).

Baseline study. The collection and analysis of data regarding the target audience or environment before an intervention. Generally, baseline data are collected to provide a point of comparison to the data collected during the intervention and at its conclusion.

Bonus weight/time. Additional advertising space or time given as a "bonus" by the media outlets for buying ad time.

Central location intercept interviews. A method for pretesting messages and materials. It involves "intercepting" potential intended audience members at a high-traffic location (such as a shopping mall), asking them a few questions to see if they fit the intended audience's characteristics, sometimes showing them a message or materials, and administering a questionnaire of predominantly closed-ended questions. Because respondents form a convenience sample, the results cannot be projected to the population. Also called mall intercept interviews.

Channels (also called vehicles). The routes or methods used to reach a target audience (e.g., mass media channels include TV, radio, newspapers, and magazines; interpersonal channels include parents and health professionals; organizational channels include faith-based organizations; community channels include community events, such as health fairs and sporting events).

Closed-ended questions. Questions worded to provide respondents with a set number of possible response choices (e.g., multiple-choice, yes/no, scales).

Communication check (or "comm check"). In advertising, a type of pretest to measure whether the messages and impressions played back by the audience after viewing the ad (the overall "take away") are as intended.

Communications plan (sometimes called media campaign plan). A written strategy document that details the framework and establishes the foundation for your communications activities. A communications or media campaign plan serves as a guide to help achieve the program goals by delineating choices made about factors such as audiences, messages, and media vehicles.

Community channel. A communications channel in which messages are disseminated at the community level (e.g., library, supermarket, house of worship, municipal swimming pool).

Concept testing. The process of 1) learning about the target audience's responses to possible concepts on which you might base your message, and 2) assessing which of the concepts is most persuasive and has the greatest likelihood of changing attitudes and behaviors. This process usually requires qualitative research such as focus groups.

Control group. A group that is randomly selected and matched to the target population according to characteristics identified in the study to permit a comparison between the changes for those who receive the intervention and those who do not.

Convenience samples. Samples of respondents in research studies who are typical of the target audience and who are easily accessible. No attempt is made to collect a probability sample, and convenience samples are not statistically representative of the entire population being studied. Therefore, findings from studies using convenience samples cannot be generalized.

Copy. The written text in print materials (e.g., ads, newspaper articles, books) or the spoken words in radio or TV (e.g., ads). This term is also used more broadly to signify a whole ad or body of ads. For example, someone might make reference to needing to develop new copy for the following year's campaign.

Copy strategy. A short and simple statement that outlines your specific communications approach for an ad or a campaign (e.g., the message to be conveyed, the intended outcome, the benefit offered to the target audience in exchange for making the desired change, and the character or tone of the advertising). The copy strategy guides the advertising agency as they develop new advertising or other materials.

Counter-advertising (or tobacco counter-advertising). Any advertising efforts aimed at countering the tobacco industry advertising and other protobacco influences. Counter-advertising seeks to counter these protobacco messages and influences with persuasive prohealth, antitobacco messages. These can take many forms, including TV, radio, billboards, print ads, outdoor and transit advertising, and cinema advertising.

Counter-marketing (or tobacco counter-marketing). Marketing and communications efforts aimed at countering the marketing efforts (including but not limited to advertising) of the tobacco industry and other protobacco influences. Counter-marketing can include efforts such as media advocacy, media relations, in-school curriculum programs, sponsorships, and promotions, as well as counter-advertising through paid media channels, such as TV, radio, billboards, the Internet, and print media.

Creative. This word is typically used as a noun in the advertising industry and has two meanings: 1) the advertising agency staff (artists and writers) who create advertising ideas and concepts are called "creatives," and 2) the body of work that the creatives produce is called "the creative" and is always used in singular form.

Creative brief. A document that guides the agency's creative team in developing concepts, messages, and materials. It includes elements such as the goal and main messages of the communications piece(s), the actions you want the target audience to take and barriers to those actions, the demographic and psychographic characteristics of the audience, and other key insights about the audience that should be considered when developing the communications piece(s).

Cultural competence. An organizational and philosophical commitment to, and actions based on, recognizing the cultural differences and similarities within, among, and between groups, including their history, culture, context, geography, and other factors.

Cultural diversity. The range of differences in race, ethnicity, religion, or nationality among various groups within a community, state, region, or nation.

Culturally appropriate. Demonstration of sensitivity to cultural similarities and differences, and effective use of cultural symbols and language to communicate messages.

Culture. The shared values, traditions, norms, customs, arts, history, folklore, and institutions of a group of people who are unified by race, ethnicity, language, nationality, or religion.

Demographics. Data, such as gender, age, ethnicity, income, or education, which can be collected from a target audience and which can be useful for defining the target audience and understanding how to communicate more effectively with them.

Earned media (also called free media or news making). Coverage of your story without paying for media placements. Examples include letters to the editor, op-eds, coverage of press conferences, appearances on talk shows or local news programs, and on-air or print interviews. Such coverage is called "earned media" because you have to develop materials (e.g., news releases, press kits), work with reporters (e.g., by holding press conferences, proactively contacting reporters), and expend resources to get it; however, you do not pay for the placement of the messages in the stories.

Executions (or creative executions). Different creative approaches for communicating the same message strategy, usually involving variations in copy, tone, casting, setting, wardrobe, music, etc. Typically each ad campaign will develop, and perhaps use, several different executions, with each execution being a unique way to communicate the same main message.

Editorial. Articles expressing opinions that appear on the editorial page of a newspaper or magazine, separate from the news stories. They are usually not signed by an individual because they are seen as representing the official position of the publication.

Flight. The period of time over which a set of ads is broadcast. For example, media campaign managers typically buy media in "flights" of 3 to 6 weeks. They may go off the air for several weeks, then return for additional flights.

Focus groups. A qualitative research method in which a skilled moderator, using a discussion guide of open-ended questions, facilitates a 1- to 2-hour discussion among 5 to 10 participants who are encouraged to talk freely and spontaneously. The discussion guide is developed on the basis of the goals of the research and on what information about the participants is sought. As new topics related to the material emerge, the moderator asks additional questions to learn more. Focus groups are often used during the planning and development stages to identify previously unknown issues or concerns, or to explore reactions to potential actions, benefits, concepts, or communications materials.

Formative evaluation. Evaluation research conducted during program development. May be used to pretest concepts, messages, and materials, and to pilot test interventions and programs.

Formative research. Research conducted during the development of a program to help decide on and describe the target audience, understand the factors that influence their behavior, and determine the best ways to reach them. It looks at behaviors, attitudes, and practices of target groups; involves exploring behavioral determinants; and uses primarily qualitative methods to collect and analyze data. Formative research may be used to complement existing epidemiologic and behavioral data to assist in program planning and design.

Framing. The process of developing a particular perspective on a news story to maximize its news value and to ensure that it is presented in a way that supports your policy goals. News coverage can provide visibility, credibility, and legitimacy to the issue being covered, and can help set public and policy agendas.

- *Framing for access*—Shaping a story to attract journalists' attention and to interest the media in covering the story.

- *Framing for content*—Shaping a story to ensure that the content supports your point of view and your policy goals.

Frequency. Used in advertising to describe the average number of times an audience is exposed to a specific media message over a certain period of time (usually 4 weeks).

Gatekeeper. An organization or individual you must work with before you can reach a target population (e.g., a schoolteacher) or accomplish a task (e.g., a TV public service director). Gatekeepers may be leaders in the community or have access to and knowledge about a group of people you are trying to reach.

Goal. The overall health improvement or other significant advance that a program, organization, or agency strives to create.

Health behavior. An action performed by an individual that can negatively or positively affect his or her health (e.g., smoking, exercising).

Health communication. The study and use of communications strategies to inform and influence individual and community decisions related to health.

Impact evaluation (also called outcome evaluation and summative evaluation). The systematic collection of information to assess the impact of a program and to measure the extent to which a program has accomplished its stated goals and objectives. This information can be used to make conclusions about the merit or worth of a program, and to make recommendations about future program direction or improvement.

In-depth individual interview. A qualitative research method that involves a one-on-one discussion during which a trained interviewer guides an individual through a discussion about selected topics, allowing the respondent to talk freely and spontaneously. The structure and interviewing style are less rigid than in quantitative, interviewer-administered surveys. This technique is often used during the planning and development stages to identify previously unknown issues or concerns, or to explore reactions to potential actions, benefits, or concepts, or communications materials.

Indicator. A specific, observable, and measurable characteristic or change that shows the progress a program is making toward achieving a specified outcome. For example, the "number of days that you smoked during the past 30 days" is an indicator of smoking behavior. Researchers often use several indicators to represent a complex concept such as behavior.

Intermediaries. Organizations, such as professional, industrial, civic, social, and fraternal groups, that act as channels for distributing program messages and materials to members of the desired target audience.

Interpersonal channel. A communications channel that involves the dissemination of messages through one-on-one communication (e.g., mentor to student, friend to friend, pharmacist to customer).

Language. Includes form and pattern of speech. It may be spoken or written, and it is used by residents or descendants of a particular area, region, or nation or by a large group of people. Language can be formal or informal and includes dialect, idiomatic speech, and slang.

Local media. Media whose coverage and circulation are confined to, or concentrated in, markets that are smaller than a state. Usually, they offer different sets of rates to national and local advertisers.

Logic model. A systematic and visual way to present the perceived relationships among the resources you have to operate the program, the activities you plan to do, and the changes or results you hope to achieve.

Marketing. The process of planning and executing the conception, promotion, and distribution of ideas, goods, and services to create exchanges that satisfy consumers.

Media. Channels for disseminating your message and materials. Mass media include TV, radio, newspapers, magazines, billboards, public transportation, direct mailings, Web sites, and others.

Media advisory. A submission to media outlets that provides basic information (who, what, when, where, why) about an upcoming event with opportunities for interviews and/or photographs. Advisories are usually not more than one page.

Media advocacy. The strategic use of media and community advocacy to advance social or policy change. Media advocacy can reframe issues; shape public discussion; or build support for a policy, point of view, or environmental change. Instead of using vehicles to send messages to the community, media advocacy works with the community to create messages to help change the environment within which the community lives.

Media alert. A short (two- to three-paragraph) announcement to the media alerting them to new information or a new development on an issue. It provides the "who, what, when, where, and how" and generally little other information.

Media campaign plan. See communications plan.

Media kit (also called press kit, press packet, or information kit). A packet (usually a folder) that includes items explaining a program or health issue to the media. It contains a lead or main press release and related elements (e.g., brochures, fact sheets, contact information, and camera-ready photographs or images) that tell a complete story to the press.

Media literacy. The ability to analyze, evaluate, and produce media in various forms. It involves the examination of the techniques, technologies, and institutions that are involved in media production, the ability to deconstruct and critically analyze media messages to identify the sponsor's motives, and the recognition of the role that audiences play in taking meaning from those messages. It also involves the ability of individuals to construct or compose media messages representing their (the intended audience's) point of view.

Media placement plan (or media buy plan or media plan). The specific schedule of paid placements that have been negotiated for an ad or set of ads. The media placement plan details the times and programs during which TV and radio ads will be aired, the locations and sizes of billboards that will be placed, the magazines, issues, and specific placements into which print ads will be placed, etc. The media placement plan also contains a summary of target audience reach and frequency, typically per 4-week period.

Media relations. Establishing a positive working relationship between individuals in your organization and members of the news media to increase the likelihood that your issue will be covered favorably, thus helping to advance your program goals. Media relations includes getting to know individual reporters (including the scope of their work and their interest areas); serving as a reliable, proactive provider of credible information about the issue; and being timely and responsive to their requests for interviews, additional contacts, and other resources.

Media tracking. The monitoring of radio, TV, and print media over a specified period of time for a specific topic or message. Data gathered can be analyzed for content, slant (positive or negative), location of placement, or trends in the amount of coverage.

Medium. Any media class used to convey a message to the public, such as TV, radio, the Internet, billboards, cable TV, newspapers, neighborhood publications, magazines, comic books, billboards, posters, music, and point-of-purchase displays.

Moderator's guide. A set of questions, probes, and discussion points used by a focus group moderator to help him or her facilitate the group. A guide can also contain reminders of which questions are most important to the research to help the moderator use the discussion time effectively.

Objectives. Quantifiable statements describing the intended program achievements necessary to reach a program goal. Objectives should be specific, measurable, achievable, relevant, and time-bound.

Op-Ed (Opinion Editorial). A letter, statement, article, or short essay submitted to a newspaper editor by a reader or a representative of an organization. Op-eds usually express a strong opinion or point of view about an issue, and are backed by well-researched and documented facts. They appear on the page opposite the editorial page.

Open-ended questions. Questions worded to allow an individual to respond freely in his or her own words, in contrast to closed-ended or fixed-choice questions.

Organizational channel. A communications channel in which messages are disseminated at the organizational level (e.g., corporate newsletters, cafeteria bulletin boards).

Outcome evaluation. See impact evaluation.

Over recruiting. Recruiting more respondents than required to compensate for expected "no shows."

Paid media (also called paid advertising). The placement of messages through advertising on TV, radio, print, outdoor media, the Internet, etc. Because you are paying for these placements, you can control the exact placement and content of the messages, making them very useful in targeting specific audience segments. However, paid advertising can be very expensive, making it difficult to use effectively with a small budget.

Partners. Individuals or organizations/agencies that contribute to the efforts initiated by a leader or a head organization/agency. Partners can have a variety of roles (e.g., contribute research data, share evaluation experience, help spread the health message).

Piggybacking. Relating your story to other breaking events in the media as a way of gaining access to the media.

Pilot testing. Implementing and evaluating the program in a limited area for a limited amount of time to make program adjustments based on the pilot experience.

Pitch letter. A brief, targeted letter or e-mail message that tries to convince a journalist to cover your story by outlining the information that you have to share and why it is valuable. Pitches can also be made by telephone.

Pretesting. A type of formative evaluation that involves assessing the target audience's reactions to your messages, materials, or both before they are finalized. This will help you determine if your messages and materials are likely to achieve the intended effect.

Primary target audience(s) (or primary audience(s)). The group(s) of individuals you determine are most important for your communications effort to reach and influence. The primary audience is a portion of a larger population selected because influencing that group will contribute most to achieving your campaign's objectives. You may also choose secondary audiences, but your greatest emphasis will be on achieving your objectives through communication with the primary target audience.

Probe. An interviewer technique that is used primarily in qualitative research (e.g., focus groups, individual in-depth interviews) to solicit additional information about a question or issue. Probes should be neutral (e.g., "What else can you tell me about _____?") rather than directive ("Do you think the pamphlet was suggesting that you take a particular step, such as changing your diet?").

Process evaluation. The systematic collection of information to document and assess how well a program is being implemented. Process evaluation includes assessments such as whether materials are being distributed to the right people and in what quantities, whether and to what extent program activities are occurring, whether and how frequently the audience is being exposed to your ads, and other measures of how and how well the program is being implemented. This information can help you determine whether the original program is being implemented as designed and can be used to improve the delivery and efficiency of the program.

Program evaluation. The systematic collection of information about a program's activities and outcomes for the purpose of making judgments about the program, improving program effectiveness, and informing decisions about future program development.

Psychographics. A set of variables that describes an individual in terms of his or her overall approach to life, including personality traits, values, beliefs, preferences, habits, and behaviors. Psychographics are not usually related to health-specific issues, but more commonly to characteristics such as consumer- or purchase-specific behaviors, beliefs, and values.

Psychosocial factors. Variables that describe an individual in terms of preferences and characteristics, such as attitudes, beliefs, values, perceived norms, self-efficacy, and intentions. In many theories of behavior, psychosocial factors are assumed to be the determinants of behaviors or the factors that influence whether a behavior is performed.

Public relations. Using various communications channels, such as earned media, paid advertising, media relations, Web sites, speakers' bureaus, and/or brochures, to help the public understand your organization, its programs, and its products and services, as well as to build a positive image of them in the community.

Public service announcement (PSA). A form of advertising that can be delivered via TV or radio and that is aired free of charge by the media. There is limited control over when or how often a PSA airs, making it difficult to effectively reach specific target audiences.

Qualitative research. Research that focuses on in-depth audience insights and information as opposed to collecting numerical measures. Qualitative research is useful for exploring reactions; collecting information about feelings, impressions, and motivations; and uncovering additional ideas, issues, or concerns. Results from qualitative research cannot be generalized to the whole target audience because the participants don't constitute a representative random sample, samples are relatively small, and not all participants are asked precisely the same questions. Focus groups and in-depth individual interviews are common types of qualitative research.

Quantitative research. Research designed to count and measure knowledge, attitudes, beliefs, and behaviors by asking a large number of people identical (and predominantly closed-ended) questions. Quantitative research yields numerical data that can be analyzed statistically. If the respondents are a representative random sample, quantitative data can be used to make statements about the intended audience as a whole. Quantitative research is useful for measuring the extent to which knowledge, attitudes, or behaviors are prevalent in an audience. Surveys are a common type of quantitative research.

Random sample. A sample of respondents in which every member of the target population has an equal chance of being included in the sample.

Rating points. Used in media buys to measure the exposure of the audience to an ad. Target rating points (TRPs) and gross rating points (GRPs) are the two main types of rating points. TRPs are obtained by multiplying the percentage of the target audience potentially reached ("reach") by the number of times that this percentage will potentially see the message ("frequency"). GRPs are a similar measure of exposure, but among the whole population, rather than just the specific target audience. Often the two terms (TRPs and GRPs) will be used interchangeably to mean exposure among the selected target audience. Rating points are usually, but not necessarily, expressed in 4-week figures. For example, an agency may recommend buying 1,200 rating points over 3 months, which means an average of 400 points per 4-week period.

Reach. Used in advertising to describe the percentage of the total target audience exposed to a specific media message during a specific period (usually 4 weeks).

Recall. The extent to which respondents remember seeing or hearing a message shown in a competitive media environment. It usually centers on the main idea or the awareness of an ad.

Schedule/flow chart. A list or graphic of the media placements that have been bought and when they are going to air or appear.

Screener. An instrument containing short-answer questions used in the recruitment process for research methods such as focus groups and central location intercept interviews. Interviewees' answers to the questions determine who is eligible to participate in the research.

Secondary target audience(s) (or secondary audience(s)). Group(s) of individuals in addition to the primary audience(s) that your communications efforts seek to reach and influence. Secondary audiences may be a subset of the primary audience (e.g., adult Hispanic/Latino smokers, if adult smokers are the primary audience); groups that may help reach or influence the primary audience (e.g., parents or teachers, if youth aged 12-17 years old is the primary audience); or other groups that are important for reaching your objectives (e.g., policy makers, if changes in policies and individual behavior are both necessary).

Self-administered questionnaires. Questionnaires that are filled out by respondents. These can be distributed by mail, handed out in person, or programmed into a computer.

Setting. A location or an environment where the target audience can be reached with a communications effort. For example, a grocery store is a setting where audience members can be reached with educational pamphlets.

Social marketing. The application and adaptation of commercial marketing concepts and techniques to the analysis, planning, implementation, and evaluation of programs designed to bring about behavior change of target audiences to improve the welfare of individuals or their society. Social marketing emphasizes thorough market research to identify and understand the intended audience and what is preventing them from adopting a certain health behavior and to then develop, monitor, and constantly adjust a program to stimulate appropriate behavior change. Social marketing programs can address any or all of the traditional marketing mix variables—product, price, place, or promotion.

Stakeholders. Individuals or organizations that are invested in the program and its outcomes. They include those involved in the campaign's operation (e.g., managers, staff, funders, partners), those served or affected by the program (e.g., advocacy groups, target group members), and those in a position to make decisions about program efforts.

Storyboard. Illustrations and accompanying scripts that represent ideas for scenes for a TV ad.

Strategy. The overall approach that a program takes. Effective strategies contribute toward achieving program goals and objectives. Strategies should be based on knowledge about effective counter-marketing; the target audience's needs and characteristics; and the program's capabilities, timelines, and resources.

Strategy statement. A written document delineating the important choices you have made that will help achieve the campaign's objectives. The strategy statement should include the target audience profile, the action audience members should take, how they will benefit (from their perspective, not necessarily from a public health perspective), and how you can reach them. This document provides the direction and consistency for all program messages and materials for this audience and is broader than a creative brief, which is used for the development of individual materials.

Style. A message quality that can be tailored to one's target audience(s). This is a general term that refers to issues such as presenting cartoon figures versus detailed graphs or using embellished text versus short or concise text.

Summative evaluation. See impact evaluation.

Surveillance. The ongoing, systematic collection, analysis, and interpretation of data essential to planning, implementation, and evaluation of public health programs. For example, this would include assessing at regular time intervals target audience beliefs, attitudes, and behaviors related to tobacco use. Surveillance efforts can also track health outcomes over time.

Tailoring. The adaptation of program components to best fit the relevant needs and characteristics of the target population.

Talking points. Prepared notes used by a speaker to guide his or her presentation. Often used in preparing for interviews or other interaction with the news media.

Target audience (target population). The group of people the program intends to involve and affect in some way. The target audience shares common characteristics that help guide decisions about program development.

Theater-style pretesting. A research method in which a large group (usually 50 to 300 people) is gathered in a theater-style setting to view and respond to audiovisual materials such as TV ads. Ads are typically shown embedded in a set of other audiovisuals (programming, other ads, or both) to replicate a more natural viewing environment and to help determine memorability of test materials when shown among other materials.

Tobacco counter-advertising. See counter-advertising.

Tobacco counter-marketing. See counter-marketing.

Tone. A message quality that can be tailored to one's target audience(s). This term refers to the manner in which a message is expressed (e.g., an authoritative tone, an alarming tone, a friendly tone).

Variable. A characteristic of an object of measurement that can take on a range of values (e.g., height, test scores, gender).

342

Appendix 2.1: Counter-Marketing Planning Worksheet

This worksheet should be used as a guide. Don't worry about filling in each item in this exact order. Developing a counter-marketing plan is an iterative process; you'll revise and improve on each step as your campaign progresses. The most important thing is that you think through each step and that every activity moves you closer to your goal. Before you complete this worksheet, it would be helpful to review Chapter 2: Planning Your Counter-Marketing Program and other relevant information in this manual. The Counter-Marketing Planning Worksheet Guidelines on the following pages provide a quick reference to use in completing the worksheet.

Tobacco Control Goal:

Problem Statement and Background:

Target Audience(s):

Counter-Marketing Program Objective(s):

Strategy Statement:

Activities and Channels:

Opportunities for Collaboration:

Evaluation Plan:

Tasks and Timeline:

Budget and Resources:

Counter-Marketing Planning Worksheet Guidelines

Tobacco Control Goal

- Base your goal(s) on research, the state's assessment, or both.

- Complete a separate Counter-Marketing Planning Worksheet for each goal, because you need a separate plan for each goal you're addressing. Make sure overlapping areas are consistent and complementary.

Problem Statement and Background

- Describe the problem you're addressing. Specify the group(s) affected, how it is affected, and the severity of the problem. Give supporting epidemiologic data from current research and scientific literature.

- Identify who might be able to positively influence this situation or the affected group(s).

- Explain why your agency is addressing the problem.

- Assess and list your program's strengths, weaknesses, opportunities, and threats (SWOTs); its assets and resources; links to or influence with the target audience(s); current activities; and gaps and barriers to achieving the needed change.

- Review relevant theories and models.

Target Audience(s)

- Define the group(s) you want to reach, the desired results, and how you'll measure those results.

- Select target audience(s). Decide which audience segments represent the highest priority for reaching your goal. Consider which audience segments are affected disproportionately by tobacco-related health problem(s), which segments can be most easily reached and influenced, and which are large enough to justify intervention.

- Describe each group you plan to reach with your campaign. Detail any knowledge you have about how each group is affected, as well as gaps in knowledge to be addressed through market research or other research. Include demographics, cultural and lifestyle characteristics, media preferences (channels, message appeals, activities, and types of involvement in the issue), and other traits that will help you understand how best to reach each group, as well as related feelings, attitudes, knowledge, and behaviors.

- Determine which secondary audience(s) can influence the behavior of your primary audience(s).

Counter-Marketing Program Objective(s)

- Set objectives that reflect the desired results of counter-marketing efforts within the given time frame and resources, and within the context of a comprehensive tobacco control program.

- Write objectives that are SMART (specific, measurable, achievable, relevant, and time-bound).

Strategy Statement

- To develop a strategy is usually an iterative process; as you learn more about one element, other elements may need to be adjusted.

- Write a strategy statement for each target audience that includes:

    - Description of the target audience

    - Description of the action you want the audience to take as a result of exposure to your program, as specified in the objectives

    - List of obstacles to taking the action

    - Description of audience's perceived benefit of taking the action

    - Explanation of why the benefit, and the audience's ability to attain it, will be credible and meaningful to the audience

    - List of potential channels and activities that will reach audience members

    - Description of image, tone, look, and feel of messages and materials most likely to reach the target audience

Activities and Channels

- Assess the current media environment related to your goal, and decide which counter-marketing approach(es) to use, such as advertising, public relations, media advocacy, grassroots marketing, and media literacy training.

- Determine for each target audience which approaches (or combination of approaches) best address the problem and your program objectives.

- Ask what is the *best* way to reach each target audience. Select channels and activities that fit your target, budget, time constraints, and resources. Consider the attributes and limitations of each type of channel.

Opportunities for Collaboration

- Determine whether you want to recruit partners for collaboration, and consider how many partners would be optimal.

- Identify organizations that have similar goals and are willing to work with you.

- Be strategic in selecting organizations as partners. Consider which community-based organizations and businesses may help you achieve your goal by providing:

    - Access to a target audience

    - Enhanced credibility for your message or program, if the target audience considers the organization to be a trusted source

    - Additional resources, either financial or in-kind

    - Added expertise

    - Cosponsorship of events

- Consider the requirements for collaboration with each partner, including time for additional approvals, minor or major changes in the program to match each partner's needs and priorities, and how these requirements fit with the direction and procedures of your organization.

Evaluation Plan

- Develop plans for formative research and evaluation, process evaluation, and outcome evaluation.

- Base the design of your evaluation plan on the objectives of the counter-marketing program. Determine the most important questions for the evaluation, the information you'll need now and in the future, how you'll gather the information, and how you'll analyze it to determine whether you've met your objectives.

- Identify evaluation experts, either internal or external to your agency, who will work with you throughout the design and implementation of your program to develop plans for the various types of evaluation.

- Perform *formative research* (research on the target audience before you develop the counter-marketing campaign) to help you gain valuable insights that will guide the development of your message and materials, as well as the channels of delivery.

- Conduct *formative evaluation* (research conducted during the development of your program to pretest and pilot test your interventions, messages, and programs) to determine (1) whether the materials you are developing effectively communicate what you intended, and (2) how the target audience will be influenced by your materials.

- Perform *process evaluation* to determine whether your program was implemented as planned. It can answer questions such as:

    - Did partners contribute as expected? Why or why not?

    - Did you have the right amount of resources?

    - Did you schedule enough time for campaign development and implementation?

    - Was your issue covered by the news media your target audience sees or reads?

    - Was your issue covered by the media in the way you had hoped? Was your approach to framing the messages reflected in the media coverage?

    - Have you become a source for journalists covering this issue?

- Conduct *outcome evaluation* to help you answer the following important questions:

    - Did your counter-marketing program achieve the outcomes you expected?

    - Did you build awareness of the ads you ran? Of the program elements?

    - Did the audience recall the campaign's main messages?

    - Did the audience increase its knowledge as desired/intended?

    - Did the audience change beliefs and attitudes as desired?

    - Did the audience change its behaviors?

    - What did the target audience think of your campaign? Did members become involved in the program?

    - Did a policy (e.g., clean indoor air ordinance or tax increase) change as desired?

Tasks and Timeline

- List all activities that need to occur before, during, and after implementation of your counter-marketing program.

- Identify major milestones, such as launch and start dates for specific activities.

- Include smaller tasks to be accomplished from the time you write the plan until the time you intend to complete the program evaluation. By building these tasks into the timeline, you'll be more likely to remember to assign the work and stay on schedule.

- Review and update your task list and timeline regularly. It is a flexible management tool that can help you track your progress.

Budget and Resources

- List all anticipated expenses, including staff time and other resources.

- Include all budget and resources available (staff, in-kind, internal, and external).

- Assess the financial and human resources available to help you anticipate funding needs, thoroughly plan your campaign to fit your budget, and make optimal use of all available resources.

- Recall that if your plan calls for efforts to lobby for a particular bill, you'll need to use funding not provided by the Centers for Disease Control and Prevention.

Appendix 3.1: Sample Recruitment Screener for Intercept Interviews on Smoking Cessation

(Interviewer instructions are in italics.)

Good morning/afternoon, my name is _____, from ____Market Research Firm, an independent market research agency. Today, we're conducting a survey in this area among people between 25 and 49 years old. Do you fit into that age group?

    Yes   ❏   *(Continue.)*
    No   ❏   *(Thank and terminate interview.)*

1. First, can I ask, do you or does anyone in your family work in any of the following areas? *(Show card A with the following items written on it.)*

    Market research   ❏ 1
    Advertising or Marketing   ❏ 2
    Media   ❏ 3
    Public relations   ❏ 4
    Auto industry   ❏ 5
    Manufacture/distribution of tobacco products   ❏ 6

(If answer is "yes" for any of these areas, except auto industry, thank and terminate interview. If answer is "no" for any of these areas, continue.)

2. Do you currently smoke cigarettes?

    Yes   ❏ 1   *(Continue.)*
    No   ❏ 2   *(Thank and terminate interview.)*

3. Since you started smoking, would you say you have smoked more than 100 cigarettes?

    Yes   ❏ 1   *(Continue.)*
    No   ❏ 2   *(Thank and terminate interview.)*

4. Please tell me how much you agree with the following statement:

"I want to stop smoking within the next 6 months."

(Show card B with the statements below written on it.)

Strongly agree	❏ 1	*(Continue.)*
Slightly agree	❏ 2	*(Continue.)*
Neither agree nor disagree	❏ 3	*(Thank and terminate interview.)*
Slightly disagree	❏ 4	*(Thank and terminate interview.)*
Strongly disagree	❏ 5	*(Thank and terminate interview.)*

5. Could you spare some time to come into the hall to answer some further questions?

(If respondents need reading glasses, check whether they have their glasses with them.)

Yes	❏ 1	*(Continue.)*
No	❏ 2	*(Thank and terminate interview.)*

(Check quotas to see whether the client has requested that there be minimum numbers of participants with certain demographics.)

6. Do you have a telephone at home or work or a cell phone where you can be reached?

Yes	❏ 1	*(Continue.)*
No	❏ 2	*(Conduct 20-minute interview.)*

7. Would you be available to take part in a further short telephone interview within the next 3 or 4 days?

Yes	❏ 1	*(Conduct 10-minute interview.)*
No	❏ 2	*(Conduct 20-minute interview.)*

Appendix 3.2: Sample Recruitment Screener for Individual Interviews To Test Advertisements and Ad Concepts

(Instructions for interviewer are in italics.)

Client: _____

Hello. My name is _____, and I'm calling on behalf of _____ (market research company) in _____ (city). We're conducting a very brief public opinion survey. If you complete the study and meet the appropriate criteria, you'll be invited to participate in a discussion about advertising in _____ (location) on _____ (date). May we ask you a few questions?

(Don't ask but do record gender. Attempt to recruit 50% males and 50% females.)

    ___ Male   ___ Female

1. Do you or anyone in your household work for any of the following types of companies: marketing, marketing research, public relations, advertising, or a tobacco company or any of its affiliates?

    ___ Yes *(Thank and terminate interview.)*

    ___ No *(Continue interview.)*

2. In which of the following age groups are you? *(Attempt to achieve a good mix of ages.)*

    ___ Younger than 25 years old *(Thank and terminate interview.)*
    ___ 25–30 years old
    ___ 31–39 years old
    ___ 40–50 years old
    ___ Older than 50 years old *(Thank and terminate interview.)*

3. Have you participated in a market research discussion group of any kind in the last 3 months?

    ___ Yes *(Thank and terminate the interview.)*
    ___ No *(Continue.)*

4. So that we can be sure that all backgrounds are represented in our study, please tell me your race or ethnic background. Are you .... ?

    ___ Caucasian/white

    ___ African American/black

    ___ Hispanic/Latino

    ___ Asian

    ___ Other

(Recruit two or three individuals per minority group.)

5. Have you smoked more than 100 cigarettes in your life?

    ___ Yes *(Continue.)*

    ___ No *(Thank and terminate the interview.)*

6. Do you currently smoke?

    ___ Yes *(Continue.)*

    ___ No *(Thank and terminate the interview.)*

7. Do you plan to quit smoking in the next 3 months?

    ___ Yes *(Continue.)*

    ___ No *(Thank and terminate the interview.)*

We are holding a discussion on _____ (date) at _____ (location). Light refreshments will be served, and you'll receive $40 (regular interviews) or $60 (floaters). *(Floaters are individuals who will be recruited for a longer period of time and will be interviewed if someone scheduled for a regular slot does not show up.)*

The topics for the focus group will be advertising and smoking.

Will you be able to join us?

    ___ Yes *(Continue.)*

    ___ No *(Thank and terminate the interview.)*

Great. Now I just need to record some information, so we can mail you a confirmation letter and directions. We'll call you the day before to confirm your attendance.

(Fill out all information on the next page.)

Recruitment Interview Summary

45-minute interview

$40 for regular times; $60 for floaters *(Floaters are individuals who will be recruited for a longer period of time and might be interviewed if someone scheduled for a regular slot does not show up. Recruiter will ask people their availability and assign them to a specific time slot. Individuals who are available for longer periods of time are typically assigned as floaters.)*

(Circle time for which participant is available and scheduled.)

Regular times: 1:00 p.m., 1:45 p.m., 2:30 p.m., 3:15 p.m., 4:00 p.m., 4:45 p.m., 5:30 p.m., 6:15 p.m., 7:00 p.m., 7:45 p.m., 8:30 p.m.

Floater times: 1:45–3:15 p.m., 4:00–5:30 p.m., 7:00–8:30 p.m.

Name _____ Date of birth _____

Address _____

City _____ State _____ ZIP _____

Telephone numbers:

Home _____

Work _____

Cell _____

Fax number _____

(Ask and record responses to the following questions after the screening interview is completed:)

When you come to the discussion, please bring a driver's license or other picture identification with your birth date for registration.

If you have any questions or need to reschedule your interview time, you may call _____ (market research company) at (xxx-xxx-xxxx).

Someone from _____ (market research company) will call you the day before the discussion in order to confirm and remind you of the time.

First name and initial of last name of phone interviewer _____

Appendix 3.3: Moderator's Guide for Focus Groups With Smokers

(Instructions for interviewer are in italics.)

Objectives for Focus Groups

This discussion guide was developed to achieve several objectives:

1. To identify potential benefits and barriers for calling a "quitline" or visiting a quitting Web site.

2. To determine which logo design most clearly conveys the purpose of the quitline and which logo elements will be most effective in getting smokers to call the quitline, to visit the Web site, or both.

3. To determine which TV and radio spots are most likely to move the target audience to take action by calling the quitline, visiting the Web site, or both.

Focus Group Discussion
Moderator's Guide

1. Warm-up, Explanations, and Introductions

Introduction and purpose

Welcome. My name is _____, and I'll be facilitating our discussion tonight.

Thanks for joining us. We do appreciate the fact that you're taking time from your day to provide us with your opinions.

What we are doing tonight is called a focus group. It's a way for us to get your opinions, much like a survey, but it's done as a group discussion rather than a lot of yes/no questions.

There are no right or wrong answers, and it's important that I hear what everyone thinks. All of your comments—both positive and negative—are important, so please speak up, even if you disagree with someone else.

Procedure

> Our discussion tonight will be videotaped and audiotaped so I don't lose any of your comments. We'll use the tapes to write a report summarizing what was said. The report won't identify any of you by name.
>
> Behind me is a one-way mirror. Some people who are interested in what you have to say will be sitting behind the glass on and off during our discussion. They aren't in the same room with us, because they can be distracting.
>
> This is a group discussion, so please don't wait for me to call on you, but please speak one at a time, so the recorder can pick up everything. It's also helpful if we give everyone in the group a chance to voice an opinion.
>
> We do have many topics to discuss in a very limited amount of time, so at times I may change the subject or move on, to keep us on schedule. I'll try to come back to earlier points at the end of our session if there's time.

Self-introductions

> Let's do a quick round of introductions. Just tell us your first name and your occupation.

2. General Information Discussion

Overview of discussion

> Tonight, we're going to talk a bit about smoking. Everyone here smokes, at least some of the time. All of you have said you want to quit. I'd like to start by asking about that.
>
> Can you tell me what good things might happen if you quit?
> *(Probe for potential benefits.)*
>
> I know most people here think it would be a good idea to stop smoking, but even things we want to do sometimes have a downside. Can you tell me what bad things might happen if you quit?
> *(Probe for unwanted consequences of quitting [e.g., more difficulty fitting in socially].)*

What makes it hard to quit?
(Probe for barriers.)

Who do you think would approve if you stopped smoking?

Who might disapprove?

When you think about quitting, whose opinion do you respect?
(Probe for trusted sources.)

Has anyone ever heard about a hotline or resource number to help you stop smoking? What have you heard? Has anyone ever called this type of number?

For those of you who haven't called, why not?

For those of you who have called, how did it work for you?

If there were a hotline like this available where you live, would you use it? Why or why not?

What would make it easier to use the number?

What makes it hard to use a hotline like that?

Has anyone ever visited a Web site to help you quit smoking or to find out more about it?
(Use follow-up questions similar to the previous five questions.)

Where would you expect to see or hear information about a hotline or Web site designed to help people quit smoking?

What would be the best way to hear about such a hotline or Web site? Why?

3. Test of Television and Radio Ads

Overview of TV testing

We'd like to show you several TV commercials on this subject. I'm going to begin by showing you a set of three commercials. I'm most interested in whether any of these ads might move you to call—or at least think about calling—a smoking cessation line, or visit a quitting Web site.

To record your individual opinions, we've provided you with a reaction sheet. Please mark your opinions individually either during the spots or immediately after you see them. We'll collect the sheets after we've completed this exercise.

(Distribute sheets, cue VCR, and run first set of spots.)

I'm now going to give you a moment to fill out your handouts. Then we're going to watch another set of three commercials.

(Allow time [a few minutes maximum] for individual responses to be completed.)

Now we're going to watch another set of three commercials. Once again, I'm most interested in whether any of these ads might move you to call—or at least think about calling—a smoking cessation line.

(Distribute sheets, cue VCR, and run second set of spots.)

Discussion of TV ads

Please take a moment to record your thoughts and pass your sheets to the front. Now I'd like to hear your feedback.

Which spots would be the most likely to catch your attention? Why?

Which spots did you like the best? Why?

Was there anything in any of the spots that upset you?
(Probe for reasons and implications.)

Overview of radio testing

I'd like to have you listen to several radio spots about smoking health, smoking cessation, or both. Each of the radio spots is 60 seconds long, and we'll be playing a total of six spots for you to review. As with the TV ads, we're most interested in hearing your feedback as to which spot or spots do the best job of motivating you to call the quitline or visit the quitting Web site.

Again, we'd like you to record your individual opinions on the sheet we're distributing and then we'll have a group discussion once the tape is finished playing.

(Distribute sheets, cue tape, and run compilation tape.)

Discussion of radio ads

> Please take a minute to record your individual thoughts on the radio spots, and pass the sheets to the front. Now I'd like to hear your feedback as to which spot or spots would make you call the quitline or visit the Web site.
>
> *(Probe as to why and why not.)*

4. Testing of Logos

Overview of logo testing

> We'd also like to get your opinions on several logo designs that are being considered. The final logo will appear on materials related to the quitline, for instance, at the end of a TV spot, on an outdoor billboard, or on a poster or handout in a physician's office.
>
> Please keep in mind that we want your feedback on which logo or logos most clearly convey what the quitline is about. As we did with the TV and radio ads, we'll be handing out a sheet to each of you. Please record your opinions, and pass your sheets to the front. Then we'll discuss your thoughts as a group.

Logo presentation and discussion

> *(Distribute sheets, present four logos, and pass around logos, display, or both for participants to review. Collect sheets.)*
>
> Which logo or logos did you like the most?
>
> Why?
>
> Which logo or logos did you like the least?
>
> Why?

5. Wrap-up

> Thank you very much for participating tonight. I'm going to see if my colleagues have anything else they'd like to ask.

(Check with staff behind the mirror if time allows.)

Thanks for sharing your opinions and your time with us tonight. This session has been extremely helpful. As you walk out, a staff member will hand you reimbursement for your time tonight. She'll also ask you to sign a form acknowledging your receipt of the compensation for this evening

Thanks again and have a good night.

Appendix 3.4: Sample Moderator's Guide for Focus Groups To Test Advertisements With Youth

(Instructions for moderator are in italics.)

1. Welcome and Ground Rules *(5 minutes)*

- There are no right or wrong answers. Give honest opinions. You're not here to decide what's good or bad.

- Everything said in the room will be confidential—only the people working on this project will know what you said, not other people in your life, such as your parents or teachers.

- We are videotaping and audiotaping all of the discussions that we are doing simply so that I don't have to take a lot of notes during this session. In addition, there may be some people interested in observing the discussion and they are seated behind that window so that they don't disturb our discussion.

2. Introductions and Warm-up *(5 minutes)*

- Give name, age, and grade in school.

- What are your favorite commercials, and why?

(Write on a flip chart. This is just an icebreaker to get respondents to think about advertising.)

3. Tobacco Knowledge *(10 minutes)*

(Explain that the purpose of this research is to better understand teens and their attitudes toward and use of tobacco. Assure respondents that they won't be judged in any way.)

- What are some of the reasons people begin to smoke cigarettes? *(Write on a flip chart.)*

- What are some of the reasons people continue to smoke cigarettes? *(Write on a flip chart.)*

- What are some of the reasons, if any, people shouldn't use tobacco? What else? What else? *(Write on a flip chart.)*

- Where did you learn about this? *(Probe for any awareness of specific advertising, media vehicles [e.g., TV, radio, magazines, billboards, Internet], or local antitobacco programs.)*

- For community and school programs: What sort of programs have you heard of or participated in at school or in your town?

- For advertising: Which of the specific ads do you remember? *(Ask to describe in detail.)*

    —What do you think they're trying to get across in these commercials?

    —What do you think are the purposes of these commercials?

4. Exposure to Ads *(45 minutes)*

(Show the ads one at a time. Rotate the order of the ads for each new group to avoid first-position bias. After showing each ad, ask respondents to write the main message on notepads that they have been given, and how much the ad makes them "stop and think about not using tobacco." Use a scale of 1 to 10. Explain that 1 means the ad doesn't make them stop and think much about not using tobacco and 10 means it really does make them stop and think about not using tobacco. Carefully explain that we're not as much interested in which ads are their favorites, but which ones are most likely to make them stop and think. Then for each ad ask the following questions before showing the next ad.)

- What do you think was the most important thing they're trying to tell you in this commercial? *(Poll the respondents and lead a brief discussion.)*

- What rating did you give this ad on the "stop and think" scale, and why? *(Ask respondents to explain their ratings.)*

- Who do you think made this commercial?

(After they have discussed each ad, ask respondents as a group to decide where each ad should be placed on a wall scale. The wall scale is simply numbers from 1 to 10 written on individual pieces of paper attached to the wall in order. It gives participants a visual way to consider each ad and compare among the ads. Explain that 1 means the ad doesn't make them stop and think much about not using tobacco and 10 means it really does make them stop and think about not using tobacco. Write the name of each ad on an index card and attach each card to the wall scale in a place the respondents think is appropriate.)

5. Wall Scale Reassessment *(10 minutes)*

(After all of the index cards have been placed on the wall scale, ask respondents to reevaluate their placement of the ads on the wall scale, now that they've seen all the ads in comparison to each other. Make any necessary changes to the order of the ads on the wall scale. Probe for reasons behind changes.)

6. Final Selection Among Ads *(10 minutes)*

Of all these ads, which do you think would most get people your age to seriously consider not using tobacco? *(Ask respondents to write the answer on their notepads, and then lead the group in a discussion.)*

7. Advice and Suggestions *(5 minutes)*

Thinking about all the things we've discussed today, what are the three pieces of advice you would give to the people who create ads to encourage people your age not to use tobacco? *(Ask respondents to write their answers on their notepads. Then lead a group discussion.)*

(Thank respondents, collect notepads from respondents, and conclude the session. Respondents will go the front desk to receive their incentives.)

Appendix 3.5: Sample Self-Administered Form To Test Fact Sheets

Pretest Questions

As you probably are aware, [name of sponsoring organization] has recently launched its tobacco control program. One component of [sponsoring organization]'s campaign is the distribution of fact sheets that convey important information about issues related to tobacco use. It's crucial that we test these fact sheets in order to ensure that we are communicating our key messages effectively.

We appreciate your willingness to share your reactions to the attached fact sheet by reading it and answering a few questions. We don't ask your name, and all information you provide will remain confidential.

Because only a few individuals are being asked to help judge this material, your response is particularly valuable.

Before you begin, please check the appropriate answers to these four questions.

1. How much would you say you know about the [sponsoring organization]'s tobacco control program?

   Nothing ____ A little ____ Some ____ A lot ____

2. Is there anything you want to know about the program?

   Yes _____ No _____   If yes, please specify.

[Note: More questions about knowledge can be added here.]

3a. Are you currently and actively involved in tobacco control and prevention?

   Yes _____ No _____

3b. Are any of your family members currently and actively involved in tobacco control and prevention?

   Yes _____ No _____

4. Are you a member of any group concerned about tobacco control and prevention?

   Yes _____ No _____

[Note: Insert page with fact sheet.]

Please turn the page and read the fact sheet.

Post-test Questions

Now that you've finished reading the fact sheet, please answer the following questions. You may refer to the fact sheet as you consider your response.

1. In your own words, what would you say is the purpose of the [sponsoring organization]'s tobacco control program?

[Note: Additional questions about knowledge can be added here.]

2. How much of the information in the fact sheet was new to you?

    Most _____ Some _____ None _____

3. Do you have questions about the [sponsoring organization]'s tobacco control program that weren't answered in the fact sheet?

    Yes _____ No _____

    If yes, please list: _____

4. Was there anything you particularly liked about the fact sheet?

    Yes _____ No _____

    If yes, what? _____

5. Was there anything you particularly disliked or found confusing about the fact sheet?

    Yes _____ No _____

    If yes, what? _____

6. This fact sheet is most appropriate for (check all that apply):

    General Public _____

    College Graduates _____

    Health Professionals _____

    Policy Makers _____

    Educators _____

    Youth _____

    Specific Populations (please list) _____

    Other (please list) _____

7. Would you recommend the fact sheet to a friend or family member?

    Yes_____ No_____

    Why or why not?

8. The following phrases describe the fact sheet. Please circle the one choice on each line that most closely reflects your opinion.

a. Very interesting	Somewhat interesting	Not at all interesting
b. Very informative	Somewhat informative	Not informative
c. Very accurate	Partially accurate	Inaccurate
d. Very clear	Somewhat clear	Confusing
e. Very useful	Somewhat useful	Not useful
f. Unbiased	Biased toward the tobacco industry	Biased toward smoker
g. Easy to read	Understandable	Hard to understand
h. Complete	Somewhat complete	Incomplete

9. Would you like to say anything else about the fact sheet? Please comment:

_____

_____

_____

_____

Thank you very much for your help in reviewing this fact sheet.

    Please return this sheet by _____ (date) to:

    [name]

    [fax #]

    [e-mail]

    If you have any questions, please contact:

    [name]

    [phone #]

    [e-mail]

Appendix 3.6: Sample Intercept Interview Questionnaire

Respondent number: _____

(Instructions for interviewer are in italics.)

Good morning/afternoon. My name is _____. Thank you for agreeing to take part in this research. I am now going to show you a short video recording. When it has finished, I will ask you some questions about what you have just seen.

(Play video of all five ads.)

1. Thinking of the video you've just seen overall, which advertisement did you like the most?

    Ad A   ❏ 1

    Ad B   ❏ 2

    Ad C   ❏ 3

    Ad D   ❏ 4

    Ad E   ❏ 5

    None   ❏ 6

1a. And why do you say that?

_____

_____

_____

_____

2. And thinking of the video you've just seen overall, which ad did you like the least?

    Ad A   ❑ 1

    Ad B   ❑ 2

    Ad C   ❑ 3

    Ad D   ❑ 4

    Ad E   ❑ 5

    None   ❑ 6

2a. And why do you say that?

_____

_____

_____

_____

(Show only test ad again.)

3. Now thinking specifically about this ad, could you tell me what you think the main message of this ad is?

_____

_____

_____

4. Again for this ad, could you tell me what you think its other messages are? Anything else?

_____

_____

_____

5. What is there that you like about this advertisement? And what else? Is there anything else at all you like about this advertisement?

_____

_____

_____

_____

6. What is there that you dislike about this advertisement? And what else? Is there anything else at all you dislike about this advertisement?

_____

_____

_____

_____

7. I'm going to read out a number of statements about the advertisement that you just viewed. For each statement I'd like to know to what extent you agree or disagree with it, using the scale on this card.

(Show card A on with scale responses.)

	Strongly Agree	Slightly Agree	Neither Agree nor Disagree	Slightly Disagree	Strongly Disagree	Don't Know
a) This advertisement has a convincing message	❑1	❑2	❑3	❑4	❑5	❑6
b) This is an attention-grabbing advertisement	❑1	❑2	❑3	❑4	❑5	❑6
c) The message of this advertisement is unclear	❑1	❑2	❑3	❑4	❑5	❑6

	Strongly Agree	Slightly Agree	Neither Agree nor Disagree	Slightly Disagree	Strongly Disagree	Don't Know
d) This advertisement is similar to other stop smoking advertisements	❏ 1	❏ 2	❏ 3	❏ 4	❏ 5	❏ 6
e) This advertisement has a persuasive message	❏ 1	❏ 2	❏ 3	❏ 4	❏ 5	❏ 6
f) This advertisement is boring	❏ 1	❏ 2	❏ 3	❏ 4	❏ 5	❏ 6

8. Can you tell me your overall opinion of this advertisement? *(Read options.)*

    Excellent   ❏ 1

    Very Good   ❏ 2

    Good   ❏ 3

    Fair   ❏ 4

    Poor   ❏ 5

9. If the ad provided a toll-free phone number, do you think you would call that number?

    Yes   ❏ 1

    No   ❏ 2

10. Overall, would this advertisement persuade you to try to quit smoking?

    Yes   ❏ 1   *(Ask question 11, then go to question 13.)*

    No   ❏ 2   *(Ask question 11, then go to question 12.)*

11. Why do you say that?

_____

_____

_____

12. *(Only ask this question if respondent answered "no" to question 10.)* What would you change about the advertisement to make it more persuasive for you to quit smoking?

_____

_____

_____

13. Have you ever tried to stop smoking before?

    Yes   ❏ 1   *(Go to question 14.)*

    No   ❏ 2   *(Go to demographics questions.)*

14. How long ago did you last try to stop smoking?

Within last 3 months	❏ 1
Over 3 months to less than 6 months	❏ 2
Over 6 months to less than 1 year	❏ 3
Over 1 year to less than 2 years	❏ 4
Over 2 years to less than 3 years	❏ 5
Over 3 years ago	❏ 6
Don't know / Can't remember	❏ 7

15. What was your main reason for trying to quit smoking on this previous occasion?

  New Year's resolution   ❑ 1

  Health reasons   ❑ 2

  Pregnancy   ❑ 3

  On medical advice   ❑ 4

  Wanted to improve fitness   ❑ 5

  To save money/couldn't afford it   ❑ 6

  Request from friend/member of family   ❑ 7

  Thought I could kick the habit   ❑ 8

Other (please specify)   ❑ 9

_____

_____

_____

Finally, these are questions for statistical purposes only.

A. In which age group do you fit?

(Show card B with age categories listed.)

  25–29   ❑ 1

  30–34   ❑ 2

  35–39   ❑ 3

  40–44   ❑ 4

  45–49   ❑ 5

B. How many people are there in your household, including yourself and children?

One	❑ 1
Two	❑ 2
Three	❑ 3
Four	❑ 4
Five	❑ 5
Six	❑ 6
Seven and above	❑ 7

C. How many children under age 16 live in your household?

None	❑ 1	*(Go to question 'E')*
One	❑ 2	
Two	❑ 3	
Three	❑ 4	
Four	❑ 5	
Five	❑ 6	
Six	❑ 7	
Seven and above	❑ 8	

D. And what are their ages?

Under 3 years	❑ 1
3 to 5 years	❑ 2
6 to 8 years	❑ 3
9 to 11 years	❑ 4
12 to 15 years	❑ 5

E. What is your employment status?

Employed full-time	❏ 1
Employed part-time	❏ 2
Self-employed	❏ 3
Student	❏ 4
Homemaker	❏ 5
Not employed	❏ 6

F. What is the highest level of education of the primary wage earner?

Primary school/none	❏ 1
Secondary school	❏ 2
High school	❏ 3
College graduate	❏ 4
Postgraduate degree	❏ 5

Thank you very much for taking part in the survey.

(Give respondent incentive.)

Appendix 5.1: Examples of Inputs, Activities, Outputs, and Outcomes for Counter-Marketing Programs

Inputs	Activities	Outputs	Short-Term Outcomes	Intermediate Outcomes	Long-Term Outcomes
Advertising					
• Funds for paid media • Advertising contractor • Advertising specialist on staff	• Conduct situational analysis to select audiences • Develop a media plan • Conduct formative research to understand audiences • Design new ads or select existing ads and pretest	Target audience is exposed to counter-marketing message via: • Spots aired on TV and radio • Posters placed in stores and on buses	Target audience is aware of ads, recalls specific messages, and has a positive reaction to the ads	Target audience has changed attitudes, beliefs, behavioral intentions or intermediate behaviors. For example: • More parents believe secondhand smoke is harmful • More adults join smoking cessation programs	Target audience has changed behavior. For example: • Fewer youth start smoking • Cessation rates are higher • Prevalence of tobacco use is reduced
Public Relations (PR)					
• PR specialist on staff • PR contractor • Health department spokespeople	• Identify stakeholders • Develop overall plan • Generate story ideas and articles • Plan and conduct press conferences • Contact media outlets • Develop and distribute newsletter • Provide spokesperson training to health department staff	Target audiences are exposed to message via: • Scheduled press conferences • Articles in newspapers • Coverage on TV news • Distribution of newsletter	Target population is aware of and understands message of stories	Target population has changed attitudes, beliefs, behavioral intentions, and intermediate behaviors. For example: • More adults join cessation programs • More smokers believe the tobacco companies engineer cigarettes to make them more addictive	Target population has changed behavior. For example: • Cessation rates are higher • Prevalence of tobacco use is reduced

Appendix 5.1: Examples of Inputs, Activities, Outputs, and Outcomes for Counter-Marketing Programs (cont.)

Inputs	Activities	Outputs	Short-Term Outcomes	Intermediate Outcomes	Long-Term Outcomes
Media Advocacy					
• Marketing staff time • Grants to community-based organizations • Funds for community coalitions	• Establish local and regional coalitions to work on adapting policies for smokefree environments • Develop plan for advocacy work • Develop news releases, stories, and strategy for pitching from policy perspective • Conduct meetings with policy makers to educate them about hazardous effects of secondhand smoke exposure and benefits of smoke-free policies • Provide spokesperson training to community members	Policy makers and restaurant and business owners are exposed to messages (e.g., hazards of secondhand smoke and the role of smokefree policies in reducing exposure) via: • News releases • Stories • Meetings	Policy makers and restaurant and business owners become more aware of the hazardous effects of secondhand smoke exposure	Policy makers and restaurant and business owners change their attitudes, beliefs, and intermediate behaviors about smokefree policies: • More policy makers and restaurant and business owners believe that secondhand smoke kills • More restaurant owners believe business would not be hurt as a result of clean indoor air policy. • Restaurant owners voluntarily adopt smokefree policies • Policy makers enact smokefree policies	Exposure to secondhand smoke is reduced

Continues

Appendix 5.1: Examples of Inputs, Activities, Outputs, and Outcomes for Counter-Marketing Programs (cont.)

Inputs	Activities	Outputs	Short-Term Outcomes	Intermediate Outcomes	Long-Term Outcomes
Grassroots Marketing					
• Marketing staff time • Funds for contests, events, and activities • Existing and available materials	• Identify whom to involve at low, medium, and high levels of engagement • Prepare brief to keep participants on strategy • Create means of communication (e.g., Web site or e-mail distribution list) for advocates • Build partnerships with key organizations • Organize college youth to collect data on advertising in stores	Targeted partners are exposed through credible interpersonal channels: • On-campus distribution of leaflets giving study results • Youth who attend concerts sponsored by tobacco industry are exposed to "truth" campaign's "Truth Truck" • Local physicians receive related messages via professional group's newsletter	Exposed youth and physicians have increased awareness of tobacco-related issues	• Youth have improved attitudes, beliefs, and intermediate behaviors (e.g., engaged youth convey message about industry's deceptive practices to others) • Physicians talk to smokers about quitting and refer them to cessation programs • More smokers join cessation programs	Target population has changed behavior. For example: • Fewer youth start smoking • Rates of successful smoking cessation are higher • Prevalence of smoking is reduced

Appendix 5.1: Examples of Inputs, Activities, Outputs, and Outcomes for Counter-Marketing Programs (cont.)

Inputs	Activities	Outputs	Short-Term Outcomes	Intermediate Outcomes	Long-Term Outcomes
Media Literacy					
• Marketing staff time • Grant funding for workshops • Existing and available materials	• Agree to hold workshops and deliver curricula • Hold workshops and presentations at sites other than schools • Offer curricula in schools	• Middle school and high school youth participate in media literacy curriculum • Youth groups participate in workshops and presentations • Adults are exposed to video presentation on secrets of tobacco advertising • Curriculum is implemented according to design	Program participants become aware of the role of media and the importance of managing and interpreting that role	Program participants develop critical viewing skills and ability to produce tobacco control messages through different forms of media. For example: • Persons who received messages of media literacy program produce tobacco control messages using different forms of media • Persons who received messages of media literacy program become involved in tobacco control campaign	• Fewer youth start smoking • Prevalence of smoking is reduced

Appendix 5.2: Key Data Collection Tools and Methods

Method	Description	Evaluation Uses and Other Consideration
Media tracking and content analysis	Systematic monitoring of the various media channels (e.g., print, radio, TV, outdoor) to identify ads, editorials, and articles relevant to the campaign and to assess messages in these ads, editorials, and articles (often with use of a professional tracking service)	• Can be used to monitor media efforts, both earned and paid, to assess quantity and quality of messages • Can be combined with data on the reach of various channels to estimate potential exposure of audience, overall and by demographics • Content analysis can be used to determine what messages are disseminated to the target audience, if those messages are on strategy, and if the messages have changed since the campaign began • Can be used to track changes in messages to determine whether they are on target and consistent with the marketing plan • Can be used to modify the media plan
Tracking requests for information	Systematic recording of the number and type of people who request information (e.g., call the quitline, visit the Web site)	• Can be used to assess the effectiveness of counter-marketing efforts that list the Web site or quitline as a source of additional information • Can be used to track simple counts of number of requests over time, to show correlation with counter-marketing efforts • Requires more effort to determine the characteristics of the population reached
Logs of events and activities	Completion of a form by the organizer of an event or activity, to describe the type of activity, where the activity happened, the number of participants, the type of participants, and comments about the event	• Can be used for rapid tracking of program activities and outputs (e.g., workshops, press conferences, summits, and community forums) for process evaluation • Can be easily entered into database, to produce summaries of activities over time and by type • Can only provide estimates of the number of participants reached and general categorization of those participants (e.g., log sheets for press events may show TV reporters vs. print reporters) • Counting of participants facilitated by sign-up sheet • Can used to determine whether program implementation is following plan

Appendix 5.2: Key Data Collection Tools and Methods (cont.)

Method	Description	Evaluation Uses and Other Consideration
Review of existing data and records	Structured analysis of information being collected for other purposes, usually on a regular basis	• Is an inexpensive source of data • Data produced may not be relevant • Requires thought and knowledge of local systems to locate relevant data
Focus group discussions	Qualitative method in which a skilled moderator uses an interview guide with open-ended questions to facilitate a 1- to 2-hour discussion among 5 to 10 participants	• Is more useful for formative evaluation than for process or outcome evaluation • Can be used diagnostically in conjunction with quantitative data to understand results • Can facilitate interaction among group members that elicits in-depth responses • Provides richer data about meanings and reactions than closed-ended questions • Can be observed, recorded, or both, to facilitate analysis • Requires a skilled moderator who understands how to manage the group process, so necessary information is collected • Can result in domination of discussion by vocal individuals • Results in findings that can't be generalized and may be biased by the unique characteristics of participants
Document analysis	Systematic assessment of the content of documents	• Can be useful if the program is expected to result in changes in documents such as local ordinances • Can be used to determine whether ordinances and policies have shifted in the desired direction
In-depth individual interviews	Qualitative data collection with a semistructured interview guide in which a limited number of respondents are asked questions (often open-ended) by a skilled interviewer	• Can be used to assess reactions to specific counter-marketing efforts • Is particularly useful to assess reactions of specific individuals (e.g., stakeholders, members of the press, station managers, and heads of key organizations) • Can be used to modify the program • Can use observation or recording of information to facilitate analysis • Requires a skilled interviewer who is knowledgeable about the reason for the interview and how the responses might be used to improve the program

Continues

Appendix 5.2: Key Data Collection Tools and Methods (cont.)

Method	Description	Evaluation Uses and Other Consideration
Participant feedback survey	Survey administered to participants in a counter-marketing event, to obtain feedback about the event	• Can be used as a simple method to describe the size and characteristics of the population reached by an event • Can be used to assess the reaction of the target population to the event • Provides insight into approaches to improve the content of and recruitment for the event • Is more useful for process evaluation than for outcome evaluation
Population-based survey	Survey of a population that follows strict sampling rules, so findings are representative of that population; administered by interviewer or self-administered	• Is likely to be used in some form to evaluate advertising efforts • Can indicate the percentage of the state population reached by counter-marketing efforts • Can be used to determine whether persons aware of the advertising or other counter-marketing efforts have improved beliefs, attitudes, and behaviors • Can be repeated at regular intervals to track changes
Random digit dialing (RDD)	Population-based survey using special telephone-dialing procedures to reach a probability sample of the state population; computer-assisted telephone interviewing is a common type of RDD	• Provides efficient, cost-effective means of generating a probability sample that can be generalized to the target population • Must use special sampling procedures to obtain sufficient samples of some populations (e.g., youth, ethnic/racial minority groups, and smokers) • See population-based survey in this table
Observation	Observation of persons in public settings or observation of physical settings, with minimal observer interaction	• In some cases, can be used to directly assess program implementation and behavior and reactions of target audience • Can also be used to determine the quantity and content of tobacco advertising, counter-advertising and promotion in physical settings • Is labor intensive and requires visits to the sites of the program and skilled observers trained to use tested protocols • May result in bias, if behaviors are influenced by the presence of the observer • May result in questioning of the ethics of observing people without their consent

Appendix 5.3: Key Variables and Sample Items To Consider Including in Survey of Target Population

Category	Variable	Sample Item
Awareness	Unaided	Describe anything you recall from recent advertising against smoking that you have seen.
	Aided	Have you recently seen an antismoking ad that shows two young men in a van who drive up to an office building and talk to a uniformed guard?
	Confirmed awareness	Can you provide more detailed information about what occurred in the ad?
	Unaided awareness of campaign or slogan	Are you aware of any antismoking campaigns now taking place in this state? What is the theme or slogan of this campaign?
Recall	Recall of ad	What happens in the ad? (List of closed-ended ad descriptions is not read, but is included for the interviewer to code responses)
	Recall of message	What do you think the main message of the ad is? (List of closed-ended ad messages is not read, but is included for the interviewer to code responses)
Reactions	Diagnostic measures	For each of the following statements, please tell me how much you agree or disagree with the statement. Do you strongly agree, agree, neither agree nor disagree, disagree, or strongly disagree? The ad was memorable. I liked the ad. The ad was believable. The ad was relevant to me. I talked with my friends about the ad.
	Open-ended measures	What specifically did you like about the ad? What did you dislike about the ad? What, if anything, was confusing about the ad? Who, if anyone, would be offended by the ad?
	Reaction to workshops and events	What specifically did you like about the workshop? What did you dislike about the workshop? Would you recommend the workshop to a friend?

Continues

Appendix 5.3: Key Variables and Sample Items To Consider Including in Survey of Target Population (cont.)

Category	Variable	Sample Item
Attitudes	Attitude toward trying cigarettes	Trying just a few cigarettes won't hurt anyone. (For all items the following response scale can be used: strongly agree, agree, disagree, strongly disagree, or no opinion.)
	Attitude toward smoking	Young people who smoke are usually "cooler" than those who don't.
	Attitude toward quitting	I can quit smoking any time I choose.
	Support for bans	Smoking in the workplace should be banned.
Beliefs	Beliefs about consequences of smoking	For each of the following statements, please tell me how much you agree or disagree with the statement. Do you strongly agree, agree, neither agree nor disagree, disagree, or strongly disagree? My smoking in the next 3 months will help me fit in. My smoking in the next 3 months is harmful to my health. My smoking in the next 3 months will make my breath smell bad. Smoking has nothing to do with whether a person is cool. Smoking causes heart disease . . . lung cancer . . . blocked arteries.
	Beliefs about the tobacco industry	For each of the following statements, please tell me how much you agree or disagree with the statement. Do you strongly agree, agree, neither agree nor disagree, disagree, or strongly disagree? Tobacco companies try to get young people to smoke because older people quit smoking or die. Tobacco companies use advertising to fool young people. If people my age knew we were being used by tobacco companies just to make money, we would never start smoking. Most people my age don't believe all the bad things we hear about tobacco companies.
	Beliefs about secondhand smoke	For each of the following statements, please tell me how much you agree or disagree with the statement. Do you strongly agree, agree, neither agree nor disagree, disagree, or strongly disagree? Secondhand smoke causes lung cancer. Secondhand smoke is an extremely important public health issue.

Appendix 5.3: Key Variables and Sample Items To Consider Including in Survey of Target Population (cont.)

Category	Variable	Sample Item
Normative beliefs	Perceptions of friends' use	How many of your close friends do you think smoke? Does your best friend smoke?
	Perception of others' use of cigarettes	How many sixth graders at this school do you think smoke cigarettes?
	Normative belief from friends	Do you strongly agree, agree, neither agree nor disagree, disagree, or strongly disagree with the following statement? My close friends think it's OK for me to smoke.
	Normative belief from parents	Do you strongly agree, agree, neither agree nor disagree, disagree, or strongly disagree with the following statement? My parents think it's OK for me to smoke.
	General normative belief	Do you strongly agree, agree, neither agree nor disagree, disagree, or strongly disagree with the following statement? Most people who are important to me think it's OK for me to smoke.
Self-efficacy	Confidence to refuse an offer	How easy or hard would it be for you to say "no" to the offer of a cigarette when you are at a party with friends? …when you are at a close friend's house and their parents are not at home? Would you say it would be very easy, easy, neither easy nor hard, hard, or very hard?
	Confidence to quit smoking	How easy or hard would it be for you to quit smoking in the next 30 days? Would you say it would be very easy, easy, neither easy nor hard, hard, or very hard?
Intention	Intention to try	Do you think that you'll try a cigarette in the next 30 days?
	Intention to refuse an offer	How likely is it that you'll refuse a cigarette the next time you're offered one? Would you say it's very likely, likely, neither likely nor unlikely, unlikely, or very unlikely?
	Intention to quit smoking	Are you planning to quit smoking in the next 30 days? How many times in the past 30 days have you thought about quitting smoking?
	Intention to avoid secondhand smoke	Would you eat at restaurants more often, as often, or less often if smoking were banned?

Continues

Appendix 5.3: Key Variables and Sample Items To Consider Including in Survey of Target Population (cont.)

Category	Variable	Sample Item
Susceptibility	Susceptibility	How many of your four best friends smoke cigarettes? (If the responses is 1 or more, respondent can be categorized as "susceptible"; if the response is "none," respondent can be categorized as "nonsusceptible")
Behavior	Initiation of smoking cigarettes	Have you ever tried cigarette smoking, even one or two puffs? (If response is "no," respondent can be categorized as "non-smoker")
	Initiation of using smokeless tobacco	Have you ever used chewing tobacco, snuff, or dip, such as Redman, Levi Garrett, Beechnut, Skoal, Skoal Bandits, or Copenhagen? (If response is "no," respondent can be categorized as "non-user of smokeless tobacco")
	Initiation of cigar smoking	Have you ever tried smoking cigars, cigarillos, or little cigars, even one or two puffs? (If response is "no," respondent can be categorized as "non-smoker")
	Never smoked, current smoker, or former smoker	Have you ever tried cigarette smoking, even one or two puffs? (If response is "no," respondent can be categorized as "non-smoker")
		Do you smoke cigarettes every day, some days, or not at all? (If response is "every day" or "some days," respondent can be categorized as "current smoker")
		During the past 30 days, on how many days did you smoke cigarettes? (If response is 1 or more days, respondent can be categorized as "current smoker")
		Have you smoked at least 100 cigarettes in your lifetime? (If response is "yes," ask next question)
		Do you smoke cigarettes every day, some days, or not at all? (If response is "not at all," respondent can be categorized as "former smoker")

Appendix 5.3: Key Variables and Sample Items To Consider Including in Survey of Target Population (cont.)

Category	Variable	Sample Item
Behavior (cont.)	No use, situational use, or established use	During the past 30 days, on the days you smoked, how many cigarettes did you smoke per day?
		(If response is "none," respondent can be categorized as "no use")
		During the past 30 days, on how many days did you smoke cigarettes?
		During the past 30 days, on the days you smoked, how many cigarettes did you smoke per day?
		(If response to first question is 6 days or fewer, and response to second question is 4 cigarettes per day or fewer, respondent can be categorized as "situational smoker")
		During the past 30 days, on how many days did you smoke cigarettes?
		During the past 30 days, on the days you smoked, how many cigarettes did you smoke per day?
		(If response to first question is 6 or more days, and response to second question is 5 or more cigarettes per day, respondent can categorized as "established smoker")
	Smoking cessation	During the past 12 months, did you ever seriously try to quit smoking cigarettes?
		How many times, if any, have you tried to quit smoking?
		When you last tried to quit, how long did you stay off cigarettes?
	Actions to avoid secondhand smoke	Have you asked an acquaintance not to smoke around you or others in the past 30 days?
		Have you asked a stranger not to smoke around you or others in the past 30 days?
		Have you avoided a smoky place in the past 30 days?
		Have you gone to a smokefree club in the past 30 days?
		If you went to a smokefree club, was part of your decision based on knowing that it was smokefree?

Appendix 6.1: Key Elements of a Request for Proposals (RFP) for a Media Campaign

Requests for Proposals (RFPs) vary significantly among states and organizations. They range in length from less than 10 pages to over a hundred pages. They also vary in terms of the elements included. The following is a list of potential elements to include in an RFP. It is not meant to be a recommendation for the structure or content of your RFP; rather, it is meant to help you in writing your RFP by providing information about elements other states have included and issues that have arisen. Your state or organization may not want to include in your RFP some of the elements listed below. Likewise, your state or organization may have additional requirements that are not addressed in this document.

General Information/Introduction

Background and Overview

What is important to know about the current situation that explains why you are issuing an RFP at this time? Did you just acquire settlement dollars? Was a tobacco tax passed whose proceeds will be going to a tobacco control program? Will a broad tobacco control program be developed at this time, or just a media/PR campaign?

Statement of Purpose/Goals/Objectives

What are you trying to achieve through the media/PR campaign? This may include a statement of work for the media campaign. If you have selected target audiences for the campaign, include those as well. Be as clear and selective as possible. The more specific you are, the more focused proposals the bidding agencies can develop. If funds are limited, you may need to focus on one goal and one or two target audiences rather than diluting your efforts by trying to influence many audiences to change behaviors.

Description of the Health Department or Program

Share relevant information about current and past tobacco control programs and describe which organizations have been involved. Describe past or existing tobacco control efforts and media campaigns. Succinctly describe what media and public relations efforts have been implemented in the past and their results, if available.

Description of Problem the Campaign Needs to Address

Share research and data specific to the state, including any important regional, demographic, or other differences.

Budget or Funding Level

Be specific about the time period for the budget, whether funds will be renewed after the first year, conditions for funding renewal, etc. If funding is uncertain, it is acceptable to include the existing conditions that have made the funding level uncertain. Also include the date when you expect to know the outcome. You may have the bidders prepare proposals at different funding levels.

Contract Period

You may want to check with your state health department's contract office to determine the types of contracts available to your program. For example, you may be able to have a contract renewable for a certain number of years, contingent upon your approval rating of the agency. Note the beginning and end dates for the contract.

Proposal Requirements

Eligibility Criteria

State who may apply for the contract. Optional requirements include the following:

- Agency based in the state. Some state government policies require hiring only in-state contractors.

- Submissions only by agencies with certain experience. For example, you may want to hire an agency with experience in one or more of the following areas: marketing, public relations, marketing research, specific ethnic group marketing, youth marketing and public education, direct marketing, new media (e.g., Internet), sports and entertainment marketing and merchandising, media buying and planning, creative development and production, grassroots organizing, crisis management, or special events.

- Annual billings within a specific range. The rationale for including this is that you might not want to hire an agency that is so small that you're concerned about it's capability to handle your account or so large that you're concerned that your account won't be so important to them.

- Lead agency may partner with other agencies that have needed experience. For example, lead agencies without ethnic marketing experience may still be considered as long as their proposals specify which ethnic marketers they would partner with.

Proposal Content and Format Requirements

- Formatting, such as white 8 1/2" x 11" paper, page numbering, limitations on number of pages, required appendices. Providing such requirements may not only make the proposals easier to read but may also help avoid the tendency of advertising and PR agencies to "out-glitz" each other by using the most creative, original formats for their proposals.

- Inclusion of specific elements and organization into specific content sections. For example, required elements might include a standard cover sheet with signature, table of contents, proposal narrative, narrative responses to questionnaire, proposed budget in standard format, work plan or action plan, nondiscrimination compliance statement, drug-free workplace certificate, etc.

- Examples of desired formats for proposal pages or appendices.

Potential or Perceived Conflict of Interest

All applicants should be required to provide a statement of disclosure regarding potential or perceived conflict of interest due to connection with the tobacco industry, and you should provide the standard format for this statement. Potential or perceived conflict of interest could include affiliation or contractual relationships, direct or indirect, with tobacco companies, owners, affiliates, subsidiaries, holding companies, or companies involved in any way in the production, processing, distribution, promotion, sale, or use of tobacco. You may choose to state in the RFP any of the following:

- Only agencies with no such affiliation within some time frame (e.g., the past five years) are allowed to apply.

- Any tobacco company affiliation disqualifies an agency from competing for the contract.

- An agency must divest itself of such affiliation prior to bidding and must submit with its bid written documentation of such divestment.

- Such affiliation doesn't necessarily disqualify agencies, but disclosure of real or apparent conflict of interest is required in the proposal.

In addition, you may require a written statement that the selected agency will not accept such relationships during the term of contract with the health department.

Applicant Questionnaire

You may ask each applicant to answer questions regarding the agency, including areas such as the following:

- Agency mission and philosophy

- List of key agency staff and agency offices

- Description of departments and staff positions within the agency

- Organizational chart

- Names of other agencies, subcontractors, and consultants to be included in submission

- Number years in business

- Annual billings

- Experience with government, nonprofit, or health-related accounts

- Antidiscrimination policy

- Past pro bono work and contacts for references

- List of top accounts (typically based on billings) and contacts for references

- Examples of accounts that demonstrate the agency's experience in changing behavior on social or public health issue (including key results)

- Information about how the agency uses research in developing, executing, and evaluating campaigns

You may ask for a narrative about how the agency plans to provide the required services. This may include more specific information about the particular agency staff who will be working on this account (e.g., titles, functions, education, experience, accounts handled at current agency, accounts handled at previous employer, level of responsibility). You may also ask about discounts, bonuses, or pro bono work the agency will offer.

Compensation

You may ask bidding agencies to recommend how they should be compensated for their work on the campaign. This will help you understand how they typically charge clients and may highlight to you some innovative approaches to compensation. In addition, you may ask for a proposal for a performance-based contract or the agency position on performance-based contracts. A performance-based contract makes the agency more accountable for bottom line outcomes of campaign; one caveat is to make sure that your expectations are realistic regarding what the potential outcomes will be. Remember that the compensation proposal is only a starting point for contract negotiations. You may choose another compensation arrangement when you negotiate the final contract with the selected agency.

Examples of Work

You may ask for examples of creative executions, especially those most relevant to the current proposal, such as materials targeted toward teens if the proposal is for a youth antitobacco campaign, materials targeted toward Hispanics/Latinos if the proposal includes a Hispanic/Latinos component, etc. Examples of materials would normally be submitted in one or more of the following forms: videotape with TV and radio ads, photos of outdoor ads, copies of print ads, examples of brochures or other educational materials, and hard copies of Web pages. You may also ask for other materials or information related to the individual campaigns (e.g., campaign results, summaries of research, target audience development, campaign strategy from one completed campaign, PR plan, samples of press materials, media plan, event plan).

Ideas for Addressing Your Campaign's Goals

Requesting the bidding agencies' ideas about approaches to your campaign will help you gauge the level of strategic and creative thinking that they can bring to your program. The description of the agency's proposed approach to addressing your campaign's goals might include information on their understanding of the problem; strategic thinking about how to address the problem; identification of target populations(s); campaign strategies and action plans; description of media buying plans and strategy; PR strategy, including media coverage, promotional events, and integration with local programs and target population(s); links to existing tobacco control efforts; how research and evaluation would be conducted; general estimate of how funds would be allocated; use of existing resources and materials (e.g., CDC's Media Campaign Resource Center, state clearinghouses); and input from external experts.

It is not recommended that you ask the bidding agencies to develop and present new creative ideas or specific advertising executions. Creative development is very time-consuming and can only be done well when agencies have full knowledge about the issue and are fully immersed in the campaign development. If you do request or allow for new creative ideas to be presented, you will want to include a statement that the health department has ownership of ideas or adaptations of ideas contained in any proposal submitted, as well as the right to copyright them.

Proposal Preparation and Submission

Schedule/Timeline
Provide information about bidder's conference and any other pertinent dates.

Application Deadlines
Include date/time of deadlines for letter of intent (confirming intent to submit full proposal) and complete proposal package.

Key Contact Information at Health Department
Provide contact information for key health department staff that may be contacted regarding the RFP process. Include instructions for how to submit questions.

Instructions for How To Submit Application
Include date and time that application is due, address where applications should be sent, and whether faxed applications will be accepted. List the number of copies of the application required. Typically, agencies are asked to submit multiple copies so that the health department does not have to make copies of the proposals for the reviewers.

Instructions for How To Withdraw Application

Provide information about how an agency can withdraw an application after it has been submitted.

Reasons for Disqualification

Possible reasons for disqualifying an application include the following:

- Incomplete or late submission
- Failure to meet requirements regarding lack of tobacco industry affiliation
- Attempts to influence a member of review panel during the review process
- Submitting application with false, inaccurate, or misleading statements
- Unwillingness or inability to fully comply with proposed contract provisions

Proposal Review/Evaluation/Selection

Criteria for Evaluation of Proposal

Proposals may be evaluated based on factors relating to the agency and staff (agency background, agency capabilities and experience, agency personnel, capabilities and experience of subcontractors), materials submitted (samples of work, strategic plan for campaign, proposed media strategies and plans, proposed budget and timeline), or quality of the proposal (clarity, creativity, innovation, quality, balance). You may choose to include in the RFP a point structure identifying the maximum number of points each section of the proposal can be awarded. You may choose to require oral presentations by some or all applicants.

Information Regarding Review of Proposals

List the stages of review process, whether the review sessions will be open sessions or closed to the public.

Award Notification and Contract Negotiation

Provide information about how (e.g., e-mail, fax) and approximately when applicants will be notified about results. You may choose to not send the final notification stating that an applicant has not been selected until after a contract is signed with the agency that is selected during the review process. If you are not able to agree on contract terms with the selected agency, then you may begin negotiating with the second choice.

Other Rules/Information/Disclaimers

Your state may choose to include some, none, or all of these stipulations:

- The health department reserves the right to negotiate and clarify before entering into contract.

- The health department reserves the right to amend the RFP prior to the proposal submission date. Applicants who have submitted a letter of intent by the required date shall be notified of amendments and will be afforded an opportunity to revise their proposal to accommodate the RFP amendment.

- In the event that the health department is unable to execute a contract with the agency selected, the health department reserves the right to continue evaluations of other agencies and select another agency.

- The RFP does not constitute commitment by the health department to award a contract.

- Deliverables and other materials provided by contractor to the health department become the property of the health department.

- A schedule of regular meetings between the agency and the health department will be required.

- Reasons for termination of contract may be listed in the RFP.

- The health department reserves the right to remove or replace subcontractors.

- The health department assumes no responsibility or liability for costs incurred by bidders prior to contract award.

- Confidentiality policies vary by state law. Some state health departments will not release information to bidders or anyone else regarding the content of any of the applications during the RFP process (or at any time). Other states require an open review process, proposals becoming public information at the end of review process, or both.

- Some states have subcontracting policies or requirements.

- Some states have affirmative action requirements.

Optional/Possible Appendices

Your state may choose to include some, none, or all of these appendices.

- Applicant Information Sheet. This might include information such as agency name and address, tax identification number, name of main contact at agency, and signed affirmation that statements contained in application package are true and complete.

- Checklist for Responding to RFP. This would clarify what key elements must be included in proposal.

- Proposal Evaluation Instrument or Evaluation Summary Sheet. This is the evaluation form used by reviewers to assess proposals.

- Standard contracts agreements/forms. Some states have specific language required in all contract agreements or forms used in all contracts.

- State contract terms and conditions (e.g., taxes, warranties, payments, indemnity, liability, insurance, termination, records maintenance, severability).

- Signature Verification Form. This would serve as notarized proof that the individual signing is authorized to execute contracts on behalf of bidder or contractor.

- Consultant/contractor submissions form/contractor data and certification form (might include information such as contractor name and address, tax identification number or social security number, contact information, and resume or statement of qualifications of key personnel).

- Reference Review Form

- Sample health department tobacco control program budget

- Conflict of Interest Statement/Statement of Disclosure of Tobacco Industry Affiliation/Statement of Assurance

- Certificate of Independent Price Determination. With this form, the bidder certifies that the prices in the proposal have been arrived at independently without consultation, communication, or agreement with any other bidder, and that the prices in the proposal have not been and will not be disclosed by the bidder, directly or indirectly, to any other bidder before bid opening or contract award unless otherwise required by law.

- Outline of proposal format

- Outline of line item project budget form

- Errata, amendments, addenda

- Instructions for oral presentations

- Q&As

Appendix 6.2: Questions and Answers on RFPs

Issues Related to RFP Process

1. How much time should the RFP process take? How much time should be allowed for each step in the process?

Each state has different rules and schedules for the RFP (Request for Proposals) process, based on variables such as state restrictions and the state funding cycle. Thus, there is no golden rule, but there are some general considerations. The key is to allow sufficient time in each step to accomplish the work required, while not delaying unnecessarily the hiring of an agency. The entire process generally takes from six weeks to three months, but much more time can be required if contract negotiations are difficult or if a bidding agency contests the award decision.

Here's a general outline of the steps involved and the approximate time needed for each step:

- **Release of RFP.** The RFP should be released as soon as possible, so an agency can be hired in a timely manner.

- **Deadline for Submission of Proposals.** In general, four to six weeks is sufficient time for the agencies to put together proposals.

- **Bidders' Conference.** The bidders' conference is a meeting held so possible applicants can obtain information they need to respond to the RFP. Enough time should be allowed to publicize the RFP and disseminate the information about this meeting to the potential bidders. The bidders' conference should be held about midway in the four- to six-week period between the release of the RFP and the proposal deadline. This schedule gives agencies sufficient time after the bidders' conference to determine whether they are still interested in submitting a proposal and, if so, to develop the proposal.

- **Technical Review of Proposals.** The technical review is conducted to ensure that the agencies making proposals meet the criteria specified in the RFP and don't need to be disqualified for any reason. This review should take place immediately after the proposals are due. Completion of the technical review by the appropriate state staff generally requires one to three days, depending on the number of proposals and the complexity of the technical requirements.

- **Review of Written Proposals.** The process for review of written proposals determines the amount of time needed to complete this review. To ensure that all reviewers are able to attend, the dates for the review of written proposals should be set well in advance.

    If the review committee reads proposals in a room together, the review of written proposals can begin immediately after the technical review and usually lasts one to four days. The amount of time necessary to read, discuss, and score the proposals depends on the number of proposals and the length of the proposals.

If the proposals are sent to the review committee to read before the committee convenes, the time required is approximately one to two weeks, including one to two days to discuss and score the proposals at the meeting.

- **Oral Presentations.** Agencies that remain in the process after the technical review and the review of written proposals are given an opportunity to make oral presentations. At least two weeks should be allowed for preparation of these presentations. These presentations might include a review of creative products from previous campaigns.

- **Final Selection of an Agency.** The final selection of the winning agency may be made after the oral presentations, on the basis of the scores calculated by the review committee. Some states require final approval by a state health department or a state contract officer. This requirement can add several days to the RFP process.

- **Signing of the Contract.** The time elapsing before the contract is signed can vary from one week to more than one month, depending on factors that include the following:

    – How much specific information about requirements (e.g., compensation and scope of work) is laid out in the RFP

    – How much negotiation with the winning agency is necessary

    – Whether the decision is contested by one of the agencies that isn't selected

    – How many levels of approval are necessary before a contract is made final.

It's advisable to wait to notify agencies that they haven't been selected for further consideration until a final contract is signed and not contested. This approach allows you to consider the second or third choices in case a problem occurs with the top choice among the agencies.

2. Should a bidders' conference be held?

Benefits of a bidders' conference include the following:

- Answers to questions can be provided at one time to all the potential applicants present.

- A transcript of the conference or a summary of the answers can be put online.

- The program manager sees the people and agencies that may be bidding and can estimate how many agencies will bid on the contract.

The greatest potential negative is the time and energy involved in setting up such a conference. You'll want the key health department staff involved in the RFP and the contracting process to be present, so scheduling a time when all are available may be difficult. In addition, you might not have all the answers to questions posed to you at the bidders' conference and you'll then have to follow up later. This problem can be avoided by asking that all questions be submitted in writing in advance. Then you can provide answers in person at the bidders, conference since you will have had time to prepare answers to questions submitted.

An alternative to a bidders' conference is to have all questions submitted in writing and provide answers online. You can announce the Web address in the RFP and make it clear that bidders can access the Web site to find updates and corrections to the RFP and answers to submitted questions.

3. How should information be disseminated to potential bidders?

Most states put the full RFP, along with information such as edits and updates to the RFP and answers to the bidders' questions, on the contracts section of the state health department Web site. When there is a high level of publicity around spending of funds for the state tobacco control program, many agencies interested in this work will be aware that an RFP is being released. Some states send a copy of the RFP to all top agencies in the state, along with a cover letter inviting them to apply. In addition, there may be publications in the state that advertise government contracts. If your contract will be large enough and you want to attract agencies from outside the state, you might consider placing an ad in advertising industry publications such as *Advertising Age*, *Ad Week*, or *Brand Week*.

4. Should health department staff perform site visits to the agencies that are bidding?

Site visits allow you to see the work space and sense the tone of the environment in which the agency staff work, and these visits may help you to better understand the technical capabilities of the agency staff. Some states and organizations have found site visits to be very beneficial, but the vast majority of states don't perform site visits, and they're probably not necessary unless extenuating circumstances exist.

5. How should the written proposals be scored?

Methods for scoring the written proposals are different in each state. Some score sheets include a number of categories that correspond to the sections of the RFP. Other score sheets include sections addressing elements such as agency experience and knowledge, technical capability, previous creative, expertise in market research, experience with media campaigns targeting a particular population, and budget management. Most states set the criteria for scoring of the proposals. In some states, however, the reviewers are given the opportunity to provide input, and the final decisions on criteria for scoring rest with the health department.

6. How should the process for review of written proposals be managed?

There are several options for managing the process for review of written proposals, and states manage this process in different ways. Some states have reviewers read the proposals in advance; others have reviewers read the proposals together. Some states allow reviewers to share scores; others explicitly prohibit sharing of scores. Some states allow reviewers to change their scores after seeing all of the presentations; others do not allow such changes. You may have some flexibility in making these decisions, but some of the decisions will be mandated by state policy. Here are some methods states use to manage the review of written proposals, along with related benefits and drawbacks for each method:

- Reviewers read proposals before meeting to discuss the proposals.

    - **Benefits.** If reviewers read the proposals before meeting, the discussion moves more quickly. Reviewers can read the proposals on their own schedule. They may be able to pay more attention to the details when they read alone than when they read in a group.

    - **Drawbacks.** Reviewers may forget the specifics of the proposals between the time they read them and the time of the meeting where the group scoring is done. Also, a large volume of proposals must be shipped or hand delivered to each reviewer. Reviewers must then bring the materials with them to the review session. In addition, some reviewers may not take the time to review the proposals before the review session. If there are a lot of proposals, review committee members may not have the time to thoroughly read each proposal. In that case, you can assign, in advance, one review committee member to report on each proposal to the group and have someone else be a second reporter, to add anything the first reporter missed. These two individuals would be responsible for reading the proposal most thoroughly, although others will read it, too.

- Reviewers read the proposals when they come together in one room.

    - **Benefits.** If the proposals are read at a meeting, they don't have to be shipped to reviewers in advance and brought back by the reviewers. Control and confidentiality of proposals are assured. Also, the information is fresh in the minds of the reviewers when they do the scoring.

    - **Drawbacks.** Reading in a group can be very distracting and tiring. Different reviewers read at different speeds, and the time devoted to each proposal may not be sufficient for adequate review. In addition, reading in a group takes longer than if reviewers come together after reading the proposals. It may be difficult for some review committee members to set aside such a large block of time from their busy schedules to participate in the reviews.

- Reviewers are allowed to share scores with the committee.

    - **Benefits.** One benefit of sharing scores is that it allows a reviewer to gauge his or her scoring against the scoring by other members of the review committee. The committee can assess whether the scoring method is consistent among all the reviewers and can make appropriate adjustments for equitable scoring, if necessary.

    - **Drawbacks.** One potential drawback of sharing scores is that one reviewer with strong opinions may influence others on the review committee.

- Reviewers are not allowed to share scores with the committee.
  - **Benefits.** A prohibition against sharing scores may ensure that reviewers are not influenced by scores of other reviewers. This approach may be more objective than the sharing of scores, and may be mandated by state contract policy.
  - **Drawbacks.** The main drawback of a prohibition against sharing scores is that different reviewers may use different methods to score proposals, and the review committee is not able to assess if scoring is inconsistent.
- Reviewers are allowed to change scores after reading, discussing, and scoring all the proposals.
  - **Benefits.** Regardless of whether scores are shared with the rest of the review committee, it's helpful for reviewers to be able change their scores after reviewing all the proposals. This is especially true for a reviewer who has never participated in an RFP review. After reading all the proposals, a reviewer has a better sense of the range of responses and can go back and view the first few proposals with a better perspective of what is good and bad in each of the proposals.
  - **Drawbacks.** Some reviewers may be unduly influenced by other committee members. Changing scores may add time to the process. In addition, changing scores may be prohibited by state contract policy.
- Review committee meets in person.
  - **Benefits.** The importance of selecting a contractor probably justifies the requirement for a meeting of the review committee. For most states, the media campaign contract involves a large amount of money and a significant portion of the budget for the tobacco control program. The discussion and interpersonal interaction are critical to the decision-making process.
  - **Drawbacks.** A meeting of the review committee requires that reviewers travel to a central location, which may involve time and travel expenses.

When there is no other alternative, one or more reviewers may participate in the review of written proposals by telephone. This option is rarely used and is not recommended, because of the value of having all the reviewers interact in person.

7. Should the bidding agencies be required to make oral presentations?

Oral presentations are very useful and should be required. They help to identify differences among the agencies that score well in the review of written proposals. Also, they often allow a better understanding of aspects of the agencies that don't always come across in a written proposal. These aspects include factors such as work flow and procedures, creativity and style, and technical capabilities.

8. Who should make the oral presentations for an agency?

If possible, you should require that the individuals who will be your day-to-day contacts make part or all of the oral presentation. You can ask that specific people be part of the presentation team (e.g., the financial person, the primary client contact, and the creative lead). The oral presentation is an opportunity for you to meet the individuals who will work on the account and to determine whether you have "chemistry" with them. You want to avoid being "wowed" by the agency head(s) or other trained presenters, only to find that you'll be working with lower-level staff once the agency is selected and contracted.

You can also specify a minimum and/or maximum number of people to participate in the oral presentation. Usually agencies will want to include more people, so providing a minimum is not usually an issue. Some states limit the number of agency staff making the presentation within a range of five to 10. Other states don't limit the number. You may choose to require that only the staff making the presentation be allowed to attend this RFP session, or you may allow additional agency staff to be present to answer questions.

In general, you want enough agency staff present to give you a clear picture of what the agency has to offer, but not too many whose presence is unnecessary. Depending on the site for the oral presentations, space may be a limiting factor.

9. How many agencies should be invited to make oral presentations?

Ideally, you'll want to invite a minimum of three qualified agencies to make oral presentations, to ensure that the review committee has an adequate number of agencies to review. In some cases, states have invited only two agencies to give oral presentations, because only two were qualified to move past the review of written proposals.

Also, you should set a maximum number of agencies to make presentations. It's not advisable to allow all the bidding agencies to give oral presentations, for several reasons:

- Depending on how the scoring is configured (i.e., how many points are assigned in each phase of the review and whether the scores from each phase are cumulative), it's usually not possible for an agency with a relatively low score after the review of written proposals to be a top scorer after the oral presentations.

- Reviewers will find it difficult to listen to too many presentations, especially if they know that some of the agencies have no chance of winning the contract.

- Preparation of an oral presentation requires an investment of time, money, and energy, so it's not fair to ask agencies that have no chance of winning the contract to put this level of effort into the oral presentation.

- Because you want to select an agency that does well in both written and oral communications, it's beneficial to eliminate agencies that don't submit a strong written proposal, even if they might be able to perform well in an oral presentation.

- If the written proposal is of low quality, you may not want to give the impression to the agency that you think their work was good enough to merit the invitation for an oral presentation.

10. How should the oral presentations be scored?

As with the scoring of the written proposals, the methods for scoring oral presentations are different in each state. In many states, reviewers are allowed to provide a combination of number scores and written comments. In other states, reviewers can provide only a number score, but the score sheets leave space for reviewers to make notes that help them to determine their scores. Depending on the laws and policies of the state, the score sheets may become public record. Reviewers should be notified of this policy in advance, so they are aware that anything they write will be accessible to the agencies and anyone else interested in examining the score sheets.

You'll need to determine how many points to allocate for each phase of the review. Another important decision you must make is whether the final selection should be based on a total score from all phases of review or whether the score in each phase is used only to determine which proposals move forward to the next phase. Some states assign points during the technical review; others don't score that phase but do eliminate proposals that don't qualify. In other states, the scores for the written proposals determine which agencies are invited to give an oral presentation, and the scores for the oral presentation determine which agency is offered the contract. In still other states, the total score from all phases of the review process (technical review, review of written proposals, review of oral presentations, and review of creative) is the only factor used to award the contract. This strategy allows one phase of the review to be given more weight by assignment of more points to that phase. However, this option should be exercised with caution. If you choose to give more weight to the review of written proposals by assigning more points to it than are assigned to the oral presentations, be aware that if the written proposals have a wide range of scores, the reviewers of the oral presentations may not be able to influence the final outcome, because they have fewer points to assign. This outcome eliminates the benefit of having additional input for decision making, based on the review of the oral presentations.

Some states don't allow the review committee to make the final decision; instead, the committee is asked to make a recommendation. Then the health department makes the final decision. The reviewers' qualitative comments can be helpful to the health department staff in their final determination, particularly when the scores are close.

11. How should the review process for the oral presentations be managed?

As with the process for review of the written proposals, there are several options for managing the process for review of oral presentations, and states manage this process differently. The comments in response to question 6 about sharing scores and changing scores are also relevant here.

You should schedule enough time for each agency to set up (at least 15 minutes) and to make the presentation (one to two hours). Additional time is required for reviewers to ask questions of the agency (30 to 60 minutes) and then to discuss and score each presentation (30 to 45 minutes). Time is also needed for activities such as breaks and meals. You'll need to provide a private and quiet room where the reviewers can talk while the next agency has access to the presentation room to set up for the oral presentation.

12. What kinds of questions should agencies be given in advance of oral presentations, and which questions should be surprises?

Providing each agency the same set of questions, either in advance or during the oral presentation, gives the reviewers some common ground for assessment and comparison of the agencies. Questions given to agencies in advance should call for responses that require planning, data gathering, alignment with agency management, or other time-consuming preparation. Surprise questions should require strategic thinking (specific choices or recommendations) related to the proposal. You should be able to ask the agency "why…?" in relation to any part of its proposal, because presumably everything in the proposal was developed with use of good strategic thinking. Some questions are appropriate either in advance or during the presentation; for example, "What potential media crises do you foresee on this account, and how would you respond?"

To demonstrate levels of creative and strategic thinking, some states ask agencies to perform tasks such as putting together initial creative ideas or developing a proposed media placement schedule. You shouldn't ask agencies to develop near-final ad executions as part of their written proposals or oral presentations. In addition to the time, cost, and energy required, such a task sets an agency in a particular direction without providing the necessary baseline data and input from the state staff.

13. What is the ideal composition of a review committee?

Many states have specific restrictions or policies that help to determine the makeup of the review committee. Such restrictions include requiring that all or a majority of the review panel live in the state or prohibiting state tobacco control staff from being on the panel. You need enough reviewers that the committee represents a range of backgrounds and expertise but not so many that the process becomes cumbersome. One member should have experience working with minority and diverse populations.

Many states invite people who manage tobacco counter-marketing contracts in other states to serve on the review committee, because they've been through the RFP process and often can offer helpful insights from experience. You can ask people in other agencies within your state government that have large advertising or marketing contracts (e.g., the lottery, tourism, or agriculture). Also, you may want to include one or two people from national organizations who have worked with other states on their counter-marketing efforts and can offer a national perspective. For example, representatives from the Health Communications Branch of the CDC's Office on Smoking and Health, the American Cancer Society, the Campaign for Tobacco-Free Kids, and other national organizations have served on review panels in a number of states. In addition, it's helpful to have people on the committee who have experience working in advertising or marketing, either for an agency or as a client. Most people with such backgrounds have an in-depth understanding of how to develop a marketing plan and advertising campaign and how to select an agency. They are also likely to be able to see through the glitz of the written and oral presentations.

14. Should the same committee review the written proposals and the oral presentations?

Sometimes state regulations and policies determine whether the same panel must review the written proposals and the oral presentations. Some states require use of the same panel for both reviews; others have no such requirement. One benefit of having the same group for both reviews is that the reviewers can follow up during the oral presentations with specific questions about the written proposals. One benefit of having different groups for both phases is that a new person added to the panel for the oral presentations comes into the process with a fresh perspective and can assess the presentations without being influenced by the written proposals.

Criteria To Aid in Selecting an Agency

1. What are some of the issues with hiring an agency based in another state or city?

Some states must select suppliers and contractors that are within the state, because government rules and policies require doing so or because if they don't, they'll be seen as giving business to other states and not supporting the local economy. In addition, if an agency from a state or city other than the location of the health department offices is selected, communications will be more difficult, because face-to-face interactions will be less frequent. Problems could result, because the state and the agency should be partners in most aspects of the campaign planning, execution, and evaluation; thus, the better the communication and interaction are, the more productive the work relationship can be. Nevertheless, it's important that every state considers the best candidates available. Effective marketing and advertising are not easy to achieve, and a local firm should not be selected at the cost of compromising the quality of the work. States should "cast the net" as broadly as possible and then choose the best candidate on the basis of specified criteria. The criteria used to select the agency should always be clear and supportable in case they are later challenged by individuals or organizations outside of the selection process.

2. What skills, experiences, and capabilities should be required of the ad agency? Of the public relations agency?

The ad agency chosen should have experience in planning, implementing, and evaluating comprehensive ad campaigns. Agency staff should be familiar with the marketing mix (product, placement, packaging, price, promotion, and politics), so they understand the importance of each element and the interrelatedness of all the elements. They should have strengths in the areas of creativity and strategic thinking (i.e., making important choices about the direction of the communications plan). The work they produce should clearly show a balance between keeping a strong strategic focus and developing products that are insightful, interesting, and deliver an impact. The ad agency should have the following functions in house: (1) account services,

(2) creative, (3) media planning and buying, and (4) research. In-house planning is optional, but more and more agencies offer this service, which is a cross between research and strategic planning. If the agency doesn't do media buying or research in-house, agency staff may have sufficient experience with the function and a strong relationship with a subcontractor to provide these services through a subcontract.

If a PR agency is to be selected, the staff of the PR agency should have experience in planning, implementing, and evaluating comprehensive PR campaigns. They must have in-depth experience interfacing with the media and should be able to show a track record of successful placements, for example, media coverage and stories that achieve high reach of target audiences, adequate frequency, exposure through major media outlets, and appropriate positioning of the issue and content covered. The staff should understand and show knowledge of the key tools for earned media (e.g., media kits, news conferences, editorial board meetings, press releases, and event planning). (See Chapter 8: Public Relations and Chapter 9: Media Advocacy for more information on these tools.) Ideally, they should understand and have experience working with ad agencies and other diverse partners. Also, if you'd like your agency to conduct media advocacy training sessions for your local coalitions, make sure that the agency staff have the necessary experience and that they understand the relationship between local coalitions and the state program.

3. When should subcontractors be used?

Subcontractors can be hired by the lead ad or PR agency when the agency doesn't have the in-house expertise or resources to manage and execute a certain part of the contract. The lead agency shouldn't subcontract major pieces of the campaign, but it may be difficult to find one agency that can meet all the needs detailed in the state's RFP. By subcontracting, a strong lead agency can do what it does well and can manage the work of the subcontractors without executing the work themselves. Common examples are subcontractors who have expertise in communication with special populations, media-buying firms, PR agencies, and research firms, as long as they're not conducting research to evaluate the effectiveness of the lead agency's outputs.

Subcontractors often report directly to the lead agency rather than the state health department, so their work is funneled through the lead agency. However, in some cases, it's important to have the subcontractors interface directly with the state, so the state can more easily assess the expertise they bring, ask questions, and develop a positive working relationship with them. In addition, it may be beneficial to structure the contract so that, in the event you aren't satisfied with the work, you're able to replace the subcontractor without having to issue a new RFP.

4. What size should the agency be?

There's no ideal size for an agency. The state must decide whether a large agency or a small agency better meets its needs. One advantage of small agencies is that you may be a large client to them, and if so, you'll get plenty of their attention, including significant involvement from personnel in upper management, who are typically the most seasoned members of the agency. If you select a very large agency, the agency's best people may not be assigned to your account, and personnel in upper management may not have time to spend on your campaign. One advantage of large agencies is that they often have more internal resources. More of the important functions (e.g., account planning, media planning and buying, and research) are in-house, so they're more directly available to you as the client. A large agency may also have a longer history and thus may have more experience in advertising and marketing. In addition, large agencies tend to be more stable, because they're less vulnerable to economic upturns and downturns. Many states select an agency that has sufficient billings and internal infrastructure to do quality work but is small enough to consider the state's account an important one.

5. Is an agency's connection with the tobacco industry acceptable? Should disclosure statements be required during the RFP process?

The acceptability of hiring an agency that has connections with the tobacco industry is controversial. One view is that no links to the tobacco industry should be allowed, so even agencies owned by a company that does business with a tobacco company subsidiary should be prohibited from competing for a contract. The contention is that any links to the tobacco industry may compromise the quality of the agency's work, because the agency will have a more important "master" to serve (i.e., management of the tobacco company). Another concern is that confidential tobacco control information that is shared with the agency could find its way into the hands of the tobacco industry.

A different viewpoint is that if the links to the tobacco industry are weak (e.g., a subsidiary connection), the agency should be allowed to compete for a contract. The argument is that if the criteria are too restrictive, the health department or another lead state agency could rule out some of the best-qualified communication firms. Many of the top firms have some loose connection with the tobacco industry, because of the industry's breadth of products and businesses. This view proposes that if the state sets high expectations for the agency (e.g., in a performance-based contract) and the agency performs well, the contract should continue. If the agency doesn't perform well or if the state suspects that agency staff are not giving the campaign their best efforts, the contract should be terminated.

Another consideration is how audiences will perceive your campaign if it's known that the agency you chose has ties to the tobacco industry, however loose they may be. You may want to determine in advance whether your campaign messages will be credible to your audience and how your legislators may respond.

Disclosure statements should be required of all agencies bidding for work on the state's counter-marketing campaign, so RFP reviewers have knowledge of any affiliation with the tobacco industry and can assess it appropriately. In addition, it's common practice to include in the contract with the ad agency a prohibition against accepting tobacco industry business while the agency is under the state contract. You must define what is meant by "accepting tobacco industry business."

6. **How heavily should experience with government programs be weighed? How important is experience with pro bono or public service programs or with campaigns related to health issues?**

The experience of an agency with government or public service programs should be considered in the RFP selection process. However, the most important strength that an ad or PR agency can bring to a contract is the ability to develop and execute effective communications.

Experience working with the government is important because agencies must understand that the government doesn't behave like most for-profit clients. State health departments are subject to many rules and administrative policies that must be followed. If an agency doesn't understand the constraints the state has, it may have a slower start, may not take into account these constraints in terms of planning timelines, may not involve the necessary people in decisions, and may become very frustrated by a system that is unfamiliar to its staff.

Pro bono experience may be considered important for at least two reasons, although neither of these reasons should make it a priority criterion for awarding a contract to an ad or PR agency. The first reason is philosophical. Pro bono experience may show the agency's level of commitment to serving the community, not just profiting from it. The second reason is based on expertise. Pro bono work may give an agency experience working on issues relevant to tobacco control (e.g., youth drug use, gambling addiction, or referendum campaigns). Agency staff may gain perspective to help them better understand how to approach prevention of youth tobacco use, smoking cessation in adults, or reduction of exposure to secondhand smoke.

Experience with a public service campaign may be important for the same reasons. In addition, if an agency has been able to secure free media placements for public service announcements, the staff may have expertise in getting the most media placements possible with limited or no funds. They may also have good relationships with media outlets and experience in acquiring bonus weight for media placement.

Experience in a campaign related to health issues may give the agency insights into ways to approach the health issue of tobacco use. The task of influencing people to change behaviors related to tobacco use can be extremely challenging, and experiences addressing other types of behavior change to improve health may be applicable. In addition, such experience may make an agency more familiar with the workings of health organizations and government agencies that focus on health issues.

Agencies bidding on a contract must do more than include in their proposals the names of campaigns they have worked on pro bono or with health organizations or government agencies. They should also be required to elaborate on how they developed and implemented the campaign(s), including the approaches they used; the insights they gleaned that helped them to create persuasive communications that had impact; the media vehicles used and why; and the results of the campaign(s).

Other RFP Issues

1. **If an ad is produced by an agency, but the creative (the ad agency person whose job is to develop ideas for advertisements) who designed the ad leaves the agency and is hired by another agency, can the ad be used as an example of the former agency's work, the work of the person who designed it, or both?**

   There's no clear answer to these questions. Agencies and agency personnel who produce creative materials will make individual decisions about which ads they'll show as examples of their work. A good ad or ad campaign comes from both the individuals who create it and the whole agency. The individual Creatives will come up with the ideas, but the management always reviews the work and provides input to it. If an agency or an individual includes ads as examples in a proposal, you can ask questions about the ads to determine how involved they were in the development process and how much of their own thinking went into the ads.

2. **What are the advantages, disadvantages, and logistic considerations of using a performance-based contract for the agency? How should such a contract be structured?**

   Performance-based contracts with agencies have been used by several states and by the American Legacy Foundation as a way to increase the accountability of the ad agencies, keep them focused on the bottom line of desired outcomes, and challenge them to achieve aggressive objectives. A performance-based contract can be developed in several ways. In the RFP, you can ask the prospective agencies how they would propose constructing the compensation package, including any performance-based elements. This request will heighten their awareness that you're considering a performance-based contract, and it will give them an opportunity to share with you methods that have worked well with other clients. You should also ask some of the states and organizations that have used performance-based contracts for information, such as the wording they used and what changes they would make if they awarded a performance-based contract again. Typically, a compensation level is established for the work provided and the performance-based aspect allows the agency to earn additional compensation if the previously established objectives of the campaign are achieved. For example, the agency might be able to earn 5% more if the campaign achieves the objectives or perhaps 5% less if none of the objectives are achieved.

   The downside to performance-based contracts is that they don't have the flexibility to take into account special circumstances. For example, the objectives may have been set too high in the face of a difficult political environment and lack of support from the legislature or the governor. On the other hand, the objectives may have been appropriate when the campaign started, but they didn't take into account other tobacco control efforts that would help the campaign to accomplish its objectives, so their achievement became too easy. The use of absolute measures to gauge success, and thus compensation, doesn't always take into account the volatility of the environment in which a campaign operates.

3. What questions should be asked to determine levels of expertise in media planning and media buying?

Most state planners of media campaigns have limited expertise in the technical area of media planning and media buying. However, questions can be asked, either in the RFP or in an oral presentation, to determine an agency's philosophy and level of expertise in media planning and media buying. Here are some of the issues to address in the questions:

- Level of experience in securing bonus time for media placement and examples of success in securing media placement at low costs

- Expertise in media buying in diverse media outlets (e.g., television, radio, outdoor, print, and the Internet)

- Strategic thinking related to which media outlets, times of the day, and programs would be most appropriate for each of the campaign's target audiences

- The reach, frequency, and duration of media presence required to achieve the campaign's awareness levels, and belief, knowledge, and attitude changes

- Examples of clients for whom the agency has purchased media

- Experience in selecting and buying media placements in all the state's counties, not just in the big media markets

The agencies submitting proposals should also clearly state whether they have the ability in-house to plan and buy media or whether they subcontract that work to outside experts.

4. What are the advantages and disadvantages of creating a "brand"? Should bidding agencies be asked to provide their thinking on a brand for this campaign?

Some states and organizations choose to develop a brand for their campaign; others choose not to develop a brand. This decision should be based on the campaign's goals. If you think that having a recognizable label, identity, or badge to tie your campaign together and help your target audience develop an allegiance to your movement will help to achieve your goals, you should consider developing a brand. However, if you think your campaign's ads should independently communicate strong messages and convey a sense of pervasiveness without being attached to an institution or organization, then a brand probably won't serve you well. For example, if the goal is to reduce exposure to secondhand smoke, there may not be a strong reason to develop a brand, as long as the advertising messages are clear and compelling. However, if the goal is to reduce youth cigarette smoking by replacing that "badge" with another one, you may choose to develop a brand to associate with a nonsmoking lifestyle. As a result, youth may choose to wear attire with your brand, assuming that it's cool, rather than choosing to pick up a cigarette when they're with their peers.

Developing a brand isn't easy. A brand needs to be clear, recognizable, and meaningful and must have positive and desirable connotations among the target audience. It must represent something with which the target audience wants to associate or identify themselves. Those criteria are challenging to achieve. The downside is that if you don't achieve one or more of these criteria, your effort may have no impact, or worse, your effort may backfire by causing the target audience to reject or make fun of your brand. It's easy to see the attraction to brands like Nike, Coke, or Britney Spears, but it's important to realize that for every brand that becomes cool or desirable, there are many, many more that are not considered cool or desirable at all.

Depending upon your campaign goals, target audience(s), and budget, you may want to ask the bidding agencies to develop and present ideas for branding, including whether or not they think branding would help or hinder achievement of the campaign's goals.

Appendix 6.3: Elements of a Creative Brief

Purposes of a Creative Brief

The creative brief includes key information gleaned from formative research and translates these research learnings into direction for the advertising agency creative staff (creatives) to develop communication materials. It serves as a link between the research and the creative process. The creative brief also helps bring everyone involved into alignment before development of materials begins. Once the individual(s) with responsibility for making the ultimate decision about creative materials has approved the creative brief, materials development can begin.

Elements of a Creative Brief

Below is a description of the most common elements included in a creative brief. There are many ways to design a creative brief, and different organizations and agencies will use formats that include some (or all) of these elements.

Project Description and Background

The specific assignment for the agency's creatives. This section provides key background information and short-term tactical thinking to help bring the long-term strategy to life in the target audience's current environment. The assignment might be a broad assignment such as the following:

- Develop comprehensive introductory advertising for a new program designed to reduce exposure to secondhand smoke.

- Develop a public education campaign designed to spur individual and community action to reduce young people's access to tobacco products, especially by building support for local enforcement efforts.

The assignment might also be as specific as the following:

- Develop a new television advertising execution (sometimes called a "pool-out") for a campaign in progress.

- Create ads for billboards to supplement existing TV and print ads.

Description of the Target Audience

Identification of the target audience you want to reach. Examples of target audiences include the following:

- Restaurant owners who smoke

- 11- to 15-year-old nonsmokers

- African-American adult male smokers

- Family members of smokers
- Policy makers

Target Audience Insights

Descriptive details about the target audience. This should include specific information about demographics, lifestyles, psychographics, and other characteristics of the target audience that help the creatives develop materials appropriate for this audience. Creative materials are most persuasive when based on one or more insights into target audience beliefs or practices related to the concept, product, attitude, or behavior being addressed. These target audience insights can be positive or negative. They are the foundation for building the content of communications materials.

One example of a target audience belief that might influence the creation of advertising executions encouraging youth not to smoke is that youth are more afraid of living a life of pain and physical problems as a result of smoking than they are afraid of dying from smoking, because their perception of death is vague and abstract.

Goal(s)

What you want the target audience to do as a result of hearing, watching, reading, or experiencing the communication. Examples include the following:

- Increase knowledge about tobacco industry marketing practices
- Change attitudes about exposing other people to secondhand smoke
- Support policies restricting smoking in public buildings
- Enter a smoking cessation program

Obstacles

Beliefs, attitudes, values, behaviors, or environmental factors that prevent the target audience from adopting the desired attitude or behavior. The obstacles are what stand between the audience and the desired attitude or behavior. Examples include the following:

- Lack of knowledge of the harmful effects of secondhand smoke
- The belief that smoking is not harmful if one smokes only occasionally in social settings
- Tobacco industry financial support of community organizations
- Smokers' belief that they must quit on their own without getting help

Key Promise/Key Benefit(s)

Statement of the key benefit(s) or reward(s) (including emotional benefits, if appropriate) that the audience will experience for adopting the desired attitudes or behavior. The key benefit is something that will make changing to the desired attitude or behavior worth it for the audience. Examples include the following:

- Ability to live long enough to see one's children grow up

- Saving oneself from great pain and suffering caused by smoking-related disease/illness

- Being a good parent by protecting one's children from secondhand smoke

Statements of Support or Reasons To Believe

A statement of support, a reason to believe, or evidence that adopting the desired attitudes or behavior will result in gaining the key benefits. These statements should be compelling enough to overcome the obstacles. Examples include the following:

- Sharing the fact that smokers who quit live an average of 15 years longer than smokers who continue smoking throughout their lives, and showing middle-aged and older nonsmokers enjoying life with their children and grandchildren

- Showing a credible portrayal of someone who became ill from smoking and revealing how difficult that smoker's life became

- Persuasively communicating the fact that children in households where smoking occurs inhale the same poisons as the smoker

Brand Character

Description of the brand's image or qualities designed to appeal to the target audience (e.g., nurturing and helpful, strong and powerful, credible and trustworthy, or rebellious and independent). Because many tobacco counter-marketing campaigns are not based on a brand, this section is often not included in a creative brief.

Copy Strategy

A short paragraph developed to succinctly summarize what the advertising needs to achieve, including who the advertising is directed to, what action is desired, the key benefit(s) of taking that action, the reason(s) to believe that benefit will be realized if the action is taken, and the brand character (if relevant). The format of a copy strategy might be something like, "The television ad will convince A (target audience) to do B (desired action) because they will believe that doing so will provide them with C (key benefit). The reason to believe will be D."

Tone

The feeling that the materials will convey (e.g., authoritative; positive and encouraging; heart-wrenching; supportive).

Media Channels/Vehicles

Media vehicle(s) for which creative materials will be produced (e.g., TV spot, radio spot, newspaper ad, billboard, transit ad, Web site, brochure, educational video).

Executional Considerations/Creative Considerations/Mandatories

Specifics that the materials should or must contain. Examples include the following:

- Materials may need to be easily adaptable for local or national use; therefore, references to names of specific towns or states should not be included.

- Materials must not alienate adults even though teens are the primary audience, because adults will be exposed to the materials as well.

- The TV advertising must include a five-second tag at the end with the quitline number.

Appendix 6.4: Creative Brief, Florida

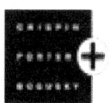

Creative Brief

This briefing document is intended to give direction and inspiration to creative. It is the beginning of the process, meant to initiate the dialogue that is an ongoing part of the development of the work. It is a guideline.

Client Florida Dept. of Health	Product "truth" TV campaign	Date 6/9/00
Why are we advertising at all? (A brief outline of our client's business situation and the problem/opportunity this ad needs to address.)	In an effort to keep the Florida Anti-Tobacco "truth" campaign fresh, we would like to produce 2-3 low-budget, teen TV spots before the end of the fiscal year (July 2000). Ultimately, the teens want to play an important part in delivering the "truth" message to their peers through our TV spots.	
What's this advertising trying to do? (What can we realistically hope to accomplish by running this ad? Be clear, be realistic, and if there's more than one objective—prioritize.)	By telling teens how the tobacco industry is manipulating them, we hope to continue to reduce tobacco use throughout the state of Florida. We want to give teens the knowledge of how the tobacco industry is manipulating them by portraying smoking as glamorous and smokers as attractive and appealing. Teens need to make their own decisions about whether or not they want to smoke. They need to control their own lives. We want to de-legitimize the tobacco industry and de-glamorize smoking.	
Whom are we talking to? (Imagine you're at a party and you run into someone from our target audience. Describe him or her.) (Whom are we not talking to?)	Teen target audience (12-17 year old males and females). Teenagers aspire to be older, so if we want to reach these teens, we must target the 25 year olds.	
What do we know about our target audience that will help us? (What is the relationship between these people and our product? How does it fit into their lives, how would their lives be different without it? What kind of language do they use to describe our product?)	Teens have the need to rebel, take risks, fit in/be liked, be independent, express themselves as individuals and feel respected. The major force behind these needs is for teens to feel in control of their lives, behaviors, their look, whom they choose to be friends with, and where they choose to hang out. Tapping into teens' need to rebel, the campaign should continue to depict tobacco use as an addictive habit marketed by an adult institution.	

Continues

Appendix 6.4: Creative Brief, Florida (cont.)

Client	Product	Date
Florida Dept. of Health	"truth" TV campaign	6/9/00
What's the main thought we need to communicate here? (Thought, not thoughts. The one thing we want them to take away that will change their behavior. This is the phrase that matters. It should be concise yet meaningful. Think of it as a billboard for the creatives.)	The tobacco industry uses deceitful, manipulative and dishonest practices to hook new users, sell more cigarettes, and make more money. We need to expose these lies and give teens the choice to make up their own minds about smoking.	
Why should they believe this? (What support do we have to show that the "main thought" matters? Relevant facts and information based on both the rational and the emotional are welcome here. Attach detail of this support if it will assist in creative development.)	Tobacco companies have, for years, worked to target and manipulate teens into smoking. They see teens as potential life-long customers. To date, "truth" has worked to replace the role tobacco plays in the lives of these teens and fulfill their needs.	
What's the best way of doing this? (Is it: a slice of life, soft sell, case histories, animated? Tonality? Give a few executional suggestions. With the emphasis on suggestions.)	To compete with the tobacco industry advertising, we need ambitious, hard-hitting, in-your-face executions. We need to continue to portray teens as rebellious activists with a sense of humor who are willing to expose the hypocrisy of adult institutions. We can show that not using tobacco can be a more rebellious and cool act than using tobacco.	
Mandatories (Things that have to be seen or heard in the advertising. Not opinions, ideas, speculations or suggestions.)	Develop scripts that include Florida teens in the spots (i.e., phone calls). The State has decided not to use the spots that were produced for the national Truth campaign (i.e., body bags, lie detector, etc.) because they do not want to run the risk of airing these spots and then having them pulled off the air. Additionally, the spots that feature teens going to the tobacco company offices also have legal implications (i.e., trespassing).	

Planning   Approval   Client
                Creative

_____   _____   _____

Appendix 6.5: Creative Brief, Centers for Disease Control and Prevention and World Health Organization

STRATEGY PLATFORM

CLIENT: World Health Organization and Centers for Disease Control and Prevention Project
PROJECT: "How To Quit" TV—Revised
DATE: 12/13/00

BACKGROUND—*what is the situation?*

The World Health Organization (WHO) and the Centers for Disease Control and Prevention (CDC) with other health organizations are committed to tobacco use reduction; making it a priority over the next three years. The goal is to reduce the use of tobacco products, thereby reducing preventable disease and death. Globally, four million deaths a year are attributed to tobacco use. If tobacco use continues, unchecked, this death rate is projected to rise to 10 million deaths annually by 2030. By 2020, 70% of tobacco-related deaths would be in developing countries. Most of the future tobacco-related deaths over the next 50 years will be those of adult smokers smoking today; thus governments concerned about making health gains for their citizens can make a significant advance by encouraging and helping adult smokers to quit.

As part of the commitment to tobacco use reduction, quit tools need to be provided to countries to assist in the fight against tobacco. As mentioned, WHO and CDC are working with other partners to develop a TV spot that educates smokers on "how to quit." There are many tools to aid quit attempts and it often takes more than one attempt to succeed.

Historically, public service announcements (or paid media TV spots) on tobacco have focused on the health risks of smoking—both for active and, more recently, passive smokers. While this remains important, in many countries the vast majority of smokers are now aware of these risks; stating that they want to quit and have tried to quit several times in the past. Unfortunately, however, the vast majority of smokers try to quit unaided, without any support (behavioral or pharmacological), despite the fact that such treatments are available and have been clinically proven to significantly increase success rates. Therefore, there is also a need to educate smokers that effective treatments do exist, that going it alone is the least successful way of quitting and to encourage them to seek out and use such treatments.

COMPETITIVE FRAMEWORK—*whom are we competing against?*

<u>General Overview</u>
The tobacco companies continue to sell tobacco and their advertising hasn't changed to include the health risks or addictiveness associated with cigarette smoking. Other than the mandated warning labels specific to

each country (each country has their own tobacco regulations) and any other enforced mandates, the industry does not disclose information about the health consequences in any of their marketing. The industry continues to expand around the world, in developed and developing countries.

Specific to Quit Attempts

In the context of helping smokers to quit, the competitor is "Cold Turkey"—the least effective, but most commonly used means of quitting.

OBJECTIVES—*what are we trying to accomplish?*

- Overcome the perception that the best way to quit is to go it alone.

- Get smokers to think about quitting with help; reinforce that quitting isn't easy and it's okay if success isn't achieved the first time.

TARGET—*whom we want to connect with (include demographics and psychographics):*
Adult smokers 18–49

Smokers' thoughts/behavior on quitting are varied:

- Some are in denial that they are addicted and that they can't quit—they feel they can quit whenever they are ready to.

- Some are ready to quit now but still may not realize they need help to succeed.

- Others feel the only way to quit is cold turkey. They are not receptive to help because they feel they should do it alone. Even if they have tried to quit before and have failed, they still feel that it's their own responsibility to quit. They want to be in control. Accepting help shows weakness and lack of control.

CURRENT RESPONSE—*what the consumer would say about the brand and/or offer before advertising:*
I know I need to quit; when I am ready I'll do it on my own.

DESIRED RESPONSE—*what we want the consumer to say after the advertising:*
I know quitting is hard and I do need help; getting help doesn't diminish my accomplishment of quitting.

KEY SELLING MESSAGE
Don't quit alone; seek out help to improve your chances of success.

MOTIVATING SUPPORT POINTS—*why should the consumer believe us?*

- Cigarette smoking is addictive and it's hard to quit. Success doesn't happen overnight. With help, it could be achieved sooner. Quit tools to consider: quitlines, pharmaceutical products, cessation programs, and web sites.

- Being in the right mindset is crucial (wanting to quit) and having the willpower is critical but getting help will significantly increase chances of success.

- Smokers have a tendency to get discouraged if success isn't immediate; they need to feel this isn't a reflection on them as a person. They need to know it's okay to attempt more than once before success is achieved.

Additional support points should be specific to the tags for pharmaceutical products or quitline support. For countries that don't have either of the above, their tags could contain a more emotional message, such as a point about how much your family cares about you and wants you to succeed in quitting—needs to be discussed further.

TONE

Understanding and Encouraging

EXECUTIONAL CONSIDERATIONS—*media/timing, unit sizes, budgets, other client directives*

- One :30 TV spot - :25/:05 split – 25 seconds dedicated to message and 5 seconds dedicated to call-to-action. Once in the creative process, the second split will more accurately be determined—the tag may need 10 seconds especially when the support points are clarified and confirmed.

- Individual tags (the 5 or 10 seconds) highlighting quitlines, web sites, cessation programs, pharmaceutical products so people know what "quit tools" are available and where to find them.

- Translations to be considered being executed by individual countries to ensure appropriate dialect/language.

- The organization's name to be included and will change by country. Each country will be responsible for inclusion when translations are done (need to discuss this portion further).

- Due to countries not being identified at this point and the fact this spot needs to globally applicable, the creative concept may need to be more visual and less talent heavy. This will be determined once creative development begins.

- Budget: (not confirmed)

- Timing: Available the week of May 7, 2001

Appendix 6.6: Creative Brief, Centers for Disease Control and Prevention

CDC/OSH Parenting Project
Creative Brief 3/24/00

Target Audience:
Less-involved parents with children ages 7 – 11 yrs.

Secondary Audience:
Less-involved parents with children ages 0 – 6 yrs.
Less-involved parents with children ages 12 – 18 yrs.

Key messages:
You have time to spend with your kids.
Here's how (tactics).

Promise:
Increased parent/child interaction will help establish protective barriers against future drug and tobacco use.
Better communication with your child.

Call to Action:
Talk/spend time with your child.

Content:
Activities and/or tactics that parents can do, with minimal effort or time, with their children.
Model desired behavior: parent/child interaction and communication.

Tone:
Fun, Simple, Casual and Friendly

Creative Considerations:
Television Commercial
Print
- Newspaper: TV Guide Section
- TV Guide Magazine, regional
- Fast Food Tray liners
- Work Posters

Radio – drive time

Testing:
Concept tested in focus groups (2).
Materials tested in 1-on-1's and with states.

Distribution:
Via CDC - through state anti-tobacco programs.

Appendix 7.1: Sample Advertising Comment Organizer

Understand

- Do you understand the layouts? What's happening in the storyboards? In the print ad? In the outdoor ad?

- Do you understand the ad agency's recommendation, if one was made?

Evaluate

Think about these questions for each creative execution.

- What is your overall reaction? Consider each entire ad.

    – Does it have stopping power?

    – Is it a fast read?

    – How would you react as a member of the target audience?

    – Is it relevant?

- Is it on strategy? If the strategy is clear and decisive, this question can be answered promptly.

- What is your reaction to the key executional elements of the ad?

    – Does it clearly communicate the key benefit?

    – Are the visuals and language provocative?

    – Is brand identification sufficient if that is a goal?

    – Is the setup or layout simple and clear?

- Are there any more details that should be considered at this time? Distracting visuals? Controversial elements? Be especially selective with any comments in this area so that you focus only on important details.

Communicate

Now it's time to organize your thoughts and communicate them to the agency clearly and positively. Test each comment in your mind to make certain it's necessary and constructive.

Give the agency your overall evaluation of the advertising and state whether you agree or disagree with its recommendation of which creative execution(s) to further develop.

Then deliver your specific comments, making sure the agency knows how strongly you feel about each comment. State specifically what you like and why, as well as what you don't like and why. Focus on important issues rather than feeling that you must address every detail.

- Strategy issues, if any
- Overall issues
    - Engagingness/stopping power (the ability to attract and keep audience attention)
    - Simplicity and clarity
    - Relevance
    - Convincingness
- Issues with key executional elements
- Comments about details (if they are important to the ad's potential effectiveness)

Overall Considerations

- **Remember, you're not the target.** The target audience doesn't have your knowledge base or experience, so what may be obvious to you may not be obvious to them.

- **Don't try to say too much.** You may be tempted to put a lot of copy points in an ad. Don't! Try to stick with communicating one main message. The more focused you are, the more likely that target audience members will take away the key point. Remember that you're competing with all other advertisers for the audience's attention.

- **Keep your production budget in mind, but remember that the quality of the final ad (production value) does matter.** Don't select an advertising execution you can't afford to produce, or it will look "homemade" and may be viewed as inferior or unprofessional to the audience, compared with other broadcast, print, or outdoor ads.

- **Take a chance.** Sometimes you need to take a leap of faith to create break-through advertising. Use your instincts. Everything you do won't be perfect, but if you always err on the side of "being safe," your work will likely reflect that attitude and ultimately won't be as effective as it can be.

Appendix 7.2: Sample Storyboard—"Carnival"

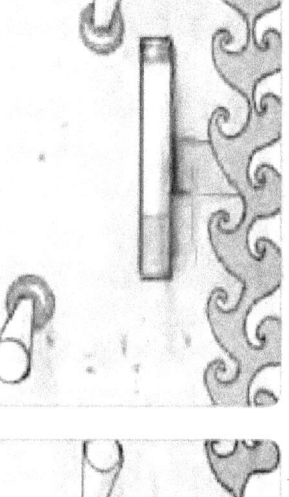

A locked off shot of a carnival target shooting game. Instead of the usual duck that goes back and forth, the target is a cigarette.

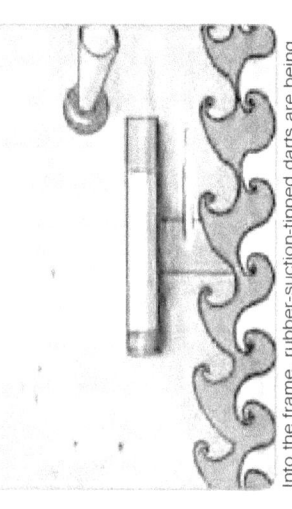

Into the frame, rubber-suction-tipped darts are being shot at the cigarette.

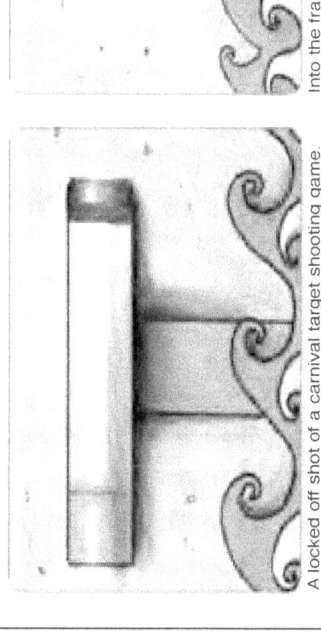

At first, the cigarette just moves back and forth like a duck target would. As some of the shots get closer the cigarette dodges out of the way. All the shots miss.

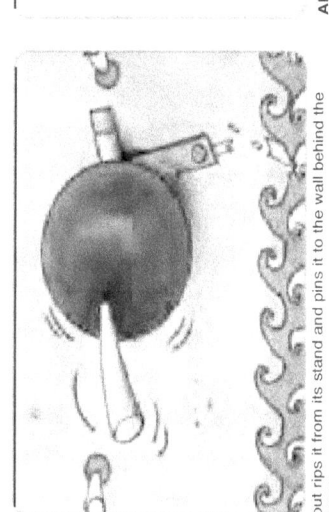

Suddenly a huge rubber-tipped dart (the size of a plunger) flies into frame and not only hits the cigarette...
VO: Unless, of course...

but rips it from its stand and pins it to the wall behind the game.
VO: you have help.

Local information goes here.

ARTCARD: For help quitting, call XXX-XXXX.

Appendix 7.3: Sample Storyboard—"Drive"

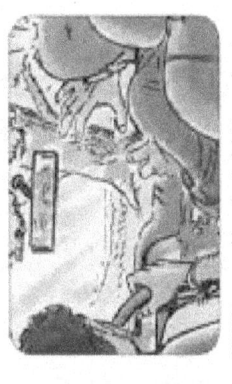

VISUAL: A man and woman are driving down the road. Not giving it any thought, the male passenger lights a cigarette in the car.

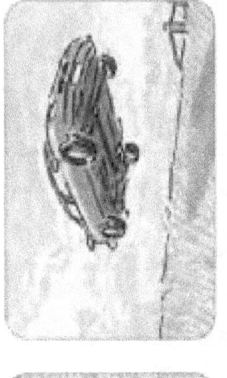

VISUAL: Female driver looks over at lit cigarette, scowls slightly, and purposely veers car off road...

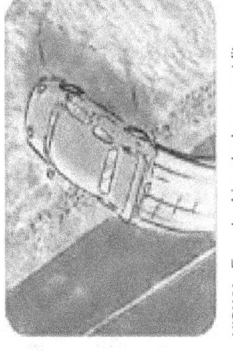

VISUAL: ... flies through a ditch...

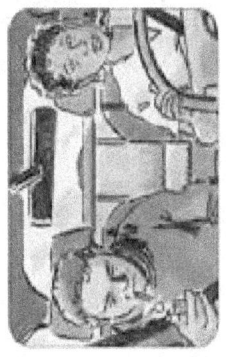

VISUAL: ... and heads straight towards a tree.

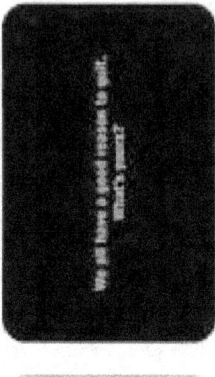

VISUAL: Male passenger is petrified.

MAN: What are you doing!?

WOMAN: (Calmly) You're endangering my life...just returning the favor.

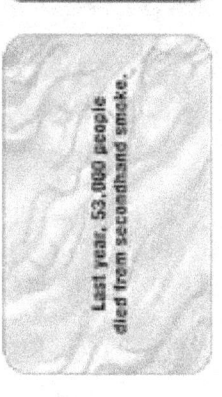

VISUAL: Car safely veers back onto road.

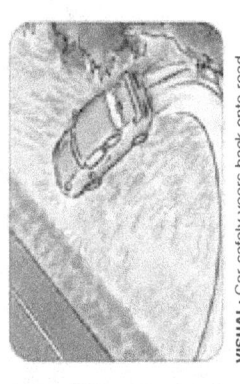

ART CARD: Last year, 53,000 people died from secondhand smoke.

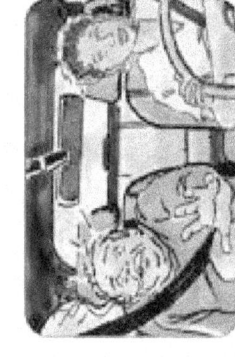

ART CARD: We all have a good reason to quit. What's yours?

Appendix 8.1: Sample Printed Campaign Newsletter

A Publication from the Colorado Department of Public Health and Environtment

Colorado Tobacco Settlement Times

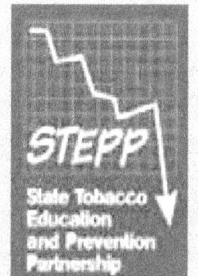

The Master Settlement Agreement: Working to Save Lives in Colorado

Building a Comprehensive Tobacco Use Prevention & Reduction Program in Colorado
Governor Announces Grants to County Nursing Services

March 2001
Issue 3

Inside This Issue

1 Governor Announces Grant Awards

2 STEPP Funds Youth Programs

 Youth Movement Gains Momentum

3 STEPP Advisory Board Convenes

 Youth Tobacco Survey Findings to be Released

 Doing Business with the State

4 STEPP Issues RFPs

State Tobacco Education and Prevention Partnership (STEPP)
Health Promotion and Disease Prevention Division
Colorado Department of Public Health and Environment
HPDP-STEPP-A5
4300 Cherry Creek Drive South
Denver, Colorado 80246-1530
303-692-2510

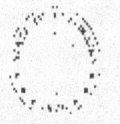

Colorado Department of Public Health and Environment

Governor Bill Owens recently announced that 28 new grants -- totaling nearly $1.4 million and covering 32 counties -- have been approved by the Colorado Board of Health and awarded to nursing services throughout the state to plan and implement local tobacco education and prevention programs.

The recipients of grants ranging from $30,000 to $60,000 are nursing services agencies representing the following counties or multi-county regions:

- Alamosa County
- Baca County
- Bent County
- Clear Creek County
- Conejos County
- Costilla County
- Crowley County
- Custer County
- Eagle County
- Fremont County
- Garfield and Pitken Counties
- Grand County
- Gunnison County
- Hinsdale County
- Jackson County
- Kiowa County
- Kit Carson, Lincoln and Cheyenne Counties
- Mineral County
- Montezuma County
- Montrose County
- Park County
- Prowers County
- Rio Grande County
- Routt and Moffat Counties
- Saguache County
- San Juan County
- Summit County
- Teller County

The grants will be used to implement the "Communities of Excellence in Tobacco Control"(CX) program developed by the American Cancer Society. The CX model provides systematic guidance to local communities for achieving critical planning outcomes specific to tobacco use prevention and reduction. Grantees will attend CX training and, working with members of their communities, implement the model in their respective areas.

"The tobacco settlement legislation passed by the Colorado Legislature emphasizes the importance of getting local programs up and running," said Karen DeLeeuw, State Tobacco Education and Prevention Partnership (STEPP) program manager.

"With the award of these 28 new grants, in addition to the 14 grants to local health departments already awarded, Colorado is well on its way to achieving our goal of having tobacco education and prevention programs in every county in the state," she added.

GRANT AWARDS, continued on page 2

1

Continues

Appendix 8.1: Sample Printed Campaign Newsletter (cont.)

Colorado Tobacco Settlement Times March 2001

GRANT AWARDS, continued

To date, STEPP has funded programs in 55 of Colorado's 63 counties, including: expansion grants to eight existing local health department programs, planning grants to an additional six local health departments and planning and implementation grants to 28 local nursing services covering 32 counties that will undertake the Communities of Excellence strategic-planning process. It has also contracted with the Alcohol and Drug Division to help enforce laws prohibiting tobacco sales to minors by conducting compliance checks and reporting violations to the Colorado Department of Revenue. In addition, a contract for the provision of cessation counseling and referral services via a statewide Quit Line is currently being negotiated. The Quit Line is expected to be operational in late June 2001.

STEPP Funds Programs to Reduce Tobacco Use Among Colorado's Youth

On Feb. 21, $37,200 was awarded to the following eight agencies for the provision of tobacco use cessation services at high school school-based health centers:

- Commerce City Community Health Services, which serves Adams City High School
- Conifer Mountain Family Medicine, which serves Platte Canyon High School

> This is the third issue of the *Colorado Tobacco Settlement Times*, a publication of the Colorado Department of Public Health and Environment's State Tobacco Education and Prevention Partnership (STEPP).
>
> The *Times* is available electronically on the STEPP website, www.cdphe.state.co.us/pp/tobacco, or in pdf format via e-mail. To add your name to the STEPP e-mail distribution list, please call Stefanie Quintana at 303-692-2516.

- Parkview Medical Center, which serves Central High School, Keating Continuing Education School, Centennial High School, South High School, and East High School in Pueblo
- Penrose-St. Francis Health Care System, which serves Fountain-Fort Carson High School and Lorraine Alternative High School
- Rocky Mountain Youth, which serves Centennial High School in Fort Collins
- Summit County Public Health Nursing Service, which serves Summit High School
- The Children's Hospital, which serves Sheridan High School

To support these programs and to provide training and technical assistance to these and subsequently funded school-based health center projects, the American Lung Association of Colorado will receive up to $20,000 in grant funding. The American Lung Association's youth cessation curriculum N-O-T (Not on Tobacco) will be used to develop and deliver cessation services at the school-based health centers.

State's Youth Movement Against Tobacco Gains Momentum

Colorado's statewide youth movement against tobacco is growing up rapidly with the establishment of 19 new coalitions.

Sixteeen community groups have been awarded American Legacy Foundation (ALF) grants of $2,000 each to launch local youth coalitions against tobacco. ALF is the non-profit organization responsible for the truth[sm] national advertising campaign - a movement launched by American youth that have united to combat tobacco. The following agencies received ALF grants:

- American Cancer Society in Colorado Springs

- Assets for Rural Youth in Norwood
- Community of Caring in Cripple Creek
- Custer County High School Student Council in Westcliffe
- Metro Gang Coalition in Denver
- Montezuma County Public Health Nursing Service
- Partners in Grand Junction
- Pueblo Central High School
- Safe and Drug-Free Schools Student Advisory Council in Grand Junction
- San Juan Basin Health Department in Durango
- San Luis Valley Community Connections
- Teller County Public Health
- The Boys and Girls Club of Larimer County
- The Family Center (Fort Collins)
- The Greater Auraria Neighborhood Affiliated for Services (GANAS)
- Youth Central-Montrose Memorial Hospital

Another three youth coalitions have been funded with tobacco settlement dollars. The agencies receiving these grants are:

- InterCept, a program of the Women's Resource Agency in Colorado Springs
- The University of Northern Colorado Lab School, Peer Education Class in Greeley
- Hinsdale County School District RE-1 in Lake City

To encourage the growth of Colorado's youth movement, settlement monies are available for the establishment of new youth coalitions. The application process for these grants Colorado is open and competitive through May 1, 2001.

"What is truly unique about this movement is that it is designed by youth, for youth," said Katy Kupecz, director of youth services for the partnership. "Even the grant application process required young people to

YOUTH MOVEMENT, continued page 3

Appendix 8.1: Sample Printed Campaign Newsletter (cont.)

Colorado Tobacco Settlement Times March 2001

YOUTH MOVEMENT, continued

write the proposals, which were submitted in formats ranging from videos to story boards to posters. Each submission was evaluated by a team of young people. Winning proposals were required to exhibit youth leadership and community readiness; reflect the community's social, ethnic and geographic diversity; and demonstrate diverse collaboration."

Youth coalition participants now will lead the way in assessing community needs, recruiting members and planning and marketing innovative strategies aimed at challenging youth to examine the truth about tobacco, she said.

"For years the tobacco industry has been targeting young people with slick advertising campaigns designed to make them believe that smoking and chewing are cool," says Kupecz. "This is an opportunity for kids to rally together, dispel the myths propagated by big tobacco and fight back."

During the first year of the Statewide Youth Movement Against Tobacco planning program, local youth coalitions will use grant funds for stipends and meeting expenses in addition to training and technical assistance. Participants also will have an opportunity to attend a Colorado Youth Tobacco Summit in April, where youth leaders from across the state will brainstorm strategies for reducing youth tobacco use in the state.

Once planning activities are completed, Colorado will be eligible to receive up to $1 million per year for three additional years from the Legacy Foundation to support a comprehensive statewide youth movement against tobacco use.

STEPP Advisory Board Meets to Discuss Long-Term Program Priorities

The STEPP Advisory Board met Feb. 9 to review progress on program funding recommendations that were outlined at its previous meeting in October and to provide advice on funding priorities and sequencing for the next four years.

Appointed by Health Department Executive Director Jane Norton, advisory board members include tobacco prevention experts and community leaders from across Colorado. The board's role is to guide STEPP in formulating program priorities and to assess the progress and effectiveness of the grant program created under SB 71.

Proceedings from the February meeting will be posted on the STEPP website in early April.

STEPP to Release Results of First-Ever Colorado Youth Tobacco Survey

On Monday, April 2, STEPP will release the results of the first-ever Youth Tobacco Survey (YTS) to be conducted in Colorado. Developed by the Centers for Disease Control and Prevention (CDC) and administered by the Colorado Department of Public Health and Environment, the results of the YTS will provide weighted data on tobacco use among middle and high school students statewide. The data will play an integral role in guiding tobacco use prevention and cessation programs aimed at youth throughout Colorado.

An executive summary of the survey will be released at a press conference at the Colorado State Capitol at 10 a.m. April 2nd. The summary, as well as all of the survey findings will be posted on the STEPP website simultaneously.

Now Online – Investing in Tobacco Control: A Guide for State Decisionmakers

On February 15, the Centers for Disease Control and Prevention's Office on Smoking and Health (CDC-OSH) and the Public Health Training Network (PHTN) hosted a nationwide satellite conference entitled "Investing in Tobacco Control: A Guide for State Decisionmakers." The broadcast is now available for viewing online.

Designed to help state decision makers learn how to invest in tobacco control programs to achieve the best results, the program features presentations by the U.S. Surgeon General and state legislators from around the country who are experienced in providing leadership in tobacco control. In addition, national and state experts describe how to establish comprehensive, sustainable, and accountable state tobacco control programs that get results and outline the short- and long-term benefits a number of state comprehensive tobacco control programs have already achieved.

To view the broadcast, visit http://www.cdc.gov/phtn/ and click on the "Calendar" option. The program can be found under the "past videoconferences" link.

Doing Business with the State

Vendors who would like to sell goods and services to the state should register on the Bid Information and Distribution System (BIDS). The annual fee for registration is $30. The following are the steps for registering with the state.

1. Log on to the Colorado Department of General Support Services and Personnel web site at http://www.gssa.state.co.us
2. Click on the "State Purchasing Office" link
3. Click on the "Doing Business with the State" link
4. Scroll to the bottom of the page, and click on the "For more information and to access BIDS, Click Here" link
5. Click on the "How to Register" link
6. Follow the onscreen instructions to register

The State Purchasing Office can also be reached at 303-866-6100.

Continues

Appendix 8.1: Sample Printed Campaign Newsletter (cont.)

Colorado Tobacco Settlement Times March 2001

STEPP Issues RFPs for Comprehensive Tobacco Use Prevention and Reduction Programs

In February, STEPP issued a series of Requests for Proposals (RFPs) aimed at implementing Colorado's Comprehensive Tobacco Use Prevention and Reduction Plan.

"We are seeking new partners throughout the state to implement evidence-based programs that will reduce the human and economic toll of tobacco use in Colorado," said Karen DeLeeuw, STEPP program manager.

Based on input from a 23-member citizen advisory board and guidance from the Centers for Disease Control and Prevention's *"Best Practices for Comprehensive Tobacco Control Programs,"* RFPs addressing the following areas were developed and issued:

- Expansion of Youth Empowerment Coalitions (application process open on continuous basis)
- Statewide Initiatives to Prevent Initiation Among Youth
- Statewide Initiatives to Reduce Exposure to Environmental Tobacco Smoke
- Needs Assessment and Development of Recommendations for Effective Tobacco Control in K-12 Public Schools
- Needs Assessment and Development of Recommendations for Effective Tobacco Control Programs Serving Eight Special Populations
- Implementation of a Statewide Training Program for Prenatal and Post Partum Care Providers
- Media Campaign to Promote Launch and Use of Quit Line
- Independent Evaluation of the State's Tobacco Education and Prevention Program

The RFPs were announced in a statewide press release and are posted on the state's website at http://www.gssa.state.co.us/BdSols.nsf/Open+Solicitations+By+Agency?OpenView and at www.CTEPA.org.

For more information, contact the tobacco prevention specialist in the local health department in your area:

Kim Hills, Program Coordinator
Boulder County Health Department
529 Coffman #225, Longmont, CO 80501; Phone: 303-678-6169; E-mail: khills@co.boulder.co.us

Bonnie Mapes
Denver Public Health
605 Bannock Street, MC 2600, Denver, CO 80204; Phone: 303-436-3046; E-mail: bmapes@dhha.org

Jason Vahling, Program Specialist
El Paso County Department of Health and Environment
301 South Union Blvd, Colorado Springs, CO 80910; Phone: 719-578-3119; E-mail: jasonvahling@elpasoco.us

Nancy Grove
Larimer County Department of Health and Environment
1525 Blue Spruce Drive, Fort Collins, CO 80524; Phone: 970-498-6753; Email: grovenl@co.larimer.co.us

Betty Mason
Mesa County Health Department North
2754 Compass Drive, Suite 240, Grand Junction, CO 81506; Phone: 970-254-4108; E-mail: bmason@co.mesa.co.us

Enid Sepulveda-Rodriguez
Pueblo City-County Health Department
151 Central Main Street, Pueblo, CO 81003; Phone: 719-583-4313; E-mail: enid.sepulveda@co.pueblo.co.us

Char Day
San Juan Basin Health Department
281 Sawyer Drive, PO Box 140, Durango, CO 81301; Phone: 970-247-5702, ext 227
E-mail: char@sjbhd.org

Marlo Rhea
Weld County Health Department
1555 North 17th Avenue, Greeley, CO 80631; Phone: 970-304-6420, ext. 2381; E-mail: mthomas@co.weld.co.us

Mia Greenhill
Delta County Health Department
255 W 6th Street, Delta, CO 81416; Phone: 970-874-2165; E-mail: mgreen@deltacounty.com

Kaysie Harrington
Otero County Department of Health
Room 11, County Courthouse, 13 West 3rd St., La Junta, CO 81050; Phone: 719-383-3040; E-mail: caysieh@holly.colostate.edu

Nancy Geha
Tri-County District Health Department
7000 E. Belleview Avenue, Suite 301, Greenwood Village, CO 80111; Phone: 303-846-6234; E-mail: geha@tchd.org

Elise Lubell
Jefferson County Department of Health
1801 19th Street, Golden, CO 80401; Phone: 303 271-5719; E-mail: elubell@co.jefferson.co.us

Ramona Gallegos
Las Animas-Huerfano Counties
412 Benedicta Avenue, Trinidad, CO 81082; Phone: 719-846-2213 X24

Statewide Tobacco Resources

The Colorado Prevention Information Center provides free access for Colorado residents to videos and print materials on a broad array of tobacco-related topics. In May 2000, STEPP contracted with the center to provide greater public access to tobacco materials.

More than 17,000 tobacco-specific items were shipped to the center for central housing and distribution, and are now available for use by interested individuals and organizations throughout Colorado.

For more information about these materials, please call Shannon Misek at (303) 239-8633, or visit the Center at 7525 W. 10th Ave., Lakewood, CO.

Appendix 8.2: Sample Online Newsletter

Online Tobacco-Free News
Current information for the Wisconsin Tobacco Control Program

Issue #28

March 7, 2002

This update has been brought to you by the Tobacco Control Resource Center for Wisconsin (TCRCW). Funding is provided by the Wisconsin Tobacco Control Board. Submissions to Online Tobacco-Free News are welcome. E-mail Emi Narita at enarita@facstaff.wisc.edu.

Table of Contents

Save the Date: April 18 & 19, 2002. The Statewide Tobacco Control Conference in Madison, WI
Theme: Taking Tobacco Control into the Future - Protecting the Investment

1) Maternal Smoking and Low Birthweight Data by County

2) FACT Introduces FACT Field Guru, Adult Advisory Panel

3) Smoke in Workplace Divides White and Blue-Collar Employees

4) The Burden of Tobacco in Wisconsin

5) Show Us the Money: An Update on the States' Allocation of the Tobacco Settlement Dollars

6) New Items from the Tobacco Control Resource Center

7) Thomas T. Melvin Youth Program Will Launch a Campaign to Promote Media Literacy

8) Evaluation Resource for Coalitions

9) 2002 National Conference on Tobacco or Health

10) State Budget Update

More information about these topics can be found at the TCRCW web site: http://www.tobwis.org

1) Maternal Smoking and Low Birthweight Data by County

   The Wisconsin Department of Health and Family Services publishes local data on infants and pregnant women. The Infants and Pregnant Women Report - 2000 has information on the number of low birthweight babies to mothers who smoked during pregnancy. Data is available for individual counties, selected cities, the five public health regions, and the state as a whole. On the same web page, you'll find the 1999 Public Health Profiles with local data on natality (such as smoking status of mother), drug-related problems, injuries, and much more. http://www.dhfs.state.wi.us/localdata/infantspgwomn/START.HTM

2) FACT Introduces FACT Field Guru, Adult Advisory Panel

   Luke Witkowski is the new Field Guru for FACT, the youth movement to fight corporate tobacco. He will attend coalition meetings to discuss FACT and work directly with the FACT members on their activism efforts. He has already traveled to many areas of the state to talk about FACT and provide support - now he wants to come to your coalition. To reach Luke, call him at 715-344-8206. The Nixon group has put together a guide for coalitions: Providing Effective FACT Support, The Coalition's Role. It can be downloaded from the tobwis web site: http://www.tobwis.org/media/coalitionrole_FACT.pdf (PDF file) In addition, a FACT Adult Advisory Panel has been created to support coalitions in their work with FACT. The panel will be made up of two to three coalition members from each region and will serve as a liaison between local and statewide efforts. Find out more at: http://www.tobwis.org/people/index.php (Go to "youth projects.")

3) Smoke in Workplace Divides White and Blue-Collar Employees

   Wisconsin employees are divided into two fairly distinct groups: blue-collar employees, subjected to secondhand smoke, and white-collar employees, who have clean air in their workplace, according to a study released this week by the University of Wisconsin's Monitoring and Evaluation Program. The study found that 40 percent of the workplaces that are traditionally considered blue-collar, allow employees to be exposed to secondhand smoke. This is compared to 13 percent of white-collar workplaces. The full report will be released in two weeks. More information on the press release:
   http://www.tobwis.org/media/WorkplacePress3_4.pdf

4) The Burden of Tobacco in Wisconsin

   Over 2,600 people in Wisconsin died of lung cancer in 2000 with 81 percent of those deaths attributed to cigarette smoking. Nearly 16 percent of all deaths in Wisconsin were attributable to cigarette smoking. The Burden of Tobacco Report describes the health and economic impact of cigarette smoking in Wisconsin. The summary of the report and press release is available at: http://www.tobwis.org/ Summary report: http://www.tobwis.org/media/BurdenFacts2_02.pdf (PDF file, 686 KB).

5) Show Us the Money: An Update on the States' Allocation of the Tobacco Settlement Dollars
The full Jan. 2002 report on the State Tobacco Settlement is online at: http://tobaccofreekids.org/reports/settlements/ -- and interestingly, shows that Wisconsin has dropped in "Rankings of States by Level of Funding for Tobacco Prevention" from 13 down to 20 in one year. It may drop even lower with the state taking away the settlement money, but we won't know how or when it will be reported. The report, entitled "Show Us the Money: An Update on the States' Allocation of the Tobacco Settlement Dollars," was released by the Campaign for Tobacco-Free Kids, American Heart Association, American Cancer Society and American Lung Association.

6) New Items from the Tobacco Control Resource Center
The Spring/Summer 2000 Tobacco Free List will be available in late March and will be available on our web site at: http://www.tobwis.org/resources/ Our staff mentioned to coalition members that we will give away novelty items such as key chains, rulers, and bookmarks, free of cost. This announcement was premature, since our supply of these specialty items is very limited. We will bring you samples of these items when we do outreach and give you a listing of places where these items can be ordered. We are sorry for any inconvenience. Emi Narita will help you find materials that the Resource Center does not have. Call her at: 608-262-7469. Look for these new items on the Free List:

TOBP015 "Butts Are Gross"

TOBP016 "Licking an Ashtray"

TOBP017 "Butts Are Gross" (Spanish)

TOB049 Mind Over Matter: The Brain's Response to Nicotine (brochure)

7) Thomas T. Melvin Youth Program Will Launch a Campaign to Promote Media Literacy
In mid-March, the Thomas T. Melvin Youth Tobacco Prevention and Education Program will launch a youth-led TV program and radio campaign to teach people about media literacy. The program will be packaged into a video and a B-Free curriculum that will be sent to all Wisconsin middle schools, as well as to the coalitions, the Wisconsin Tobacco Control Board members, and the regional public health offices. The curriculum will help youth explore issues introduced by the video, such as peer pressure and media tricks. It also raises issues implied by the theme of freedom from tobacco, such as addiction. Check out the new B-Free web site: http://www.be-free.org

8) Evaluation Resource for Coalitions
The Monitoring and Evaluation Program (MEP) has published a resource titled "Collecting Evaluation Data: An Overview of Sources and Methods". MEP has more specific evaluation resources, but this is a good starting point for doing evaluation. It will help you answer questions like: who will use the information and how? What will they or we want to know? The publication can be found at:

http://cf.uwex.edu/ces/pubs/pdf/G3658_4.PDF This document can be downloaded, and there are bound, hard copies at UW-Extension. Other evaluation materials:
http://www.uwex.edu/ces/tobaccoeval/manual.htm

9) 2002 National Conference on Tobacco or Health
November 19-21, 2002 • Hilton San Francisco • Call for abstracts deadline: March 25, 2002
Submit your abstract online at http://www.tobaccocontrolconference.org
The 2002 National Conference is looking for abstracts of presentations and workshops that will provide current scientific and practical information on effective tobacco control strategies and developments. All abstracts must be submitted online.

10) State Budget Update
Joint Finance voted on the budget yesterday. Like the Governor's proposal, the Republican plan uses the money the state will get from the tobacco settlement to pay for shared revenue. The Republican plan would shift $214 million from the tobacco endowment to the state's general fund. McCallum's plan would have used all the endowment. News article:
http://wisconsinstatejournal.com/local/21684.html Budget Adjustment paper:
http://www.legis.state.wi.us/lfb/2001-03BudgetAdjustment/Papers/1250.pdf

Smoke Free Wisconsin and other partners will sponsor a training on how to "Develop Long-Term Relationships With Policymakers." Trainings will be held in each region beginning in March. More details: http://www.tobwis.org/events/

End Issue #28

Send to Friends and Colleagues

We encourage you to pass along this issue on Online Tobacco-Free News to your colleagues. If you received this issue from someone you know, and you wish to have your own subscription, please send a message to Emi Narita at enarita@facstaff.wisc.edu.

Suggested citation:

The Online Tobacco-Free News was reprinted with permission from the Wisconsin Clearinghouse for Prevention Resources/Tobacco Control Resource Center for Wisconsin. Funding was provided by the Wisconsin Tobacco Control Board.

Appendix 8.3: Sample Editorial

USA Today Editorial
February 13, 2002

Triple Threat to Teen Smoking

States are suddenly lining up to hit the tobacco industry where it hurts, and teen smokers where it just might help — right in the wallet.

In recent months, five states have raised cigarette taxes significantly, four of them to $1 or more per pack. Now, 18 more states, from Connecticut to New Mexico, are considering tax hikes, too, according to the American Lung Association, which releases its state tobacco report today.

Tax increases are one of the most promising ways to deter smoking, especially among price-sensitive teens. When Oregon raised its cigarette tax 60% to 78 cents per pack in 1997, consumption dropped 20% in the next two years. Among eighth-graders, smoking plummeted 30% in 1999, according to the Centers for Disease Control and Prevention.

Typically, smoking deterrence is not the lure when states hike cigarette taxes. This year, just as in 2001, most states are driven by budget deficits. Cigarette taxes are simply a politically convenient target.

If states were serious about public health, they'd use at least some of the proceeds to deter this deadly habit. Few do, even though teens are most likely to avoid cigarettes when states use a triple strategy: making cigarettes less affordable, less alluring and less available. That requires combining high-priced cigarettes with anti-smoking-ad campaigns and local programs to enforce laws against selling tobacco to minors.

The trifecta works. California and Massachusetts, which used it, have seen the most sustained reductions in tobacco use in the nation.

When states hike taxes without spending money to help their citizens quit smoking, they're simply taxing the addicts of today. Worse, they stop short of keeping teens from becoming the addicts of tomorrow.

© Copyright 2002 USA TODAY, a division of Gannett Co. Inc.

Appendix 8.4: Sample Letter to the Editor

Tuesday, April 2, 2002

Comments on today's editorial and letters can be sent to The Guardian at letters@chg.southam.ca

We must do more to help smokers

Editor:

Smoking has been well-established as harmful, not only to those who engage in it, but also to the health of those around the smokers. Smoking has great costs, not only in dollars to purchase the cigarettes, but also to health-decreased lung capacity, increased risks of cancer, smaller birth weight of babies, and a long list of other detrimental health effects. Smokers' homes and clothes require increased cleaning time and energy over those of non-smokers. Those who work, live or happen to be passing though environments where smoking is permitted are at risk from the smoke. Families and the health-care system bear any costs of this addiction. The P.E.I.* Home Economics Association respectfully urges the government of P.E.I. to enact legislation to make all public spaces on P.E.I. smoke-free. Studies show this should lower the overall consumption of cigarettes. The government of P.E.I. has established a 'Quit-Smoking Line' (1-888-818-6300) to help smokers find cessation programs. P.E.I. and Islanders could only benefit from fewer people smoking. We also need to put increased resources into helping people quit smoking discouraging youth from beginning to smoke. Islanders would find it difficult to find someone who was happy to have started smoking or who was sad to have quit. What can we, as Islanders, do to lower the numbers of people smoking? Increased taxes, fewer places where smoking is allowed, subsidized or free smoking cessation programs, and counselling for lifestyle changes? We obviously have to do more than we are doing now.

Shari MacDonald
President, P.E.I. Home Economics Association

* Prince Edward Island, Canada

Appendix 8.5: Sample Op-Ed

Pioneer Planet

Published: Thursday, September 27, 2001

VIEWPOINT   State teens reaching peers with anti-smoking message

BY JAN K. MALCOLM
Guest Columnist

Last month, teens from Minnesota's teen-led Target Market campaign released survey results telling us that young people across the state are hearing Target Market's anti-tobacco industry message. As a result, teen behaviors and attitudes toward the industry and tobacco use are changing—for the first time in more than a decade. The news from Target Market is an exciting sign that, after just one year, the campaign is doing precisely what Minnesota's youth designed it to do—reduce the number of underage smokers.

The changes in attitude highlighted in the survey are important precursors to long-term reductions in youth tobacco use. If the trend continues, as we hope it will, it will be a real success story for the Target Market campaign and the state's broader Youth Tobacco Prevention Initiative.

When legislators and Gov. Jesse Ventura created the tobacco prevention endowment in 1999, they gave the Minnesota Health Department an important charge to use the resources wisely to produce long-term health gains for Minnesota's youth. The stakes are high—in lives we can save and in future health care costs we can avoid.

Our department took a very different approach from prior tobacco prevention campaigns. This time we empowered Minnesota youth themselves to lead a marketing effort that could speak credibly to young people about tobacco. That credibility requires that teens deliver the message peer-to-peer in their own voice, which is not always a voice adults understand.

The survey results tell us that in just one year, Target Market's edgy campaign has already successfully reached Minnesota kids. Ninety-three percent of Minnesota teens are aware of Target Market's central message about the tobacco industry's manipulation of youth. That's an awareness level most consumer brands would envy. About three-quarters of the youth surveyed did not want to be targets of the tobacco companies, and more than half say they now feel they have the power to fight back and resist tobacco company marketing.

Does the campaign really work? Will it lead to a long-term decline in Minnesota's rates of youth tobacco use? We think it will, as long as the effort can be sustained over time. The survey results are an important first indication that youth smoking rates in Minnesota are on the decline. Compared to a survey conducted before the Target Market campaign began, the number of committed non-smokers increased by 20 percent in the past year, and the number of teens who said they might try smoking someday decreased by 25 percent. After more than a decade of significantly increasing youth tobacco use rates (which have been about 4 percent higher than the national average), the survey suggests the trend is on its way downward.

Changing the social climate around tobacco use is the primary purpose of the Minnesota Youth Tobacco Prevention Initiative of which Target Market is a part.

The Target Market campaign is the most visible part of these efforts, but statewide grants and grants to community coalitions working to help young smokers quit, making sure kids cannot buy cigarettes and providing education in schools are vital parts of what the Centers for Disease Control and Prevention recommend for an effective and comprehensive tobacco control program. Each strategy plays an important role in reshaping and reinforcing the attitudes our kids have toward smoking.

The survey results indicate a phenomenal success for Target Market and the entire initiative. It tells those involved in Target Market and those working statewide and on the community level that their efforts are paying off. Our work, however, is far from done.

The tobacco industry continues to spend millions each year on marketing its products in Minnesota. To reach the goal the Legislature and governor set for us to decrease youth smoking rates by 30 percent by 2005, we will have to continue to be aggressive, innovative and responsive to the evidence of what works.

While the public health community is still David to the Goliath tobacco industry, the results from Target Market are exciting indications that these efforts can succeed. However, to turn these results into a sustained trend and long-term decreases in youth tobacco use, we must maintain our commitment to Target Market and all of the innovative, statewide strategies and community-based approaches we're taking to decrease the number of Minnesota kids who use tobacco.

We have an unprecedented opportunity to reduce the human and economic consequences that tobacco use has on our youth and our communities. When we succeed, it will be one of the best public health investments we've ever made.

Malcolm is Minnesota commissioner of health. Contact her by e-mail at commissioner@health.state.mn.us.

Appendix 8.6: Sample Spokesperson Profile Sheet

If you are interested in serving as a spokesperson for the [INSERT NAME OF PROGRAM], please complete the form below.

The information will be shared with members of the [NAME OF PROGRAM] media subcommittee and [NAME OF PR FIRM] public relations firm. A special spokesperson kit containing key talking points, background information, a full press kit about [YOUR STATE]'s tobacco settlement – as well as public speaking guidelines – will be sent to each spokesperson when asked to speak.

Name: _____
             First   Middle   Last

Title: _____

Organization: _____

Address: _____

_____

Telephone: Business: _____ Home: _____

                Pager: _____ Cellular: _____

Fax: _____ E-mail: _____

Gender: ❏ Male   ❏ Female   Year of birth: _____

Ethnicity:
- ❏ African American
- ❏ Asian American
- ❏ Caucasian
- ❏ Hispanic/Latino
- ❏ Native American
- ❏ Other _____

(please check one)
- ❏ I can speak on behalf of my organization
- ❏ I can speak as a private citizen

(please check one)
- ❏ I am available to speak to broadcast media or newspaper editorial boards.
    I will need ____ days lead time.
- ❏ I have limited time to speak. Please call me to check my availability.
- ❏ You can sign my name to a letter to the editor for a local newspaper.

Spokesperson Profile (page 2)

Topics that I can speak on: *(check as many as apply)*

❏ Medical information about health risks associated with tobacco use

___ general ___ pregnant women ___ smoking and children

❏ Statistical data about tobacco use in [STATE]
❏ Personal testimony about the impact of tobacco product use
❏ Youth perspective about the impact of tobacco use
❏ Minority communities and the impact of tobacco use
❏ General information about tobacco settlement monies and the importance of prevention, cessation, and education programs

Briefly describe your public speaking experience:

_____
_____

Name(s) of your local community newspaper. Describe any relationship or experience that you have with the paper.

1. _____ 2. _____
3. _____ 4. _____

TV/radio/news talk show in your area: Name of show: _____
Host: _____ Phone: _____

Name of your U.S. congressional delegate: _____ District: _____
❏ know very well
❏ know marginally
❏ do not know

Name of state senator: _____ District: _____
_____ ❏ know very well
❏ know marginally
❏ do not know

Name of state representative: _____ District: _____
❏ know very well
❏ know marginally
❏ do not know

If you have additional questions about this form, please call [NAME] at [PHONE NUMBER].
Please fax this form to [CONTACT NAME] at [FAX NUMBER] by [DATE].

Appendix 8.7: Sample Pitch Letter

(Type pitch letters on your organization's letterhead. Adapt to reflect local data before sending to a reporter. Use to introduce an idea, to make an interview offer, or as a cover sheet for additional information that accompanies the letter.)

[DATE]

Dear [NAME OF NEWS DIRECTOR or REPORTER],

Every day, more than 2,000 of our American youth become regular tobacco smokers. Roughly 28 percent of U.S. high school students and nearly 13 percent of middle school students currently smoke. Right here in [INSERT LOCAL DATA and/or ANECDOTE HERE TO LOCALIZE THE ISSUE.]

In an effort to prevent youth smoking in our community, [ORGANIZATION NAME] is launching a youth tobacco counter-marketing program. Our goal is to increase awareness about how the tobacco industry influences our youth, parents, and others who work with youth in [CITY OR COMMUNITY NAME], and how we can all work together to prevent that negative influence.

[NAME], [ORGANIZATION] director, will be available for interviews on this issue, and we would like to schedule a time when he/she could talk with someone from [THEIR NEWS ORGANIZATION]. I will contact you in the next few days to make arrangements for the interview.

If you have any questions, please call me at [PHONE]. I look forward to working with you.

Sincerely,

[YOUR NAME]
[TITLE]

For more help on crafting pitch letters, visit http://www.altonmiller.com/pitch.htm.

Appendix 8.8: Sample News Release

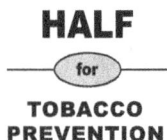

FOR IMMEDIATE RELEASE

POLL SHOWS ILLINOIS VOTERS SUPPORT TOBACCO PREVENTION SPENDING

(Springfield, IL - November 17, 1999) Ninety-one percent of Illinoisans favor spending a portion of the settlement funds on programs that help children and teenagers stop smoking and prevent others from starting to smoke, says a poll released today by the **Half for Tobacco Prevention** campaign. Additionally, 79 percent support spending on programs to help adults quit smoking.

"The people of Illinois want this money spent on tobacco prevention," said Ronald Johnson, M.D., President-Elect of the Illinois Academy of Family Physicians. "An overwhelming majority of people see this tobacco settlement windfall for what it really is – a once-in-a-lifetime opportunity to undo the damage done by the tobacco industry over the last few decades."

The poll also revealed that nearly half of registered voters would be less likely to vote for a candidate who opposes programs that advocate tobacco control, smoking prevention and that help people stop smoking.

Today's announcement comes as part of "Operation Half the Pie," a campaign designed to educate the public and key leaders on the importance of establishing a comprehensive tobacco control and prevention plan in Illinois. Another aspect of today's event was the delivery of half of a pumpkin pie to every member of the General Assembly to illustrate what the campaign is asking for – half of the settlement "pie" put exclusively towards tobacco control and prevention.

Why half? According to recommendations from the U.S. Centers for Disease Control and Prevention, that's what is necessary in order to provide an effective tobacco control and prevention program in Illinois, including:

- a media and public awareness campaign that will deglamorize tobacco use, especially among youth
- strengthening and continuing to develop effective community-based programs
- cessation services for those who want to stop smoking
- a strong surveillance, evaluation and research component to ensure that funds are being put to the best use possible
- a funds administration system so that the money is secure, accessible and free of the tobacco industry's influence
- enforcement of public policies that restrict the sales and marketing of tobacco products to youth

"Another fact that this survey revealed is that more than half of the smokers in our state are either currently trying to quit smoking, or have tried in the past," said Dr. Johnson. "But the state spends just 2.4 cents per person per year on tobacco control and prevention. Why should anyone be surprised to hear that nearly twenty thousand Illinoisans die each year because of smoking-related diseases? It's time for the General Assembly to listen to the medical and public health community of this state, as well as the people, and use this money to make a real impact on tobacco use."

The poll was conducted October 26-28 by McKeon & Associates, asking Illinoisans statewide about their views on the state's tobacco settlement and possible spending options for the funds. The sampling error is +/- 3.8 percentage points.

Backed by more than 65 public health organizations and physicians associations across the state, **Half for Tobacco** Prevention includes the American Heart Association, American Lung Association, American Cancer Society, Illinois State Medical Society, Illinois Academy of Family Physicians, Illinois Association of Public Health Administrators and the American Academy of Pediatrics, Illinois Chapter among its members.

###

To schedule an interview with a campaign member, please call Citigate Communications at 312-895-4715.

Appendix 8.9: Sample Fact Sheet

TOBACCO-FREE TOOL KIT — FACT SHEET

KNOW THE FACTS ABOUT SECONDHAND SMOKE

Secondhand smoke, also referred to as environmental tobacco smoke (ETS), is a complex mixture of chemicals emitted from a lit tobacco product (cigar, cigarette, pipe) and from smoke exhaled by a smoker.

Exposure to secondhand smoke is often involuntary or considered passive smoking because nonsmokers can inhale the chemicals, poisons and known cancer-causing agents from the smoke in the same way smokers do. Some of these poisons are nicotine, ammonia, formaldehyde, hydrogen cyanide, carbon monoxide and benzene.

Secondhand smoke knows no boundaries. Simply creating separate smoking and nonsmoking areas in a business, workplace or home won't prevent nonsmokers from being exposed to secondhand smoke.

FACT
It is estimated that only 15% of cigarette smoke gets inhaled by the smoker.
The remaining 85% lingers in the air for everyone to breathe.

SOURCE Irish Cancer Society, Irish Heart Foundation. "Second-hand Smoke is Dangerous." Online. Internet. 13 February 1997. Available: smoke-free.eire.org/secondhand.htm

---

FACT
Nine out of 10 nonsmoking Americans are exposed to secondhand smoke at least once every two to three days.

SOURCE U.S. Centers for Disease Control (CDC), April 1996.

FACT
If a person spends two hours in a room where someone is smoking, the nonsmoker inhales the equivalent of four cigarettes.

SOURCE Katharine Hammond, Ph.D., University of California, Berkeley, School of Public Health.

FACT
Secondhand smoke contains 43 cancer-causing agents.

SOURCE American Cancer Society. "Clean Indoor Air." Online. Internet. 30 October 2000. Available: cancer.org/tobacco/air.html

---

FACT
Secondhand smoke contains 200 poisons.

SOURCE American Lung Association. "Fact Sheet: Secondhand Smoke." Online. Internet. September 2000. Available: lungusa.org/tobacco/secondhand_factsheet99.html

---

FACT
Cigarettes kill one in three smokers.

SOURCE CDC. "Projected Smoking-Related Deaths Among Youth-United States. Morbidity and Mortality Weekly Report, November 8, 1996.

Appendix 8.9: Sample Fact Sheet (cont.)

TOBACCO-FREE TOOL KIT

FACT SHEET CONTINUED

FACT
For every eight smokers who die from smoking, one nonsmoker dies from secondhand smoke.

SOURCE National Cancer Institute. Health Effects of Exposure to Environmental Tobacco Smoke: The Report of the California Environmental Protection Agency. Smoking and Tobacco Control Monograph no. 10. Bethesda, MD. U.S. Department of Health and Human Services, National Institutes of Health, National Cancer Institute, NIH Pub. No. 99-4645, 1999.
Centers for Disease Control and Prevention. Smoking-attributable mortality and years of potential life lost – United States, 1990. Morbidity and Mortality Weekly Report 1993; 42 (33):645-8.

FACT
53,000 nonsmokers die every year from secondhand smoke.

SOURCE American Cancer Society. "Clean Indoor Air." Online. Internet. 30 October 2000. Available: cancer.org/tobacco/air.html. National Cancer Institute. Health Effects of Exposure to Environmental Tobacco Smoke: The Report of the California Environmental Protection Agency. Smoking and Tobacco Control Monograph no. 10. Bethesda, MD. U.S. Department of Health and Human Services, National Institutes of Health, National Cancer Institute, NIH Pub. No. 99-4645, 1999.

FACT
43,510 people die annually from motor vehicle accidents.

SOURCE Murphy, Sherry L. "Deaths: Final Data for 1998." National Vital Statistics Reports vol. 48 no. 11. Maryland: National Center for Health Statistics, 2000.

FACT
In 1998, there were 683 deaths due to aviation accidents in the US.

SOURCE National Transportation Safety Board. "Transportation Fatalities Drop in 1998." Online. Internet. Available: NTSB.GOV/pressrel/1999/990909.htm

FACT
30,575 people commit suicide annually.

SOURCE Murphy, Sherry L. "Deaths: Final Data for 1998." National Vital Statistics Reports vol. 48 no. 11. Maryland: National Center for Health Statistics, 2000.

FACT
18,272 people are murdered annually.

SOURCE Murphy, Sherry L. "Deaths: Final Data for 1998." National Vital Statistics Reports vol. 48 no. 11. Maryland: National Center for Health Statistics, 2000.

FACT
6,926 people suffer drug-induced deaths annually.

SOURCE Murphy, Sherry L. "Deaths: Final Data for 1998." National Vital Statistics Reports vol. 48 no. 11. Maryland: National Center for Health Statistics, 2000.

Continues

Appendix 8.9: Sample Fact Sheet (cont.)

TOBACCO-FREE TOOL KIT — FACT SHEET CONTINUED

FACT
15,935 people die in drunk driving accidents annually.

SOURCE U.S. Department of Transportation. "Traffic Safety Facts 1998: Alcohol." Online. Internet. Available: http://www.nhtsa.dot.gov/people/ncsa/FactPrev/pdf/Alcohol98.pdf

---

FACT
13,426 people die from AIDS annually.

SOURCE Murphy, Sherry L. "Deaths: Final Data for 1998." National Vital Statistics Reports vol. 48 no. 11. Maryland: National Center for Health Statistics, 2000.

FACT
Secondhand smoke kills more people than murder, drugs and AIDS combined.

SOURCE Murphy, Sherry L. "Deaths: Final Data for 1998." National Vital Statistics Reports vol. 48 no. 11. Maryland: National Center for Health Statistics, 2000.

FACT
Annually, 15 million American children are exposed to secondhand smoke.

SOURCE U.S. Centers for Disease Control (CDC), April 1996.

FACT
Children of parents who smoke can inhale the equivalent of 102 packs of cigarettes by age 5.

SOURCE Hammond, S. K., G. Sorensen, R. Youngstrom, and J.K. Ockene. "Occupational Exposure to Environmental Tobacco Smoke." JAMA 274 (1995): 956–960.

FACT
Children of smoking parents have 70 percent more respiratory problems.

SOURCE World Health Organization. International Consultation on Environmental Tobacco Smoke (ETS) and Child Health. Switzerland: 1999.

FACT
Each year, secondhand smoke is responsible for up to 300,000 cases of bronchitis and pneumo in children and hundreds of thousands of ear infections and other respiratory ailments.

SOURCE National Cancer Institute. Health Effects of Exposure to Environmental Tobacco Smoke: The Report of the California Environmental Protection Agency. Smoking and Tobacco Control Monograph no. 10. Bethesda, MD. U.S. Department of Health and Human Services, National Institutes of Health, National Cancer Institute, NIH Pub. No. 99-4645, 1999.

FACT
Each year, up to 26,000 kids develop asthma from secondhand smoke.

SOURCE National Cancer Institute. Health Effects of Exposure to Environmental Tobacco Smoke: The Report of the California Environmental Protection Agency. Smoking and Tobacco Control Monograph no. 10. Bethesda, MD. U.S. Department of Health and Human Services, National Institutes of Health, National Cancer Institute, NIH Pub. No. 99-4645, 1999.

Appendix 8.9: Sample Fact Sheet (cont.)

TOBACCO-FREE TOOL KIT — FACT SHEET CONTINUED

FACT
Children of parents who smoke suffer more from middle ear infections.

SOURCE National Cancer Institute. *Health Effects of Exposure to Environmental Tobacco Smoke: The Report of the California Environmental Protection Agency. Smoking and Tobacco Control Monograph no. 10.* Bethesda, MD: U.S. Department of Health and Human Services, National Institutes of Health, National Cancer Institute, NIH Pub. No. 99-4645, 1999.

FACT
Infants exposed to secondhand smoke are four times more likely to die from Sudden Infant Death Syndrome (SIDS).

SOURCE World Health Organization. *International Consultation on Environmental Tobacco Smoke (ETS) and Child Health.* Switzerland: 1999.

FACT
Children of parents who smoke miss more school days.

SOURCE U.S. Environmental Protection Agency. "Air they breathe." Online. Internet. 19 January 2000. Available: epa.gov/children/air.htm#tobacco

FACT
Children of parents who smoke are hospitalized more frequently.

SOURCE National Cancer Institute. *Health Effects of Exposure to Environmental Tobacco Smoke: The Report of the California Environmental Protection Agency. Smoking and Tobacco Control Monograph no. 10.* Bethesda, MD: U.S. Department of Health and Human Services, National Institutes of Health, National Cancer Institute, NIH Pub. No. 99-4645, 1999.

FACT
Secondhand smoke has been linked to lung cancer and heart disease.

SOURCE National Cancer Institute. *Health Effects of Exposure to Environmental Tobacco Smoke: The Report of the California Environmental Protection Agency. Smoking and Tobacco Control Monograph no. 10.* Bethesda, MD: U.S. Department of Health and Human Services, National Institutes of Health, National Cancer Institute, NIH Pub. No. 99-4645, 1999.

FACT
About 60,000 Americans develop heart disease from secondhand smoke annually.

SOURCE National Cancer Institute. *Health Effects of Exposure to Environmental Tobacco Smoke: The Report of the California Environmental Protection Agency. Smoking and Tobacco Control Monograph no. 10.* Bethesda, MD: U.S. Department of Health and Human Services, National Institutes of Health, National Cancer Institute, NIH Pub. No. 99-4645, 1999.

FACT
Women married to smokers have twice the risk of dying from lung cancer.

SOURCE National Research Council. *Indoor Pollutants.* Washington: National Academy Press, 1981.

Continues

Appendix 8.9: Sample Fact Sheet (cont.)

TOBACCO-FREE TOOL KIT — FACT SHEET CONTINUED

FACT
Heart disease is the leading cause of death for women.

SOURCE Murphy, Sherry L. "Deaths: Final Data for 1998." National Vital Statistics Reports vol. 48 no. 11. Maryland: National Center for Health Statistics, 2000.

FACT
Women who live with a smoker have a 91 percent greater risk of heart disease.

SOURCE Kawachi et al. "A Prospective Study of Passive Smoking and Coronary Heart Disease." Circulation 1997, 95: 2374-2379.

FACT
Nonsmoking women who are only occasionally exposed to secondhand smoke have a 58 percent higher risk of heart attack and death.

SOURCE Kawachi et al. "A Prospective Study of Passive Smoking and Coronary Heart Disease." Circulation 1997, 95: 2374-2379.

FACT
Heart disease is the leading cause of death among African Americans, American Indians, Asian Americans and Hispanics.

SOURCE US Department of Health and Human Services. Tobacco Use Among US Racial/Ethnic Minority Groups, African Americans, American Indians and Alaskan Natives, Asian Americans and Pacific Islanders and Hispanics: A Report of the Surgeon General. Atlanta: US Department of Health and Human Services, Centers for Disease Control and Prevention, 1998. www.cdc.gov/tobacco/sgr/sgr_1998/sgr-min-fs-asi.htm

FACT
Lung cancer is the leading cause of cancer-related death among African Americans, American Indians, Asian Americans and Hispanics.

SOURCE US Department of Health and Human Services. Tobacco Use Among US Racial/Ethnic Minority Groups, African Americans, American Indians and Alaskan Natives, Asian Americans and Pacific Islanders and Hispanics: A Report of the Surgeon General. Atlanta: US Department of Health and Human Services, Centers for Disease Control and Prevention, 1998. www.cdc.gov/tobacco/sgr/sgr_1998/sgr-min-fs-asi.htm

FACT
Twenty minutes after you quit, your blood pressure drops. Twenty-four hours after, your chance of a heart attack decreases. And three months after, your lung function increases up to 30 percent.

SOURCE American Cancer Society. "Quitting Smoking." Online. Internet. 2 November 2000. Available: cancer.org/tobacco/quitting.html

Appendix 8.10: Media Contact Record

Date of contact: _____ Time: _____

Handled by: _____

Name of Contact/Editor/Reporter: _____

Title: _____

Name of Publication/TV Station/Radio Station: _____

Address: _____

Telephone Number(s): _____ Fax Number(s): _____

Circulation/Audience/Reach: _____

Deadline/Schedule: _____

Purpose of call: _____

circle one: incoming call   outgoing call

Response provided over phone: _____

Mailed/faxed/e-mailed the following information: _____

Arranged interview with: _____

Additional follow-up required: _____

Date story ran/will run: _____

Other Comments/Miscellaneous Information:

_____

_____

_____

_____

_____

Appendix 10.1: Georgia Burden of Tobacco Brochure

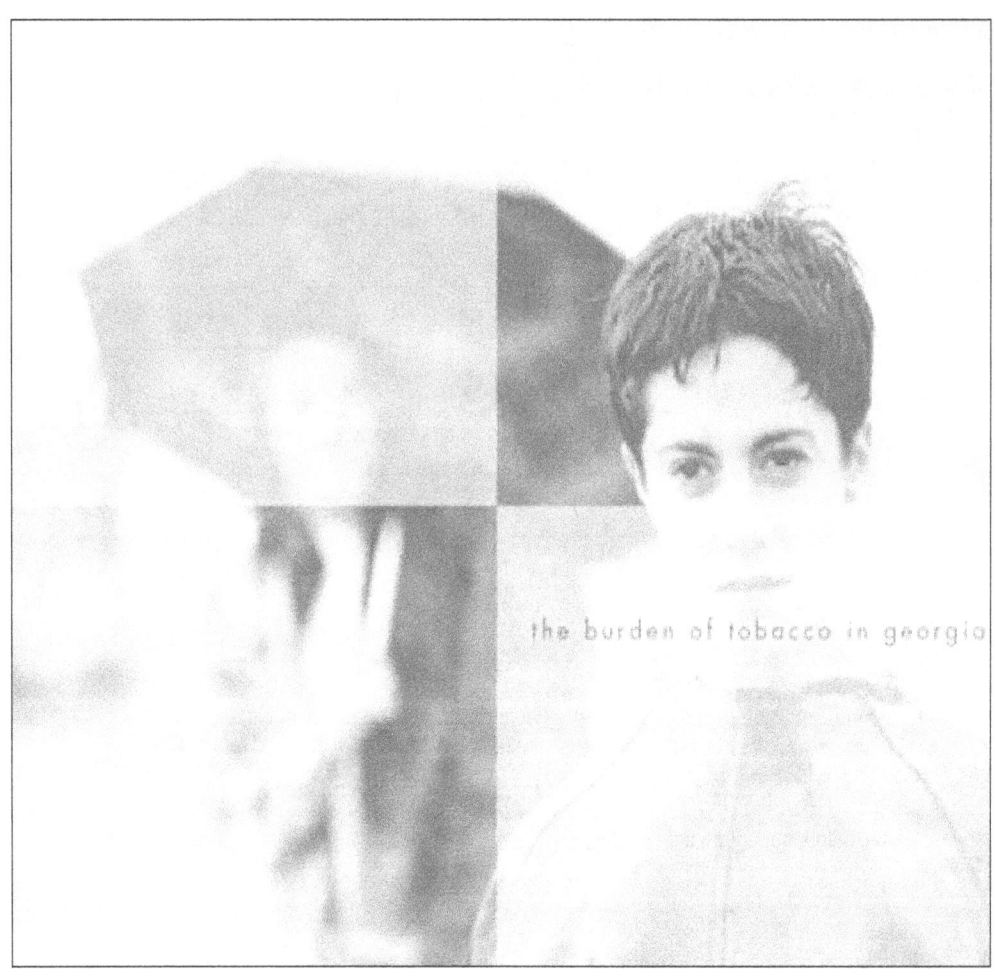

Appendix 10.1: Georgia Burden of Tobacco Brochure (cont.)

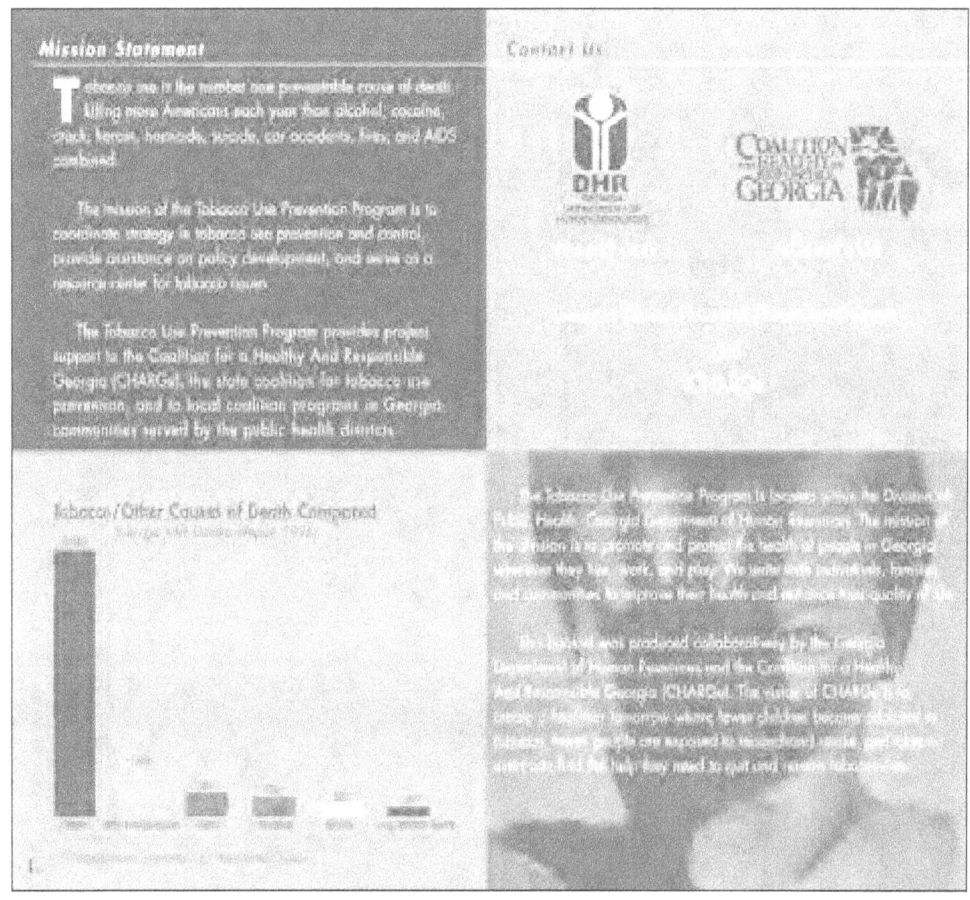

Continues

Appendix 10.1: Georgia Burden of Tobacco Brochure (cont.)

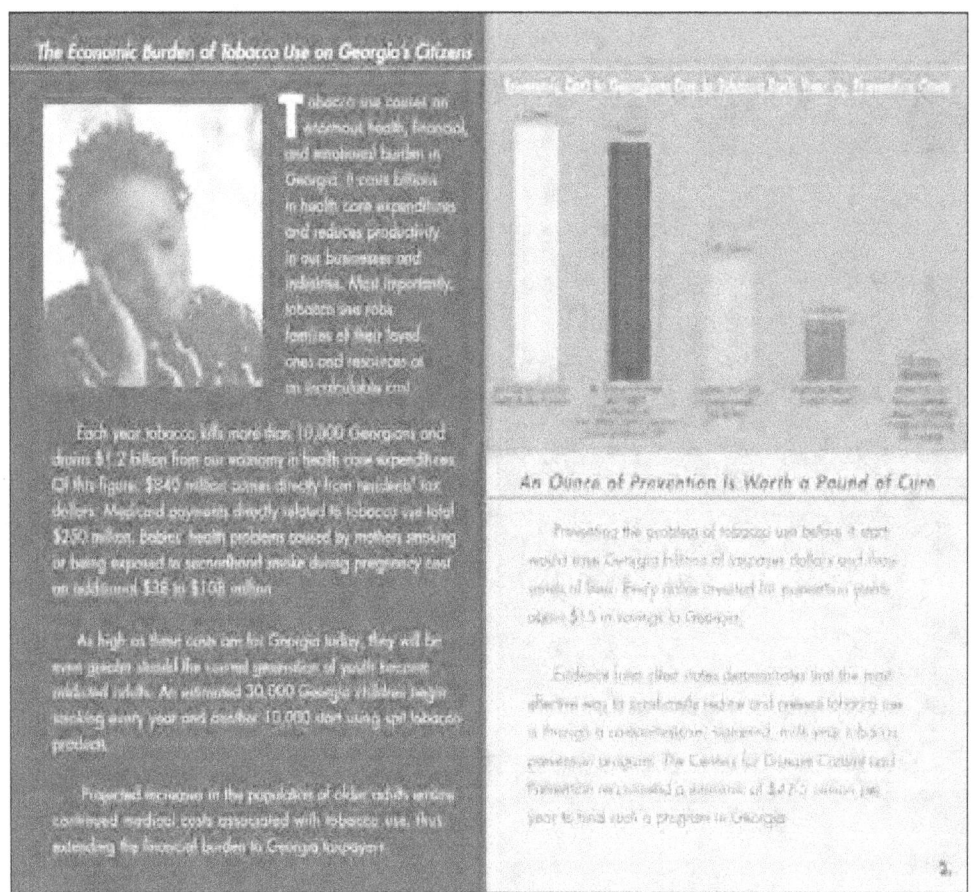

Appendix 10.1: Georgia Burden of Tobacco Brochure (cont.)

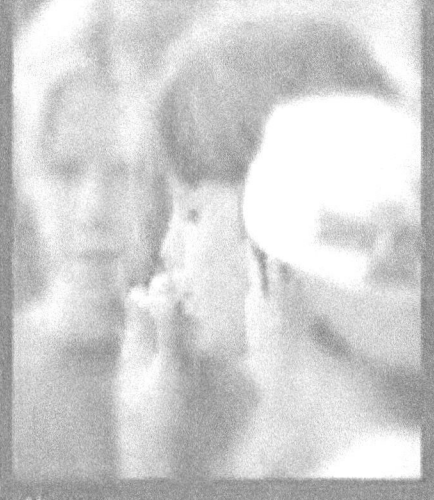

Continues

Appendix 10.1: Georgia Burden of Tobacco Brochure (cont.)

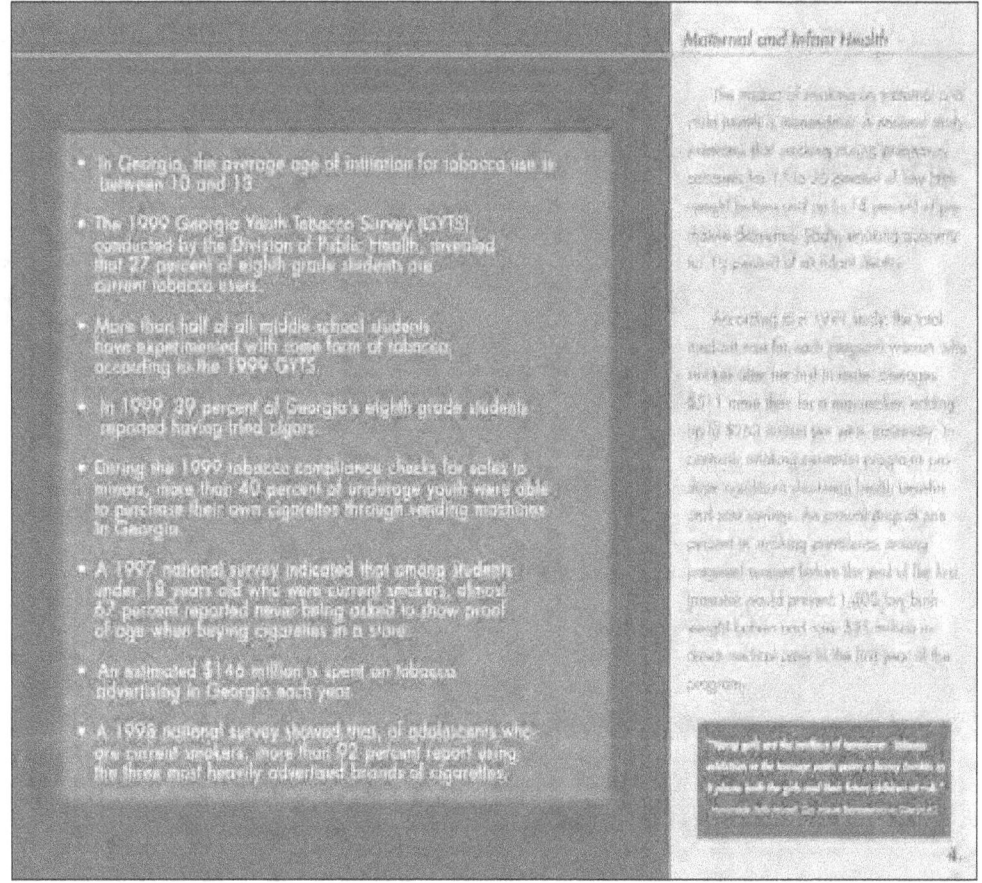

Appendix 10.1: Georgia Burden of Tobacco Brochure (cont.)

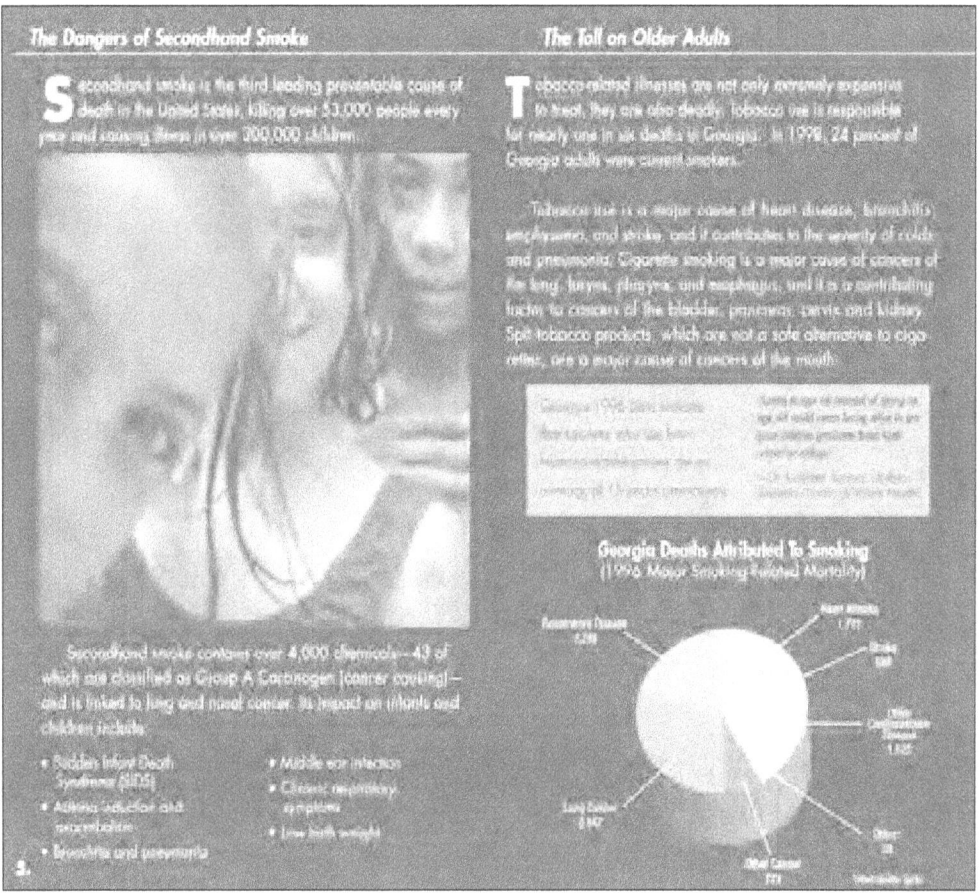

Continues

Appendix 10.1: Georgia Burden of Tobacco Brochure (cont.)

Appendix 10.1: Georgia Burden of Tobacco Brochure (cont.)

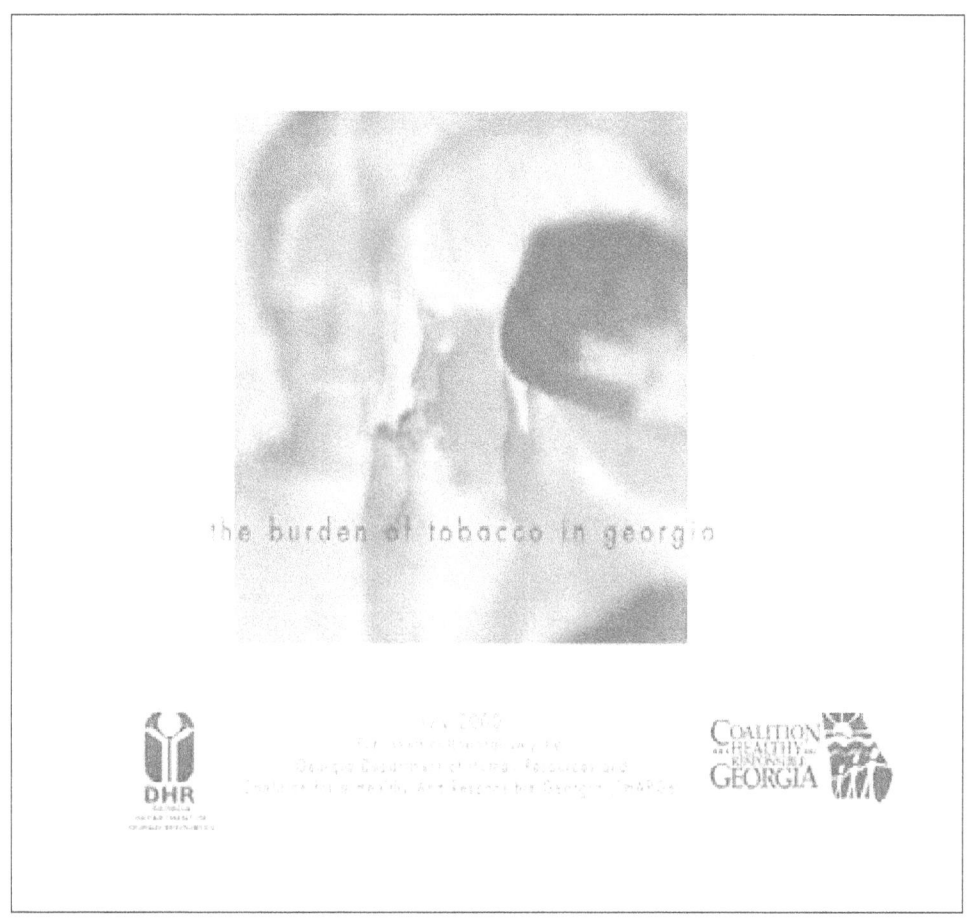

Notes

Feedback Form

The Centers for Disease Control and Prevention would like to hear from you about your experience with *Designing and Implementing an Effective Tobacco Counter-Marketing Campaign.*

To prepare future editions of this manual, we would appreciate any comments or suggestions. To share your opinions, please complete the tear-out card on the next page and drop it in the mail. If you prefer to send comments via e-mail, please send them to CampaignManualFeedback@cdc.gov.

To order additional copies of *Designing and Implementing an Effective Tobacco Counter-Marketing Campaign*, please contact the CDC Media Campaign Resource Center at mcrc@cdc.gov or call 770-488-5705, press 2.

Thank you.

Feedback Form

To share your comments or suggestions about *Designing and Implementing an Effective Tobacco Counter-Marketing Campaign*, answer the questions on this form, carefully tear the form out of the manual, fold it in half, tape it closed, and drop it in the mail. Thank you!

1. **Overall, how useful did you find the manual?** (Please check one.)

    ❏ very useful   ❏ somewhat useful   ❏ not useful

    Why? _____

    _____

2. **Did you find the book to be:**

a. well organized?	❏ yes	❏ no	c. up to date?	❏ yes	❏ no
b. easy to read?	❏ yes	❏ no	d. relevant to your work?	❏ yes	❏ no

3. **If you answered "no" in question 2, please explain.** _____

    _____

4. **Please mark which chapters of the manual you have read:**

    ❏ Introduction

    ❏ Chapter 1: Overview

    ❏ Chapter 2: Planning Your Counter-Marketing Program

    ❏ Chapter 3: Gaining and Using Target Audience Insights

    ❏ Chapter 4: Reaching Specific Populations

    ❏ Chapter 5: Evaluation

    ❏ Chapter 6: Managing and Implementing Your Counter-Marketing Program

    ❏ Chapter 7: Advertising

    ❏ Chapter 8: Public Relations

    ❏ Chapter 9: Media Advocacy

    ❏ Chapter 10: Grassroots Marketing

    ❏ Chapter 11: Media Literacy

5. **Which chapters, if any, did not meet you needs? Why?** _____

    _____

6. **How useful did you find the following sections in the back of the manual?**

Resources and Tools:	❏ very useful	❏ somewhat useful	❏ not useful	❏ didn't review
Glossary:	❏ very useful	❏ somewhat useful	❏ not useful	❏ didn't review
Appendices:	❏ very useful	❏ somewhat useful	❏ not useful	❏ didn't review

7. **What was most useful in the manual? Why?** _____

    _____

8. **What was least useful? Why?** _____

    _____

9. **What best describes the scope of your work?** (Check all that apply.)

    ❏ local   ❏ state   ❏ national   ❏ international   ❏ non-U.S.

10. **What kind of organization do you work for?** (Check all that apply.)

    ❏ tobacco control program

    ❏ market research firm

    ❏ tobacco control coalition

    ❏ non-profit/voluntary organization/network

    ❏ university

    ❏ independent consultant

    ❏ advertising/public relations firm

    ❏ other _____

11. **What other resources or Web sites should be included in the manual?** _____

    _____

12. **How might this manual be improved?** _____

    _____

Tear Along Perforation

www.ingramcontent.com/pod-product-compliance
Lightning Source LLC
Chambersburg PA
CBHW081715170526
45167CB00009B/3584